The Complete Idiot's R

tear here

Jourdan's Ten-Minu Hard-Body Wor

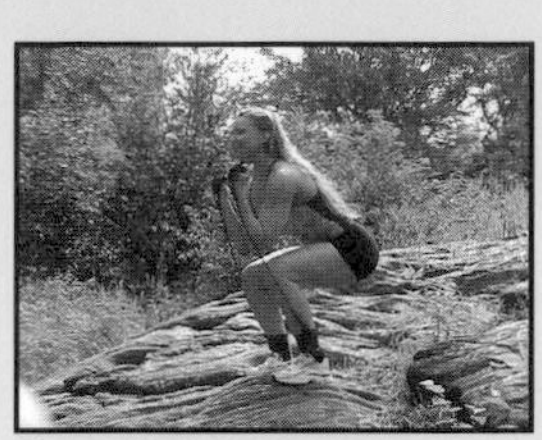

Step 1.

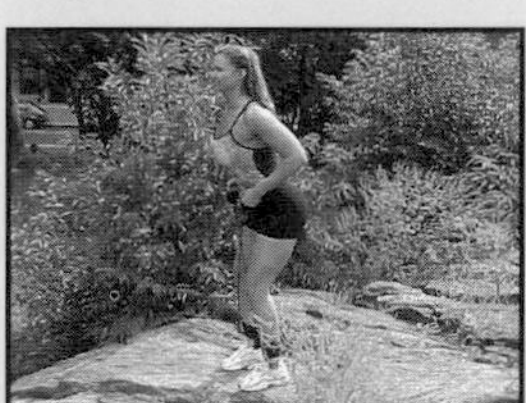

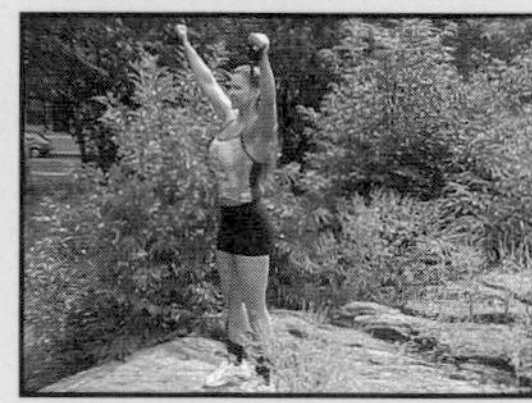

Step 2.

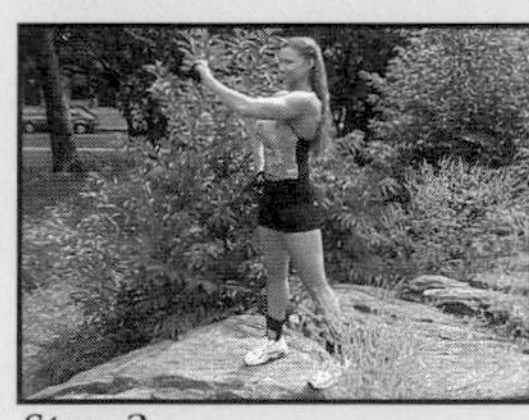

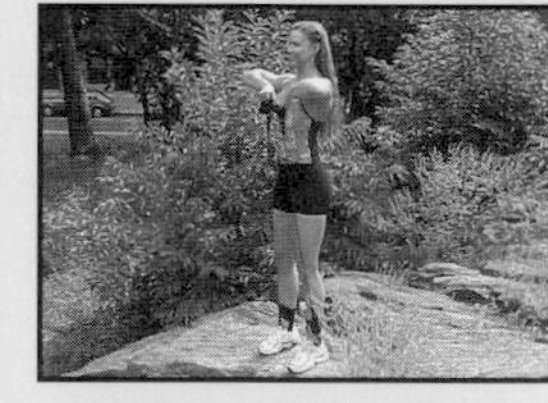

Step 3.

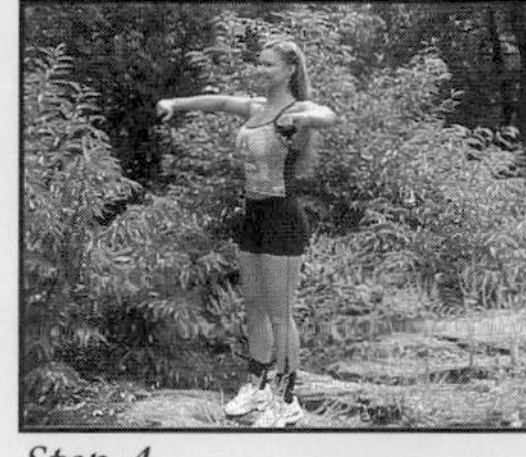

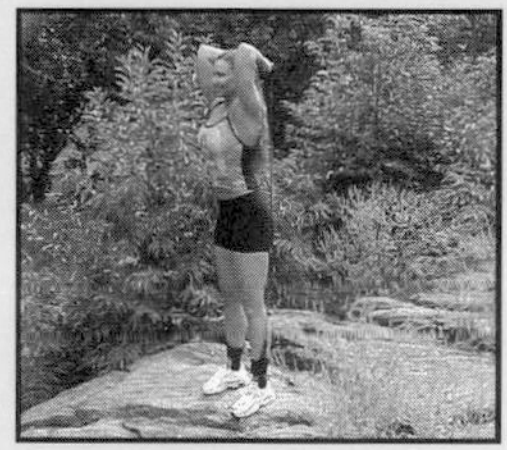

Step 4.

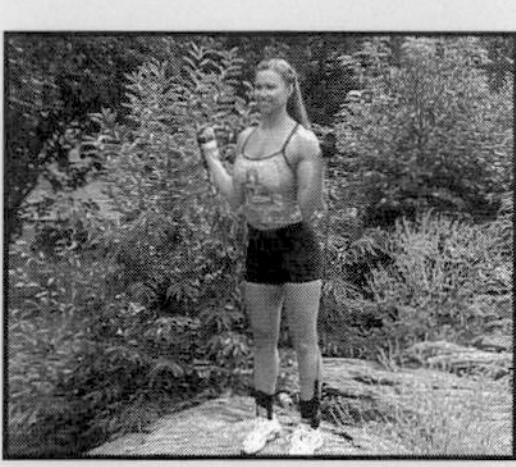

Step 5.

alpha books

Jourdan's Ten-Minute Home Hard-Body Workout

This time-saver routine gives your muscles the perfect pump in less then 10 minutes. Do the exercises in the order shown, with no rest in between, to get a cardio workout and a resistance workout in one. Work up to 20 reps for each move.

Step 1 Squat press Stand hip-width apart with the "Burke Spencer's Personal Trainer" attached to your legs, and with your arms by your sides, holding the ends of the bands. With shoulders back and chest forward, inhale and squat back while curling your arms to your shoulders. Exhale and rise, extending your arms overhead while turning your palms until they face forward. Lower slowly, and repeat for desired reps.

Step 2 Row/x-cross Stand with feet hip-width apart and back straight, bending forward from waist. Cross the band in front and pull up and back, contract back, and lower to starting position. Then stand up straight and extend your arms up and out. The band should be in the shape of a giant X. Lower slowly, and repeat for desired reps.

Step 3 Chest lift With your back straight, place one hand on your hip and the other by your side, palm up. Exhale and extend the straight arm up across your body to your opposite shoulder. Lower slowly, and repeat for desired reps. Switch arms and repeat on your other side.

Step 4 Lateral raise Raise the band out to the side until you reach shoulder height. Lower slowly to the starting position, and repeat for desired reps.

Step 5 Overhead press Raise the band up so that your arms are straight above your head, yet unlocked. Lower the band behind your head until you feel a stretch in your triceps. Exhale and straighten your arms while contracting your triceps. Repeat for desired reps.

For my latest fitness information and routines check out my site at www.teamjourdan.com.

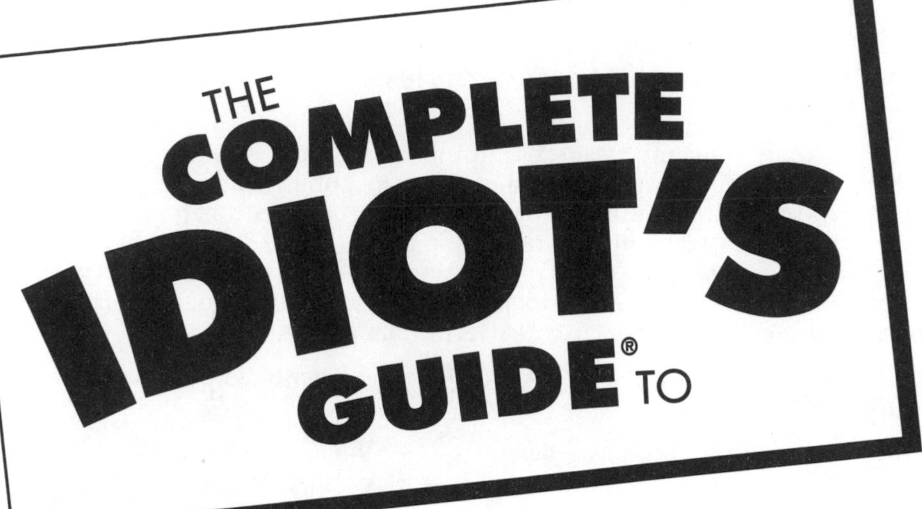

Working Out at Home

by Jourdan Zayles

alpha books

Macmillan USA, Inc.
201 West 103rd Street
Indianapolis, IN 46290

A Pearson Education Company

To my mom, who gave me the passion and strength to do anything I set my mind to.

International Standard Book Number: 0-02-863959-6
Library of Congress Catalog Card Number: Available upon request.

03 02 01 8 7 6 5 4 3 2 1

Interpretation of the printing code: The rightmost number of the first series of numbers is the year of the book's printing; the rightmost number of the second series of numbers is the number of the book's printing. For example, a printing code of 01-1 shows that the first printing occurred in 2001.

Printed in the United States of America

All photos in Chapters 5, 6, 7, 8, and 12, and all photos of the author in Chapter 11, were provided by John Puric. Lisa George was the makeup artist for all chapters except Chapters 13, 18, and 19.

Publisher
Marie Butler-Knight

Product Manager
Phil Kitchel

Managing Editor
Cari Luna

Acquisitions Editor
Amy Zavatto

Development Editor
Tom Stevens

Production Editors
JoAnna Kremer
Christy Wagner

Copy Editor
Krista Hansing

Illustrator
Brian Moyer

Cover Designers
Mike Freeland
Kevin Spear

Book Designers
Scott Cook and Amy Adams of DesignLab

Indexer
Lisa Wilson

Layout/Proofreading
Angela Calvert
Mary Hunt

Contents at a Glance

Contents

Foreword

Although a few lucky people keep up the exercise habit naturally and effortlessly, the rest of us need to be guided, goaded, and loaded with motivation. So we turn to personal trainers, fitness magazines, and fit friends. What are we looking for? Optimism. Confidence. Passion. Athletic discipline. For most of us, these things are hot commodities. When we find something that provides us with that precious can-do energy, we want to share the secret with everyone who will listen. That's why I'm promoting this book.

As both an exerciser who needs an extra boost and someone who aims to inspire the masses (as editor-in-chief of *FIT* magazine) I know something about the art of motivation. And I know firsthand the number-one biggest obstacle when attempting to motivate: keeping it real. It's easy to inspire people with bogus lines like "Lose 20 Pounds in One Month" or "Get in Perfect Shape in Just Five Minutes a Day." Jourdan, however, the wise author of this book, has managed to steer clear of inflated pipe-dreams while providing endless encouragement. She combines hardcore realism with endless doses of uplifting, joyous, and empowering motivation.

From figuring out your present condition and your body type to designing a completely personalized workout schedule, this book is nothing if not medically and physiologically sound and realistic. That means that if you follow Jourdan's advice, you're going to get in great shape and you're not going to get hurt or discouraged or be asked to spend an unreasonable amount of time devoted to your fitness goals. In a world of hooks, scams, and thrilling claims, this book is just plain sensible. Yet Jourdan's contagious spirit shines through on every page, making it exciting, never boring, and igniting the reader with the will and the passion to follow through and actually do it. A realistic plan combined with the right attitude will get you to your fitness dreams. That combination of down-to-earth realism and sky-high inspiration is what makes this book so valuable.

Plus, Jourdan's coverage of fitness is 100 percent thorough. Jourdan covers every single aspect of cardiovascular training, weight lifting, and toning and stretching. Whether you need tips on working out while on vacation, yoga, or pampering yourself, Jourdan provides you with the straightforward information you need.

Also, to make sure you follow through on your plan, Jourdan provides you with exercise logs that you can simply make copies of and place in your fitness binder. I've interviewed many professional athletes, fitness competitors, and countless women who have gone from overweight and unhealthy to fit and fabulous. The one constant that unites all these success stories is their use of exercise logs. They're a great way to check up on yourself, give yourself a great pat on the back, and note all your gains and achievements.

To summarize, this book gives you all the tools and knowledge to get you into the best shape of your life, while inspiring you to actually stick with it on a day-to-day basis.

Lisa Klugman

Lisa Klugman has been on the editorial staff of *FIT* magazine for 10 years. For the past four years, she has been editor-in-chief and has reshaped the editorial content to reflect her down-to-earth and often humorous view of health and fitness.

Introduction

Getting a great body from the comfort of your own home is easy when you know what to do and how to do it. As your personal coach, motivator, and friend, I invite you to join me on a journey to feeling and looking better than you ever have. Your desire, combined with the information in this book, gives you everything you need to succeed.

What You'll Find Inside

This book is divided into four parts that serve as your guide to getting and keeping your best home hard body. The following is a quick summary.

Part 1, "Motivation Starts in the Home," is dedicated to doing the groundwork necessary to turn your home-body fixer-upper into a head-turning, hard-body hacienda. A solid foundation makes it possible for you to get your hard body in the safest and most effective way.

Part 2, "Home Hard-Body Training Tricks," complete with exercise and stretching encyclopedias, has what it takes to give you maximum results in minimal time.

Part 3, "Body and Soul: Keeping Your Hard Work Hard," gives you the knowledge you need to maintain your hard body at its peak performance level.

Part 4, "Expanding Your Hard-Body Horizons," shows you that your hard-body training doesn't have to stop at your front door. Cross-training in the park and travel routines can keep you on top of your hard-body game wherever you go.

Extras

This book also contains sidebars that give you my hard-body training tips, fitness definitions, warnings, and interesting information that would fall under the "bet you didn't know this" category. Check them out as you cruise through this book.

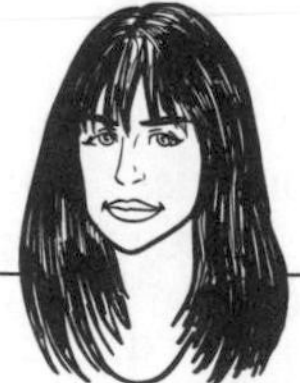

Jourdan's Gems

These boxes contain my training tips that'll maximize your results in minimal time and make training more enjoyable along the way.

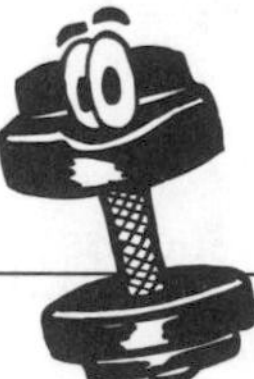

Hard-Body Headliners

Here you'll find interesting fitness information that you might not know or that you might be misinformed about.

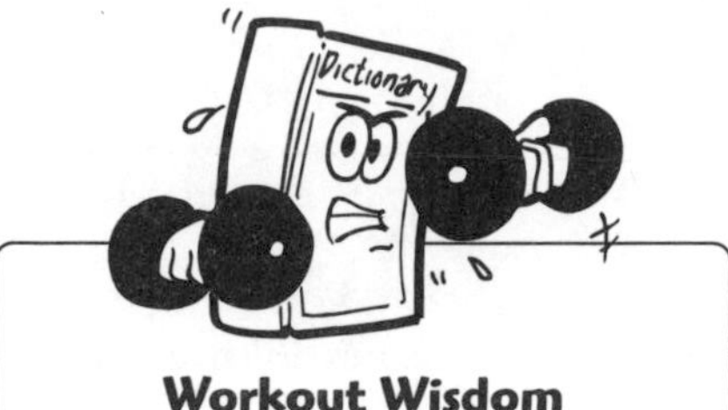

Workout Wisdom

Brush up on your workout vocabulary and definitions here so that you can talk the hard-body training talk.

Safety Scoop

These boxes contain warnings that'll keep your hard body safe.

Acknowledgments

I'd like to thank all the people who helped make this book everything you see here.

Special thanks to Claudette Jimerson for the use of her beautiful home for photos, and to her daughter Courtney for her great work in designing the muscle diagrams. I'd like to thank photographers John Puric and John Field for their great work, and Lisa George for making me look beautiful while sweating.

Last, but far from least, I'd like to thank my family and friends for all their love and support. A big thanks goes to my friend Kelly for her late-night computer help in making my manuscript deadline.

Special Thanks to the Technical Reviewer

The Complete Idiot's Guide to Working Out at Home was reviewed by an expert who double-checked the accuracy of what you'll learn here, to help us ensure that this book gives you everything you need to know about working out at home. Special thanks are extended to Pierre Romaine.

Trademarks

Part 1

Motivation Starts in the Home

Part 1 covers the groundwork necessary to turn your home body fixer-upper into a head-turning, hard-body hacienda. A solid foundation will make it possible for you to get your hard body in the safest and most effective way.

Chapter 1, "Home Bodies Unite," gets your head in the right place to renovate. Making a commitment in writing to do what it takes will get you on the road to hard-body success. Your hard-body home team will be in your corner to cheer you on every step of the way.

Once in the hard-body frame of mind, you're ready to break ground. Determining your body type and evaluating your current fitness level in Chapter 2, "Do Your Homework!" gives you a solid foundation to start building your best home hard body.

Even the best workouts won't work if you don't do them, so Chapter 3, "Punch the (Alarm) Clock," shows you how to create a user-friendly schedule that gives you the feeling of creating time, not doing time.

When you've finished testing and have your schedule in order it's time to gear up. In Chapter 4, "Home Grown," I help you find the equipment that's right for you and your budget.

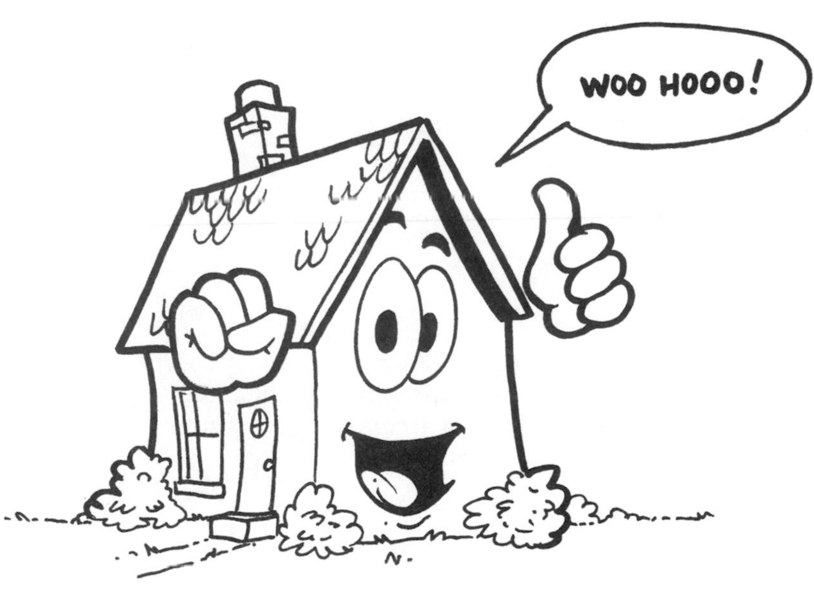

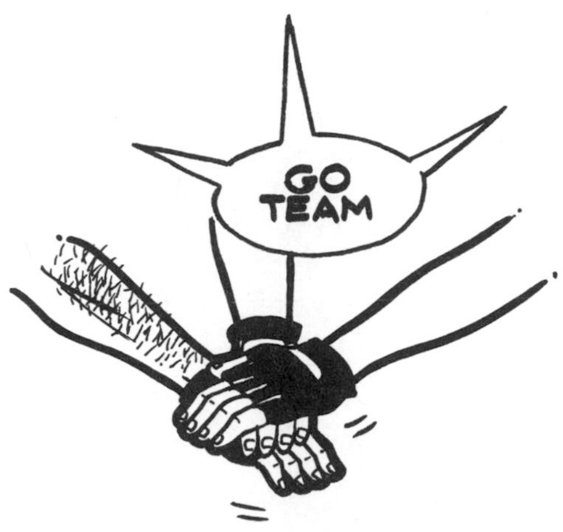

Chapter 1

Home Bodies Unite

In This Chapter

- Hard-body thinking
- Committing to get fit
- Home Hard-Body Journal
- Hard-body home team

The little engine that said, "I think I can," made it over the mountain because he knew he could do it. He succeeded because he busted his caboose, rain or shine, and didn't know the meaning of the word "quit." He stuck with it because whatever pain he felt during the journey paled in comparison to how amazing he knew he would feel after he achieved his goal. The physical soreness soon became a distant memory, but the empowering feeling of achievement burned brightly throughout his life.

Most people fail not because they don't believe they can do it. They fail because they're not willing to do what it sometimes takes to succeed. Your level of commitment will determine whether you run on rocket fuel or run at all. Making a commitment to yourself is the first step to creating your life and living your dreams. Your Home Hard-Body Journal will help you stay on your "commit to get fit" track, keep track of your progress so that you can achieve your maximum potential in minimal time, and make the journey fun along the way.

When you get discouraged, remember that you're not alone on your fitness quest. You have your friends, your family, your personal coach (me), and your hard-body home team (confidence, pride, and enthusiasm). With us in your corner to back you up, you can get ready to sport the hard body of your dreams.

Think, Act, and Win

If you think that I must have always been thin and athletic growing up, think again. I am a member of the genetically challenged endomorphs. (See Chapter 2, "Do Your Homework!" for body type descriptions.) That means that if I don't work out, I'll fill out. I started working out with weights when I was 28, and I know what it's like to start at the bottom of the fitness ladder. At 37, I feel and look better now than I ever have. I'm here to tell you that if I can do it, I know you can, too.

Reading this book will help you to avoid the mistakes that I made and let you in on some of the secrets I discovered along the way that speed up the process. I've broken out my only fat picture (I've burned the rest) to show you that anything is possible.

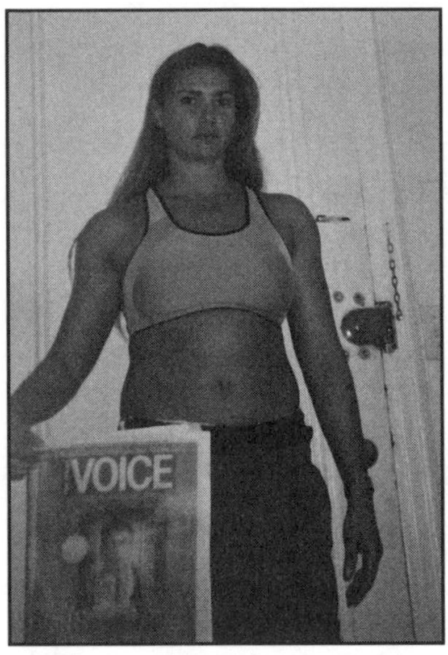

This picture was taken in March of 2000, during a traumatic period in my life. I'm holding the newspaper to prove the date.

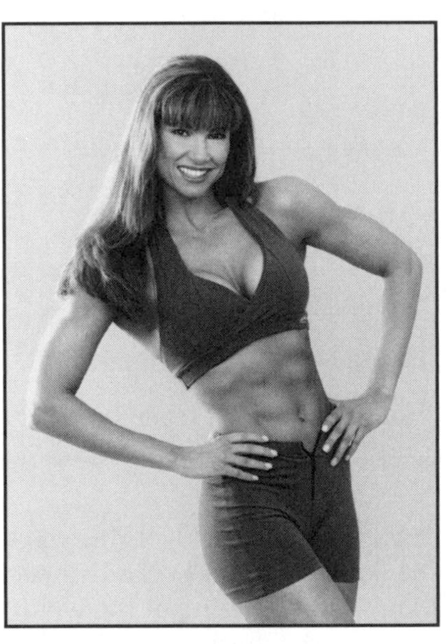

This is what I now look like, after removing all stressful situations from my life and following my exercise program.

Commit to Get Fit

Now is the best time to make a *commitment* to yourself to feel better, look better, and have more energy then you ever did. Go beyond the short-term goal of just losing the weight, and dare to commit the rest of your life to living the life that you were meant to live.

Fill in your Hard Body Commitment certificate right now, and make it official. As your personal coach, motivator, and friend, I'm here to tell you that you can do it. The first step is to take action and commit to living your dreams.

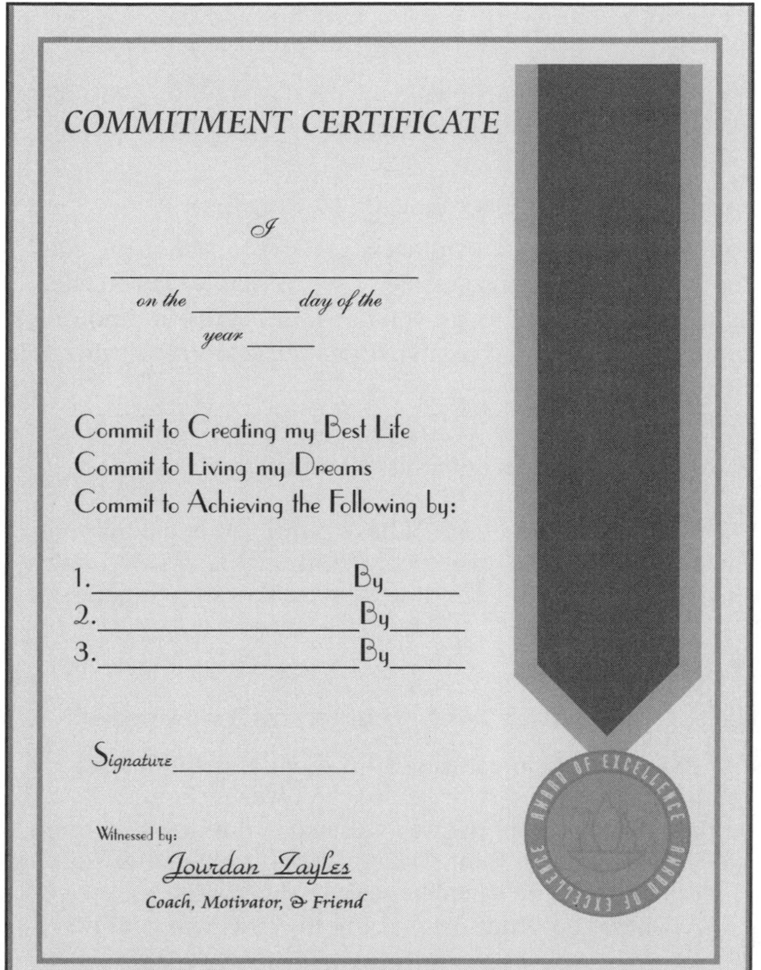

COMMITMENT CERTIFICATE

I

____

on the ________ day of the

year ______

Commit to Creating my Best Life
Commit to Living my Dreams
Commit to Achieving the Following by:

1.____________________ By______
2.____________________ By______
3.____________________ By______

Signature______________

Witnessed by:
Jourdan Zayles
Coach, Motivator, & Friend

Fill in your name, today's date, goals you will achieve, and the dates you will achieve them by.

Your Home Hard-Body Journal

Your Home Hard-Body Journal will document your hard-body journey. Personalize it and make it your own. Carry this with you during the day so that you can add entries at mealtime or anytime you feel like writing down your thoughts.

Start by filling in the dates for one month. This will be your 30-day body enlightenment period. During this time, you will exchange old, draining thoughts for new empowering and success-oriented ones. Use tabs to separate your journal into the following sections:

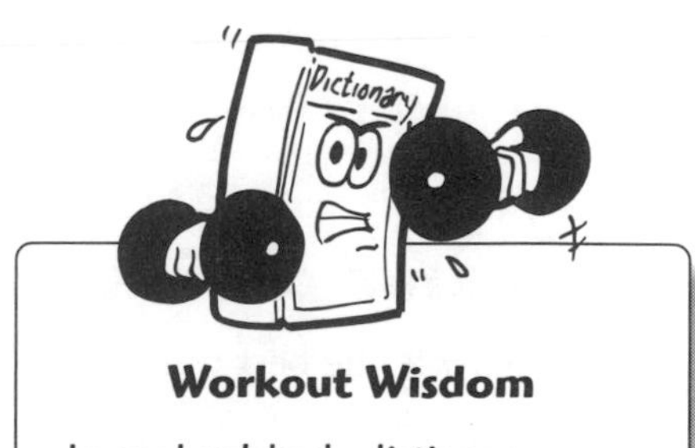

Workout Wisdom

In my hard-body dictionary, **commitment** means "no matter what."

- **Weekly schedules.** Contains your weekly training schedule and your weekly meal planner.
- **Daily events.** Contains your daily events planner. Each day should have a place for today's priorities, business goals, and personal goals. Do at least one thing each day toward your business and personal goals.
- **Strength/cardio training logs.** Contains your daily training logs.
- **Daily food logs.** Contains your daily food intake logs. Leave space at the bottom of each page for comments. Here make note of meals that leave you energized and feeling light, and those that weigh you down or bloat you. Knowing how your body responds to certain food combinations is the secret to being able to control your weight at will.
- **Extra charts.** Contains all other charts that are valuable to keep at your fingertips, such as energy expenditure charts and food calorie charts.

See Chapter 17, "Dear Diary," for sample log pages. I have put together a 30-day Home Hard-Body Journal complete with daily motivational thoughts, if you'd rather start with a journal that's already set up. You can order it at www.teamjourdan.com.

Hard-Body Homework

You will have one hard-body "Power Builder" assignment for this 30-day period.

Make room to receive your good. Start by organizing your room and eliminating everything that you do not use, wear, or need. (If you haven't worn it or seen it in six months, it's out.) Getting these things out of the way will make room for the things that you do want. The old things only clutter your life and take up valuable space that you need for all the new good stuff that's going to come into your life.

Also take time to re-evaluate your current relationships to see if any drain your valuable energy and remove instead of add value to your life. If you have a question, affirm, "I let go of all my old negative living, working, and relationship habits. I am open to receiving only my best life, work, and relationships."

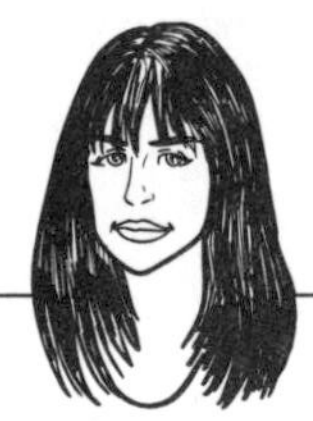

Jourdan's Gems

Take 15 minutes at the start of your day to go over your daily goals. Take 15 minutes at the end of your day to see how you did. Your immediate goal should be to accomplish everything on your daily list.

The Hard-Body Home Team

When doubt comes knocking at your door or the world with all its challenges seems too big to handle, remember the home team in your corner. Your hard-body crew consists of confidence, pride, and enthusiasm. Confidence will make it possible to do anything. Pride will make sure that you always do your best, and enthusiasm will give the whole thing meaning.

Enthusiasm will be the secret to your success. It's your faith in action. Kids use this all the time to shoot for the moon because they believe that they can get there. Even if they don't reach the moon, by giving it their all, they'll definitely be among the stars. Somehow along the way, our light of enthusiasm began to fade as we got older, complaining became our favorite pastime, and pity parties became a regular event. Everything you do can become a task of love with the magic of enthusiasm. With this power, you're able to see beyond your current situation to the big picture, and you can see that even menial tasks serve a purpose in attaining your desires.

It's time to release the darkness of doubt and embrace the light of your spirit to see the endless possibilities that your life has to offer. Decide now to deal the cards and create your life so that you can live your dreams. (On the way to realizing your dreams, don't forget to play like you've never played before.)

The Least You Need to Know

- An idea is great only when followed up with action.
- Make the commitment to yourself today (in writing) to achieve your goals.
- When in doubt, call on the home team: confidence, pride, and enthusiasm.
- You have the power to deal the cards if you don't like the ones you've been dealt.

Chapter 2

Do Your Homework!

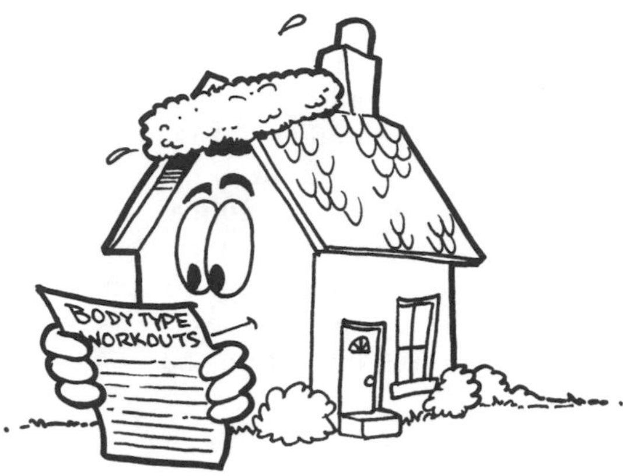

In This Chapter

- Home health history review
- Figuring out your body type
- Assessing your fitness level
- Creating your home hard-body fitness profile

It's time to see whether you're ready for the black diamonds or the bunny slopes. Before you say anything, let me tell you that everyone who has ever skied a black diamond run has at one time been a bunny slope mayor. I rather enjoyed and met many new friends during my extended term. Yes, you can be born with natural talent, but you become an expert only with practice and hard work.

The bottom line is, if you're not honest with your health history, body type, and starting level, you will waste time training incorrectly and will risk possible injury. Not doing too much too soon will also help you avoid the unbearable soreness that'll trap you in your bed and quickly discourage you from continuing your fitness quest.

Taking my simple assessment test and completing your fitness profile will give you a solid foundation from which you can build your best home hard body in the quickest and safest way possible.

Getting Your Building Permit

Before you start construction on your home hard body, you first need to get your building permit. If you've already had a physical with a clean bill of health within the last year and no major illness or accidents since, you should be okay to gradually start up a new exercise program. If you haven't had a recent physical, the Physical Activity Readiness Questionnaire (PAR-Q) is a generally accepted minimal self-assessment questionnaire that lets you know whether you're ready to break ground or whether you need a doc's once-over first. This does not take the place of a physical, so if you have any nagging aches, answer "yes" to any of the questions, or are over 69 years old, you need to see your doctor and get checked out before you start your new program.

PAR-Q and You

The PAR-Q is designed to help you help yourself. Many health benefits are associated with regular exercise, and the completion of PAR-Q is a sensible first step to take if you are planning to increase the amount of physical activity in your life.

For most people, physical activity should not pose any problem or hazard. PAR-Q has been designed to identify the small number of adults for whom physical activity might be inappropriate or those who should have medical advice concerning the type of activity most suitable for them.

Common sense is your best guide in answering these few questions. Please read them carefully and check the right answer as it applies to you.

Yes	No	
❑	❑	1. Has your doctor ever said that you have heart trouble?
❑	❑	2. Do you frequently have pains in your heart and chest?
❑	❑	3. Do you often feel faint or have spells of severe dizziness?
❑	❑	4. Has a doctor ever said that your blood pressure was too high?
❑	❑	5. Has your doctor ever told you that you have a bone or joint problem, such as arthritis, that has been aggravated by exercise or that might be made worse with exercise?
❑	❑	6. Is there a good physical reason not mentioned here why you should not follow an activity program even if you wanted to?
❑	❑	7. Are you over age 65 and not accustomed to vigorous exercise?

Yes to One or More Questions

If you have not recently done so, consult with your personal physician by telephone or in person before increasing your physical activity or taking a fitness appraisal. Tell your physician what questions you answered "yes" to on the PAR-Q, or present your PAR-Q copy.

Programs

After medical evaluation, seek advice from your physician as to your suitability for the following:

- Unrestricted physical activity, starting off easily and progressing gradually.
- Restricted or supervised activity to meet your specific needs, at least on an initial basis. Check in your community for special programs or services.

No to All Questions

If you have answered PAR-Q accurately, you have reasonable assurance of your present suitability for the following:

- **A graduated exercise program** A gradual increase in proper exercise promotes good fitness development while minimizing or eliminating discomfort.
- **A fitness appraisal** Canadian Standardized Test of Fitness (CSTF). Take a fitness appraisal. This is an excellent way to determine your current fitness level so you can safely and effectively increase your activity level.

Delay Increasing Your Activity Level

If you don't feel well because of a temporary illness such as a cold or a fever, wait until you feel better.

Know Your Type

It's important to know your body type and to develop your exercise program with your type in mind. Looking at the shape of your parents will give you a good idea of your genetic makeup. Knowing your body type's characteristics will let you know how your body will respond to certain exercises and to determine what sports will be a natural fit. (You don't see many ballet dancers built like linebackers leaping over Swan Lake.)

It is very common to have characteristics of more then one body type. If you fall into this category, you are predominately one type (primary type) with traits of another (secondary type)—that is, an *ectomorph* with some *mesomorph* traits.)

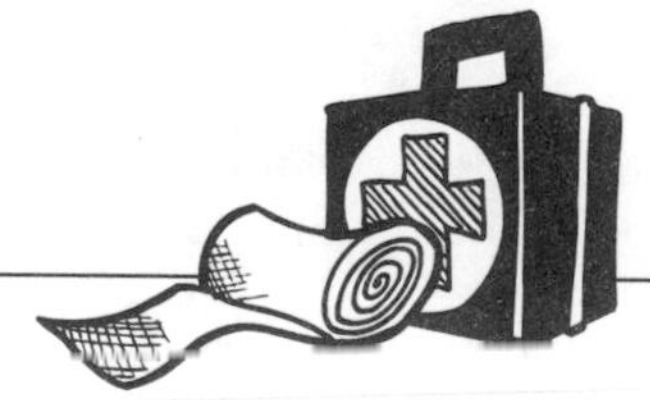

Safety Scoop

Remember that even if you answer "no" to all the questions in the PAR-Q and already exercise, it's important to start all new programs slowly, doing the basics first. How fast you progress will be determined by your starting level and how quickly you master the basics.

This information will prove to be critical to your exercise selection if you want to make changes to your current body shape. With the right exercises and emphasis on creating angular illusions (finally a use for geometry), it is possible to change your body shape.

Stick House

If you look in the mirror and see a person whose physique resembles a ruler, you fall into the ectomorph category. A classic ectomorph has a slender build, small bones, narrow hips, and long arms and legs, and is naturally flexible.

Ectomorphs maintain a lean physique easily because their naturally fast metabolism burns the most calories of all the body types. Yes, that makes you one of the people that other body types love to hate because you can eat pizza and Ben & Jerry's ice cream while still losing weight. A classic ectomorph has a very difficult time gaining weight. This might seem more like a prize instead of a problem, but that also means that ectomorphs have a very difficult time building muscle. I had a training partner that was an ectomorph, and that was a real problem he dealt with. I admit that it burned my *endomorph* hide when he ate huge plates of bread and pasta in front of me while I feasted on grilled chicken and steamed spinach, but I managed to get even in the gym when I lifted more and built muscle quicker.

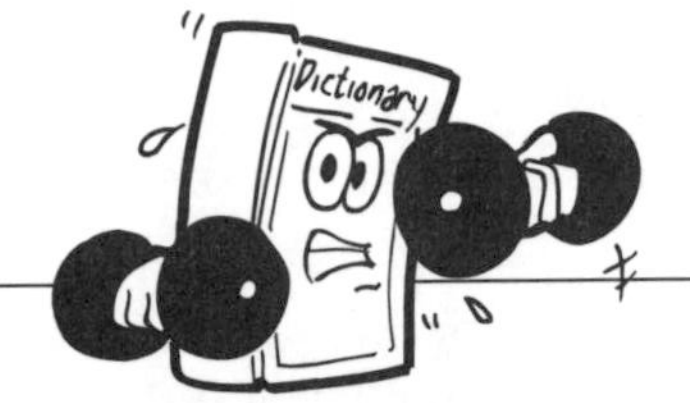

Workout Wisdom

An **ectomorph** is a body type that is naturally slender with small bones, narrow hips, and long arms and legs.

A **mesomorph** is a body type that is naturally athletic looking with broader shoulders, larger bones and thick muscles.

An ectomorph's workout should include weight training and *cardiovascular* (cardio) and stretching exercises, with the emphasis on weight training. A good program to give your ruler shape some symmetry would be a four-day split routine, as shown in Chapter 9, "Custom Home Hard Bodies," exercising each body part once a week except for the abdominals (abs) and calves. Do these two to three times a week. Raising the intensity of your upper back and shoulder workout with techniques such as *drop setting* or *super setting* will increase the width of your shoulders and back, and give your now vertical physique that sought after V-shape.

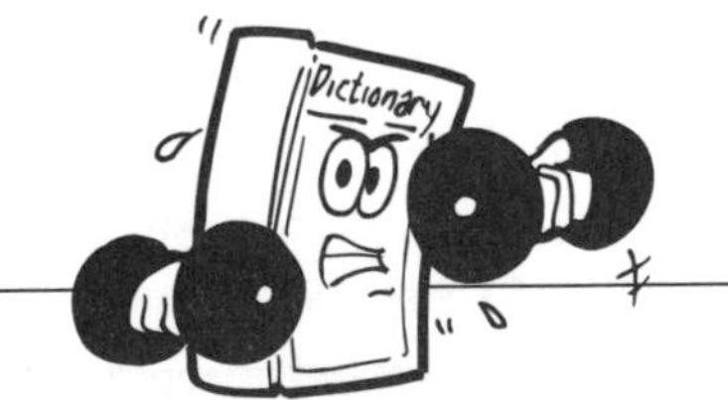

Workout Wisdom

An **endomorph** is a body type that is naturally curvy in shape and puts on weight easily.

The only time that ectomorphs gain muscle easily is when they also possess some mesomorph traits. This would mean that you have the best of both worlds, so feel blessed and be supportive to rest of us who have to put in overtime sweatin' to the oldies. (The good news for the rest of us is that there is truth to the saying, "If it comes too easy, it won't mean as much.")

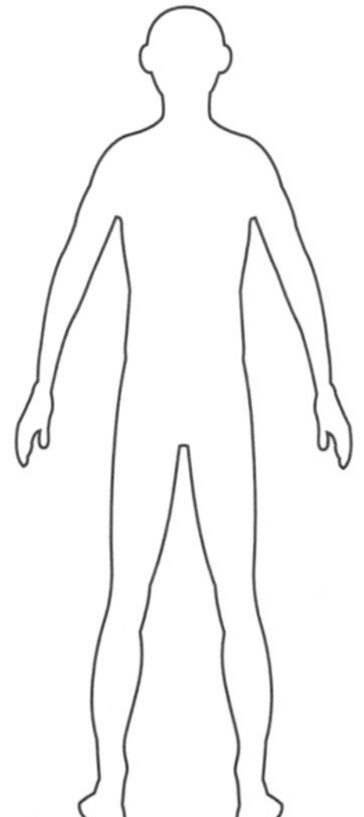

The typical ectomorph shape.

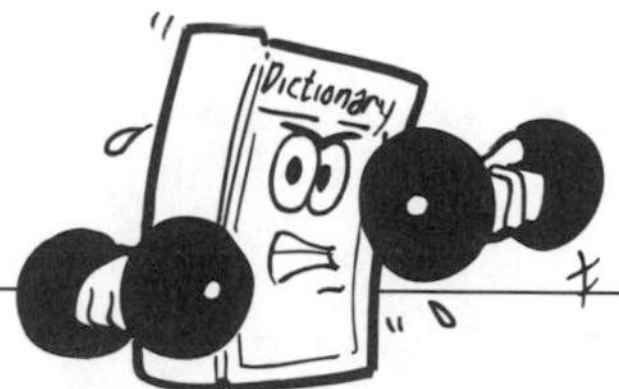

Workout Wisdom

Cardiovascular (cardio) exercise is a type of exercise, the main functions of which are to strengthen the heart and lungs and burn excess body fat.

Drop setting is a technique used to raise the intensity of an exercise set. You do as many repetitions (reps) as possible (AMRAP) while maintaining perfect form of the exercise at one weight. When you can't do another repetition, instead of stopping you drop down to a lighter weight (such as starting with 10 lb. and then dropping to 5 lb.) and do AMRAP at that weight.

Super setting is a technique used to raise the intensity of an exercise set. You do two exercises back to back, with no rest, for the same or the opposite muscle group.

Ectomorphs are naturally suited for endurance activities that require speed, agility, and precision. The following sports are naturally suited to an ectomorph:

- Long-distance running
- Track and field events such as hurdles and the long jump

- Volleyball
- Dancing
- Cycling
- Basketball

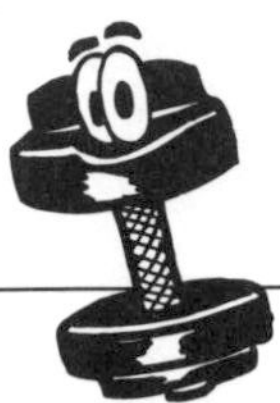

Hard-Body Headliners

Just because you're thin on the outside doesn't mean that you're thin on the inside. If you don't exercise and you eat a lot of fat, you will have a high percentage of body fat that could lead to insulin resistance, high blood pressure, and obesity.

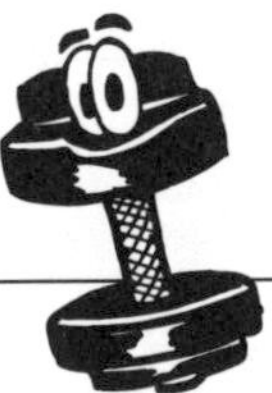

Hard-Body Headliners

Increasing your muscle mass will increase your metabolism and your bone density. An increased metabolism will burn more calories (and body fat) working, playing, and even snoozing. Stronger bones will prevent osteoporosis and injury from happening as you get older.

Brick House

If you are a mesomorph, you have an athletic-looking body. The classic mesomorph body has a rectangular shape, broader shoulders, a well-defined chest, larger bones, and thick muscles. Mesomorphs build muscle mass easily and gain weight evenly throughout their body. Because of their body structure, flexibility doesn't come easy, and a regular stretching program is needed to increase their range of motion. Being a mesomorph doesn't mean that you can keep those perfect pectorals (pecs) without exercise. Your brick house will easily turn into a big house if you're the armchair aerobics king and if eating like Henry VIII is your royal pastime.

Besides the possibility of having some ectomorph traits, the mesomorph can also have endomorph traits. This would mean that you would have the tendency to carry extra body fat. That just means that you need to up your cardio work to stay lean.

Mesomorph workouts should consist of weight training, cardio exercise, and stretching. For toning, you can do a full-body or upper and lower split routines, as shown in Chapter 9, three to four times a week. To increase your workout intensity and change the shape of certain muscle groups, four sessions a week are recommended. Each muscle group should be worked once, except for abs and calves, which can be worked two to three times a week. Mesomorphs should balance weight training and cardio unless they have some endomorph traits; then some extra cardio sessions will be needed. To increase their range of motion and have better muscular development, mesomorphs need to stretch during and after weight training. I recommend a warm-up and light stretching before cardio sessions and deep stretching afterward.

Mesomorphs are suited for sports that require strength and short bursts of power. The following sports are naturally suited to a mesomorph:

- ➤ Boxing
- ➤ Wrestling
- ➤ Weight lifting
- ➤ Football
- ➤ Baseball
- ➤ Gymnastics

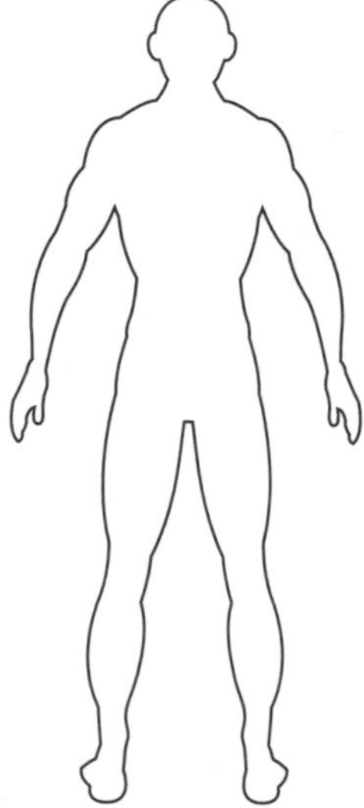

The typical mesomorph shape.

Thick House

When we think of endomorphs, we picture someone soft and curvy. Endomorphs, unfortunately, are the "lucky" ones who put on body fat easily. The extra body fat is stored either in the midsection "spare tire" or in the hip and butt area "pyramid."

I know you've heard the saying "If it doesn't kill you, it makes you stronger." (This saying is my endomorph battle cry each time that I want to stop before finishing my set or when I want to skip cardio and watch *Friends* instead. I solved my dilemma by taping *Friends* and watching it after my cardio session.) The great part about being an endomorph (of which I am a proud member) is that we are strong—we're lifting weights 24 hours a day—and can build muscle easily. Okay, we have to watch what we eat and do a lot of cardio, but we can turn the thick house into a brick house.

Before you throw in the towel because this sounds like way too much work, remember my earlier saying: "If it comes too easily, it won't mean as much." Just take a moment and think how good you will feel and how much confidence you will have by knowing that you can do anything that you set your mind to. Soon, exercise will stop being work and will start becoming a part of loving yourself. I speak from experience when I say that you will love the way you feel, love the way you look, and love all the extra energy that you will get. (I'm sure you'll be able to find many uses for this extra energy.)

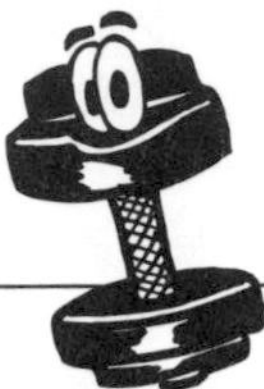

Hard-Body Headliners

You burn more body fat if you do your cardio session after weight training. Intense weight training for 45 to 60 minutes should deplete your glucose supply so that you can get down to the business of fat burning. Because your heart rate is already elevated, you will also reach your fat-burning threshold quicker than if you started your session cold. If you start cold, you first have to elevate your heart rate slowly for 10–15 minutes and then burn up your remaining glucose supply before you start to make a dent in your body fat.

An endomorph's workout should consist of weight training, cardio, and stretching. For toning, you can start by doing a full-body routine, as shown in Chapter 9, three times a week. As your strength level increases, you can switch to an upper and lower split routine four times a week doing lower body training on Monday and Thursday, upper body training on Tuesday and Friday, and resting on Wednesday and Saturday. To change your shape and build muscle, you can start with the same beginning routine that I used to change my shape. (I have included my beginner through advanced training routines in Chapter 9.) As your strength increases, you can switch to my intermediate routine and finally to my advanced routine. Include stretching during and after your weight workouts. Your emphasis should be on cardio, and you will need five to six sessions a week for weight loss. By using my cardio maximizer tips found in Chapter 10, "Home Is Where the Heart Gets Fit," you can make the most of each session and get results fast and safe.

Endomorphs are very strong and have a lot of lower-body power. The following sports are naturally suited to an endomorph:

- Football
- Baseball
- Martial arts
- Tennis
- Weight lifting
- Wrestling

Building a Solid Foundation

To make sure that you start your renovation project with the routine that's best suited to your current fitness level, you need to be assessed in the following four areas.

- **Body composition.** The ratio of fat tissue to other tissue in your body.
- **Cardio fitness.** Ability of your body to take in and utilize oxygen to create energy.
- **Muscular strength.** Strength and endurance of your muscles.
- **Flexibility.** Ability to bend joints and stretch muscles through a full range of motion.

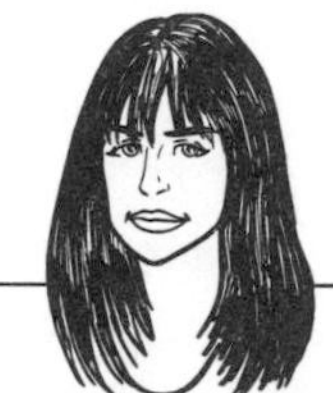

Jourdan's Gems

I carry my before photo in the back of my daily organizer and look at it when I need a motivating boost to show how far I've come. I also look at it when I'm tempted to skip workouts or cheat badly on my diet to show me where I never want to be again.

The dress code is workout gear or loose-fitting, comfortable clothing and a pair of good athletic shoes. Getting a friend in on the action will make doing your evaluations easier and more fun than doing it alone. If you do the assessments with a friend, take turns doing the tests while the other runs the stopwatch and logs the scores. The tests are set up so that they can be done alone as well. Getting a good caliper reading by yourself is the only thing that might be kind of tricky, so have this test redone as soon as possible by a friend or a fitness professional just to double-check the results.

After completing each test, log your results in your Home Hard-Body Profile that's found in the following table. Copy the profile and put it in the front section of your Home Hard-Body Journal. You will also need to take a photo of yourself in workout clothes or a bathing suit. Write the start date on a separate page, and tape this photo under that heading.

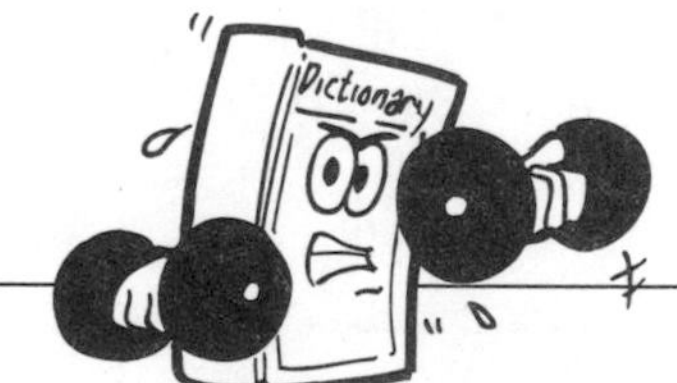

Workout Wisdom

Adipose tissue is another word for fatty tissue. Your total body mass is divided into fat-free mass (bone, muscle, and organs) and fat mass, which is composed of adipose tissue.

This may not be fun now, but it'll be really fun when you see proof of your progress in your follow-up photos. Retest and take new photos (in the same outfit as before) every four weeks to check your progress in each fitness area.

Home Hard-Body Fitness Profile

Fitness Assessment	Start Date	4th Week	8th Week	12th Week
Body composition	______	______	______	______
Body weight	______	______	______	______
BMI	______	______	______	______
Weight category	______	______	______	______
Body fat percentage	______	______	______	______
Body fat percentage category	______	______	______	______
Measurements				
Arm	______	______	______	______
Chest	______	______	______	______
Waist	______	______	______	______
Hip	______	______	______	______
Thigh	______	______	______	______
Calf	______	______	______	______
Cardio Fitness				
Step test	______	______	______	______
Cardio level	______	______	______	______
Muscular Strength				
Push-up test	______	______	______	______
Strength level	______	______	______	______
Flexibility				
Sit-and-reach test	______	______	______	______
Flexibility level	______	______	______	______

Body Composition

You will be using two methods to determine the ratio of *adipose* tissue to other tissue in your body. You will need a scale to weigh yourself and calipers to do the "pinch an inch" test.

To determine your body mass index, follow these steps:

1. Weigh yourself, and log your weight on your Home Hard Body Fitness Profile chart.
2. Use the body mass index (BMI) chart that follows, and find your weight in pounds in the left column and your height in inches in the top row.
3. Trace a line across from your weight and a line down from your height. The number where both lines intersect is your BMI.

4. Use the BMI reference chart following the body mass index chart to determine your weight category. Log your results in your Home Hard Body Fitness Profile chart.

Body Mass Index Chart (BMI)

	19	20	21	22	23	24	25	26	27	28	29	30	35	40
Height (Inches)						*Weight (Pounds)*								
58	91	85	100	105	110	115	119	124	129	134	138	143	167	191
59	94	99	104	109	114	119	124	128	133	138	143	148	173	198
60	97	102	107	112	118	123	128	133	138	143	148	153	179	204
61	100	106	111	116	121	127	132	137	143	148	153	158	185	211
62	104	109	115	120	125	131	136	142	147	153	158	164	191	218
63	107	113	118	124	130	135	141	146	152	158	163	169	197	225
64	110	116	122	128	134	140	145	151	157	163	169	174	203	233
65	114	120	126	132	138	144	150	156	162	168	174	180	210	240
66	117	124	130	136	142	148	155	161	167	173	179	185	216	247
67	121	127	134	140	147	153	159	166	172	178	185	191	223	255
68	125	131	138	144	151	158	164	171	177	184	190	197	230	263
69	128	135	142	149	155	162	169	176	182	189	196	203	237	270
70	132	139	146	153	160	167	174	181	188	195	202	209	243	278
71	136	143	150	157	165	172	179	186	193	200	207	215	250	286
72	140	147	155	162	169	177	184	191	199	206	213	221	258	294
73	144	151	159	166	174	182	189	197	204	212	219	227	265	303
74	148	155	163	171	179	187	194	202	210	218	225	233	272	311
75	152	160	168	176	184	192	200	208	216	224	232	240	279	319
76	156	164	172	180	189	197	205	213	221	230	238	246	287	328

BMI Reference Chart

Weight Category	BMI Range	Percent Above Normal Weight
Normal weight	19–25	0%
Overweight	26–30	20–40%
Obese	31–35	41–100%
Seriously obese	Over 35	Over 100%

To get a more accurate body fat percentage measurement, especially if you currently work out, I also suggest that you do a pinch test using calipers. You can purchase calipers from Power Systems, ranging in price from $19.95 for the basic model to $200 for the professional model. I have used both successfully—the only difference is that the less expensive model is made of plastic, and the professional

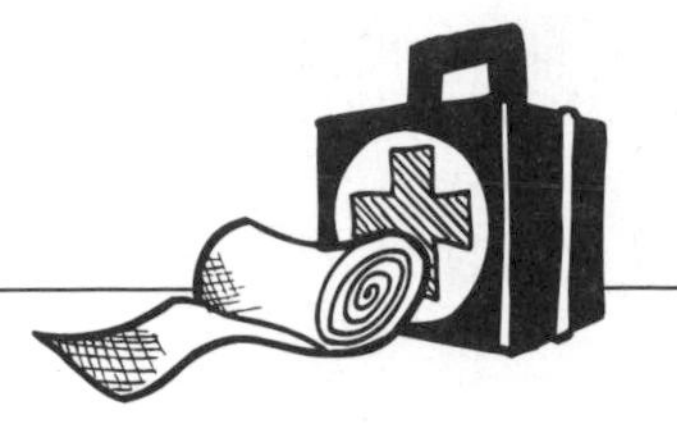

Safety Scoop

The BMI might be way off base if you have a strength-training background. Because the BMI is calculated with a person's total body weight, it can't tell the difference between someone with too much body fat and an athlete with more muscle.

model is metal and comes with a fancy case. All caliper measurements have a degree of inaccuracy of about 3 percent. Because the basic model is just as accurate, I'd put the $180 difference toward something that you really need, such as a new outfit to show off your new hard body. You can contact Power Systems at 1-800-321-6975 or log onto the company's Web site at www.power-systems.com.

You will be taking measurements from three different sites. Women will take measurements from their triceps, abdomen, and thigh. Men will be measuring their chest, abdomen, and thigh. For continuity, use the left side of the body for all test measuring.

Add the three measurements. Using the appropriate body fat percentage chart, locate the number that intersects your score with your age. This is your current body fat percentage. Use the following table to determine your current level. Log all results in your profile.

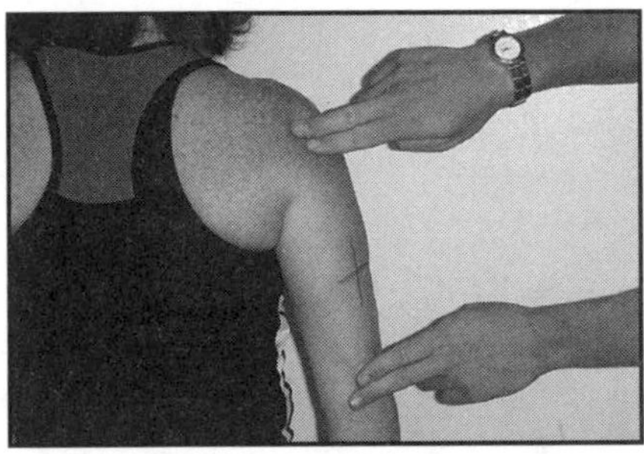

Locate the site midway between the shoulder and elbow.

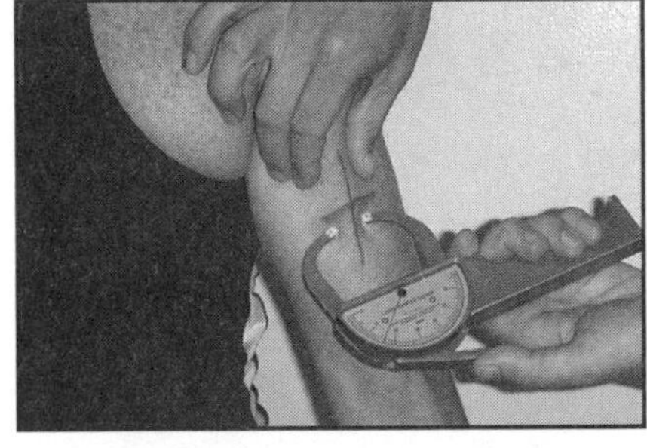

Grasp a vertical fold, and pull it away from the muscle.

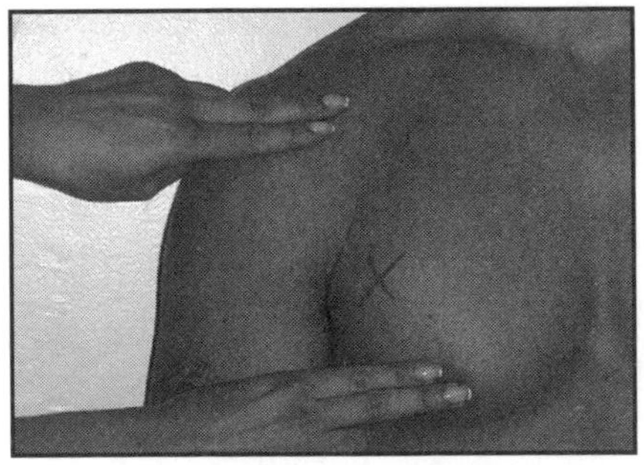

Locate the site midway between the anterior line and the nipple.

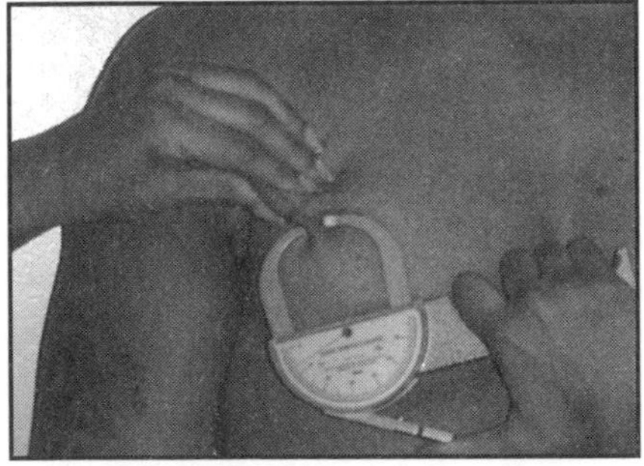

Grasp a vertical fold, and pull it away from the muscle.

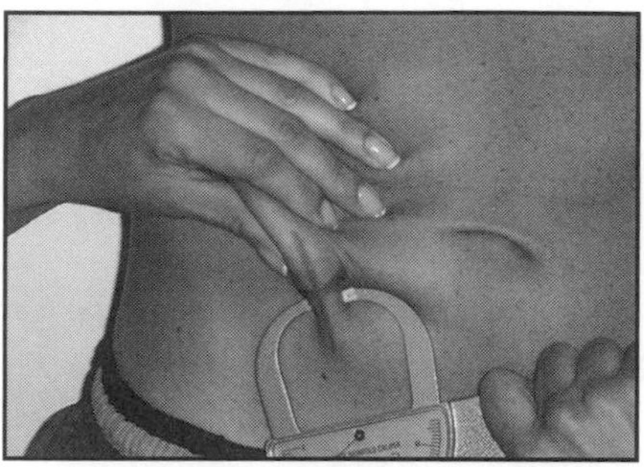

Locate the site midway between the hipbone and the navel.

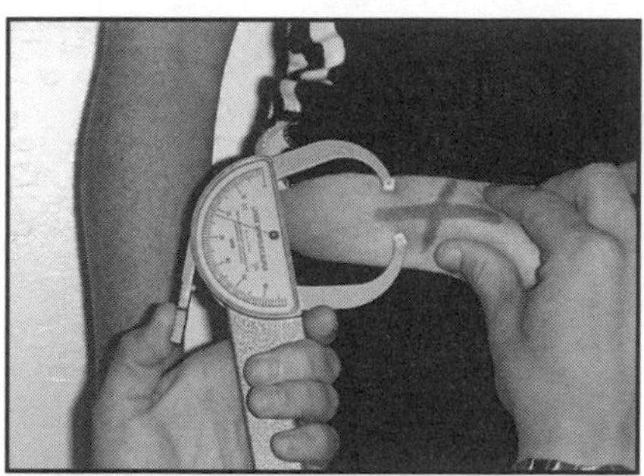

Grasp a vertical fold, and pull it away from the muscle.

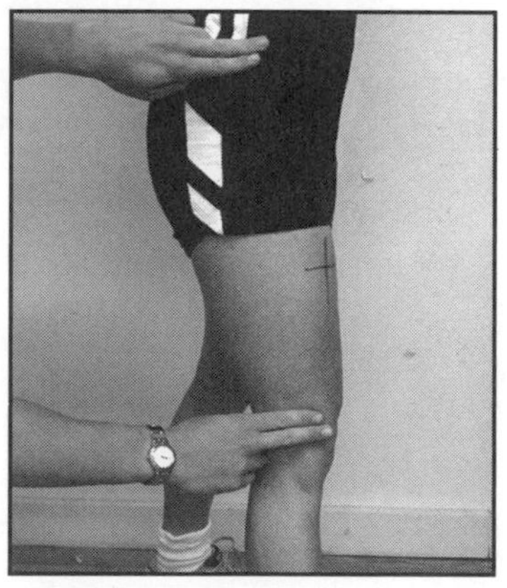

Locate the site midway between the hip and knee joints.

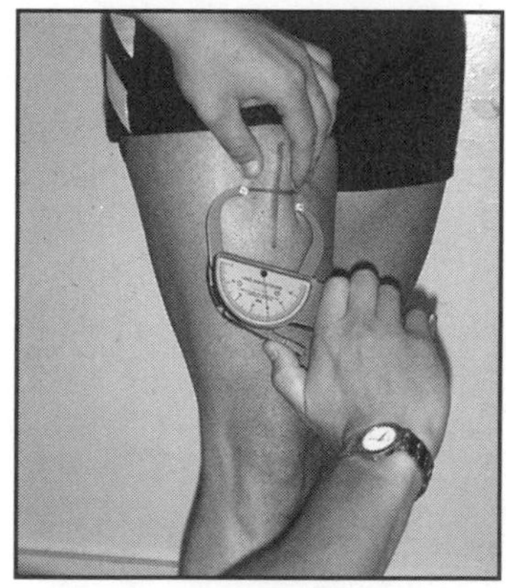

Grasp a vertical skin fold, and pull away from the muscle.

Percent Body Fat Estimations for Women—Jackson and Pollock Formula

Sum of Skinfolds (mm)	Age Groups Under 22	23–27	28–32	33–37	38–42	43–47	48–52	53–57	Over 57
23–25	9.7	9.9	10.2	10.4	10.7	10.9	11.2	11.4	11.7
26–28	11.0	11.2	11.5	11.7	12.0	12.3	12.5	12.7	13.0
29–31	12.3	12.5	12.8	13.0	13.3	13.5	13.8	14.0	14.3
32–34	13.6	13.8	14.0	14.3	14.5	14.8	15.0	15.3	15.5

continues

Percent Body Fat Estimations for Women—Jackson and Pollock Formula (continued)

Sum of Skinfolds (mm)	Age Groups Under 22	23–27	28–32	33–37	38–42	43–47	48–52	53–57	Over 57
35–37	14.8	15.0	15.3	15.5	15.8	16.0	16.3	16.5	16.8
38–40	16.0	16.3	16.5	16.7	17.0	17.2	17.5	17.7	18.0
41–43	17.2	17.4	17.7	17.9	18.2	18.4	18.7	18.9	19.2
44–46	18.3	18.6	18.8	19.1	19.3	19.6	19.8	20.1	20.3
47–49	19.5	19.7	20.0	20.2	20.5	20.7	21.0	21.2	21.5
50–52	20.6	20.8	21.1	21.3	21.6	21.8	22.1	22.3	22.6
53–55	21.7	21.9	22.1	22.4	22.6	22.9	23.1	23.4	23.6
56–58	22.7	23.0	23.2	23.4	23.7	23.9	24.2	24.4	24.7
59–61	23.7	24.0	24.2	24.5	24.7	25.0	25.2	25.5	25.7
62–64	24.7	25.0	25.2	25.5	25.7	26.0	26.7	26.4	26.7
65–67	25.7	25.9	26.2	26.4	26.7	25.9	27.2	27.4	27.7
68–70	26.6	26.9	27.1	27.4	27.6	27.9	28.1	28.4	28.6
71–73	27.5	27.8	28.0	28.3	28.5	28.8	29.0	29.3	29.5
74–76	28.4	28.7	28.9	29.2	29.4	29.7	29.9	30.2	30.4
77–79	29.3	29.5	29.8	30.0	30.3	30.5	30.8	31.0	31.3
80–82	30.1	30.4	30.6	30.9	31.1	31.4	31.6	31.9	32.1
83–85	30.9	31.2	31.4	31.7	31.9	32.2	32.4	32.7	32.9
86–88	31.7	32.0	32.2	32.5	32.7	32.9	33.2	33.4	33.7
89–91	32.5	32.7	33.0	33.2	33.5	33.7	33.9	34.2	34.4
92–94	33.2	33.4	33.7	33.9	34.2	34.4	34.7	34.9	35.2
95–97	33.9	34.1	34.4	34.6	34.9	35.1	35.4	35.6	35.9
98–100	34.6	34.8	35.1	35.3	35.5	35.8	36.0	36.3	36.5
101–103	35.3	35.4	35.7	35.9	36.2	36.4	36.7	36.9	37.2
104–106	35.8	36.1	36.3	36.6	36.8	37.1	37.3	37.5	37.8
107–109	36.4	36.7	36.9	37.1	37.4	37.6	37.9	38.1	38.4
110–112	37.0	37.2	37.5	37.7	38.0	38.2	38.5	38.7	38.9
113–115	37.5	37.8	38.0	38.2	38.5	38.7	39.0	39.2	39.5
116–118	38.0	38.3	38.5	38.8	39.0	39.3	39.5	39.7	40.0
119–121	38.5	38.7	39.0	39.2	39.5	39.7	40.0	40.2	40.5
122–124	39.0	39.2	39.4	39.7	39.9	40.2	40.4	40.7	40.9
125–127	39.4	39.6	39.9	40.1	40.4	40.6	40.9	41.1	41.4
128–130	39.8	40.0	40.3	40.5	40.8	41.0	41.3	41.5	41.8

Source: Reprinted by permission from Andrew Jackson, PED, et al., Practical Assessment of Body Composition: The Physician and Sportsmedicine, *vol. 13, no. 5. (May 1985).*

Percent Body Fat Estimations for Men—Jackson and Pollock Formula

Sum of Skinfolds (mm)	Under 22	Age Groups 23–27	28–32	33–37	38–42	43–47	48–52	53–57	Over 57
8–10	1.3	1.8	2.3	2.9	3.4	3.9	4.5	5.0	5.5
11–13	2.2	2.8	3.3	3.9	4.4	4.9	5.5	6.0	6.5
14–16	3.2	3.8	4.3	4.8	5.4	5.9	6.4	7.0	7.5
17–19	4.2	4.7	5.3	5.8	6.3	6.9	7.4	8.0	8.5
20–22	5.1	5.7	6.2	6.8	7.3	7.9	8.4	8.9	9.5
23–25	6.1	6.6	7.2	7.7	8.3	8.8	9.4	9.9	10.5
26–28	7.0	7.6	8.1	8.7	9.2	9.8	10.3	10.9	11.4
29–31	8.0	8.5	9.1	9.6	10.2	10.7	11.3	11.8	12.4
32–34	8.9	9.4	10.4	10.5	11.1	11.6	12.2	12.8	13.3
35–37	9.8	10.4	10.9	11.5	12.0	12.6	13.1	13.7	14.3
38–40	10.7	11.3	11.8	12.4	12.9	13.5	14.1	14.6	15.2
41–43	11.6	12.2	12.7	13.3	13.8	14.4	15.0	15.5	16.1
44–46	12.5	13.1	13.6	14.2	14.7	15.3	15.9	16.4	17.0
47–49	13.4	13.9	14.5	15.1	15.6	16.2	16.8	17.3	17.9
50–52	14.3	14.8	15.4	15.9	16.5	17.1	17.6	18.2	18.8
53–55	15.1	15.7	16.2	16.8	17.4	17.9	18.5	19.1	19.7
56–58	16.0	16.5	17.1	17.7	18.2	18.8	19.4	20.0	20.5
59–61	16.9	17.4	17.9	18.5	19.1	19.7	20.2	20.8	21.4
62–64	17.6	18.2	18.8	19.4	19.9	20.5	21.1	21.7	22.2
65–67	18.5	19.0	19.6	20.2	20.8	21.3	21.9	22.5	23.1
68–70	19.3	19.9	20.4	21.0	21.6	22.2	22.7	23.3	23.9
71–73	20.1	20.7	21.2	21.8	22.4	23.0	23.6	24.1	24.7
74–76	20.9	21.5	22.0	22.6	23.2	23.8	24.4	25.0	25.5
77–79	21.7	22.2	22.8	23.4	24.0	24.6	25.2	25.8	26.3
80–82	22.4	23.0	23.6	24.2	24.8	25.4	25.9	26.5	27.1
83–85	23.2	23.8	24.4	25.0	25.5	26.1	26.7	27.3	27.9
86–88	24.0	24.5	25.1	25.7	26.3	26.9	27.5	28.1	28.7
89–91	24.7	25.3	25.9	26.5	27.1	27.6	28.2	28.8	29.4
92–94	25.4	26.0	26.6	27.2	27.8	28.4	29.0	29.6	30.2
95–97	26.1	26.7	27.3	27.9	28.5	29.1	29.7	30.3	30.9
98–100	26.9	27.4	28.0	28.6	29.2	29.8	30.4	31.0	31.6
101–103	27.5	28.1	28.7	29.3	29.9	30.5	31.1	31.7	32.3
104–106	28.2	28.8	29.4	30.0	30.6	31.2	31.8	32.4	33.0
107–109	28.9	29.5	30.1	30.7	31.1	31.9	32.5	33.1	33.7
110–112	29.6	30.2	30.8	31.4	32.0	32.6	33.2	33.8	34.4

continues

Percent Body Fat Estimations for Men—Jackson and Pollock Formula (continued)

Sum of Skinfolds (mm)	Under 22	23–27	28–32	33–37	38–42	43–47	48–52	53–57	Over 57
113–115	30.2	30.8	31.4	32.0	32.6	33.2	33.8	34.5	35.1
116–118	30.9	31.5	32.1	32.7	33.3	33.9	34.5	35.1	35.74
119–121	31.5	32.1	32.7	33.3	33.9	34.5	35.1	35.7	36.4
122–124	32.1	32.7	33.3	33.9	34.5	35.1	35.8	36.4	37.0
125–127	32.7	33.3	33.9	34.5	35.1	35.8	36.4	37.0	37.6

Source: Reprinted by permission from Andrew Jackson, PED, et al., Practical Assessment of Body Composition: The Physician and Sportsmedicine, *vol. 13, no. 5. (May 1985).*

Body Fat Percentage Categories

Classification	Women (% fat)	Men (% fat)
Essential fat	11–14%	3–5%
Athletes	12–22%	5–13%
Fitness	16–25%	12–18%
Possible risk	26–31%	19–24%
Obese	32% and higher	25% and higher

Source: Reprinted by permission from E. Howley and B. Franks, Health Fitness Instructor's Handbook, 3rd ed. *(Champaign, IL Human Kinetics, 1997), 166.*

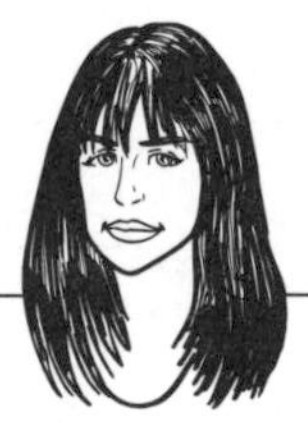

Jourdan's Gems

For a creative timer, heat some water for three minutes in the microwave oven while you do your step test. When the timer goes off, stop stepping. Steep your favorite herbal tea while you do the last two tests. You've worked hard, so savor each sip as you design the home hard-body workout that's perfect for you.

Use a tape measure to measure the following locations and log the measurements in your fitness profile:

- Arm (left side)
- Chest
- Waist
- Hips
- Thigh (left side)
- Calf (left side)

Cardio Fitness

Now that we've been pinched and measured, it's time to move on to the cardio section of your home-body assessment. For this section, you need a stopwatch and a step with risers. If you don't have a step, you can use a sturdy milk crate or footstool. A watch with a second hand or a stove timer can take the place of a stopwatch.

Start stepping up and down for three minutes, as shown in the accompanying photo. Wait 5 seconds, and then take a 15-second pulse reading. Multiply that number by 4 to get your beats per minute. Log this number in your log, along with your fitness level, which can be found in one of the two following tables, depending on your gender.

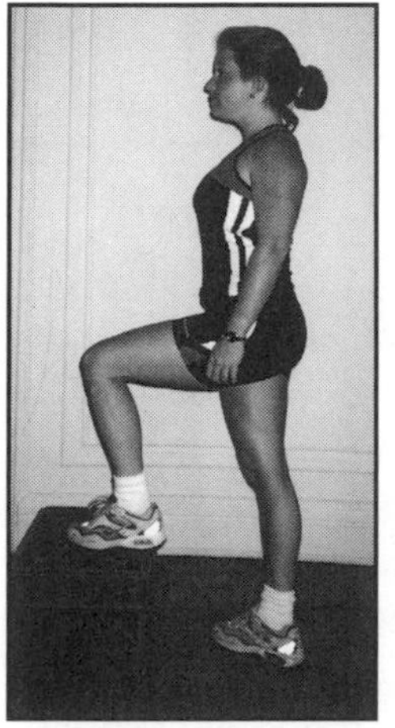
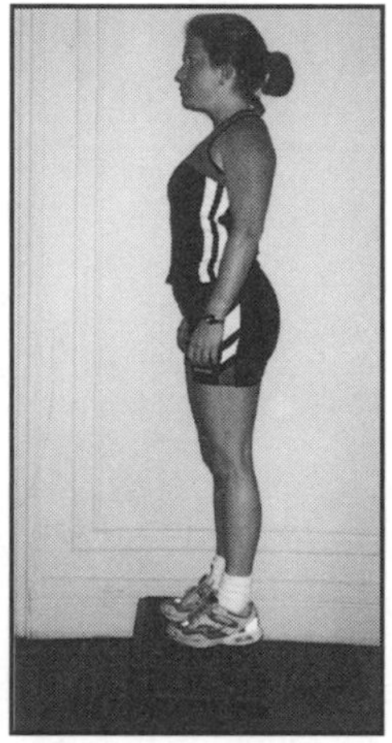
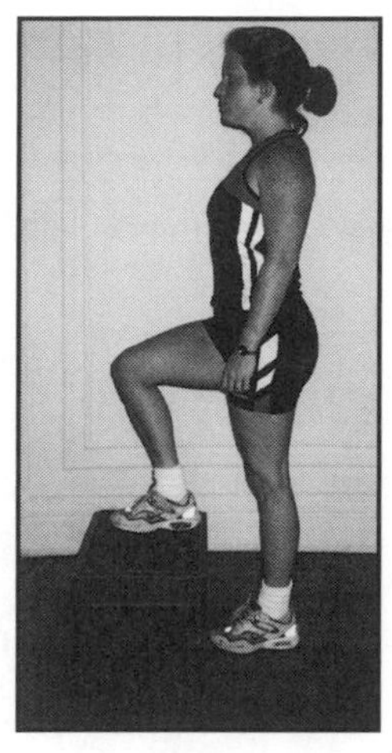
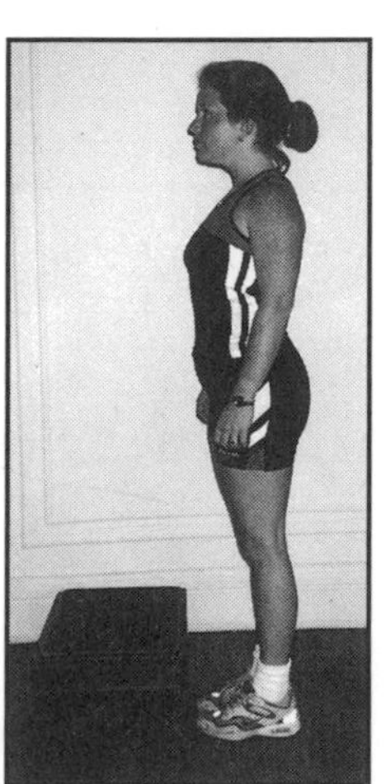

These photos show the correct form for the Three-Minute Step Test.

Male Norms for the Three-Minute Step Test (with Age in Years)

Cardio Level	18–25	26–35	36–45	46–55	56–65	65+
Excellent	50–76	51–76	49–76	56–82	60–77	59–81
Good	79–84	79–85	80–88	87–93	86–94	87–92
Above average	88–93	88–94	92–98	95–101	97–100	94–102
Average	95–100	96–102	100–105	103–111	103–109	104–110
Below average	102–107	104–110	108–113	113–119	111–117	114–118
Poor	111–119	114–121	116–124	121–126	119–128	121–126
Very poor	124–157	126–161	130–163	131–159	131–154	130–151

Source: Reprinted by permission from the YMCA of the USA, YMCA Fitness Testing and Assessment Manual, 4th ed. *Lawrence A. Golding, editor (Chicago).*

Female Norms for the Three-Minute Step Test (with Age in Years)

Cardio Level	18–25	26–35	36–45	46–55	56–65	65+
Excellent	52–81	58–80	51–84	63–91	60–92	70–92
Good	85–93	85–92	89–96	95–101	97–103	96–101
Above average	96–102	95–101	100–104	104–110	106–111	104–111
Average	104–110	104–110	107–112	113–118	113–118	116–121
Below average	113–120	113–119	115–120	120–124	119–127	123–126
Poor	122–131	122–129	124–132	126–132	129–135	128–133
Very poor	135–169	134–171	137–169	137–171	141–174	135–155

Source: Reprinted by permission from the YMCA of the USA, YMCA Fitness Testing and Assessment Manual, 4th ed. *Lawrence A. Golding, editor (Chicago).*

Muscular Strength

Your muscular strength and endurance are determined by doing as many push-ups as you can before you poop out. Women can do a modified push-up on their knees. Because we are assessing upper-body muscle strength, individuals with less upper-body strength should use the modified push-up. Guys, don't even think about it. You'll be doing the regular version on your toes. Use one of the following tables, depending on your gender, to find your fitness level and record both on your profile.

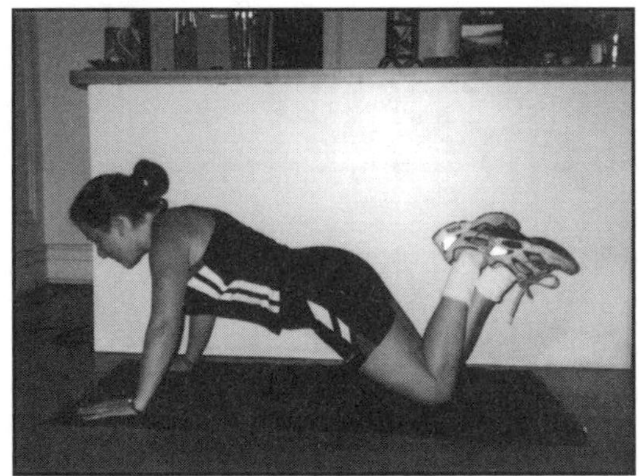

This shows the correct form for modified push-ups.

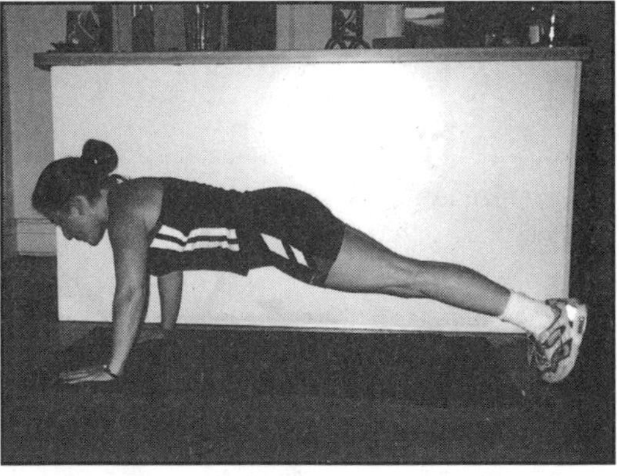

This shows the correct form for straight-leg push-ups.

Male Norms for Push-Up Test (Number Completed)

Age (Years)	20–29	30–39	40–49	50–59	60–69
Rating					
Above average	29–35	22–29	17–21	13–20	11–17
Average	22–28	17–21	13–16	10–12	8–10
Below average	17–21	12–16	10–12	7–9	5–7
Low	16	11	9	6	4

Source: Reprinted by permission from David C. Nieman, Exercise Testing and Prescription: A Health-Related Approach, 4th ed. *(Mayfield Publishing Company, 1999).*

Female Norms for Push-Up Test (Number Completed)

Age (Years)	20–29	30–39	40–49	50–59	60–69
Rating					
Above average	21–29	20–26	15–23	11–20	12–16
Average	15–20	13–19	11–14	7–10	5–11
Below average	10–14	8–12	5–10	2–6	1–4
Low	9	7	4	1	1

Source: Reprinted by permission from David C. Nieman, Exercise Testing and Prescription: A Health-Related Approach, 4th ed. *(Mayfield Publishing Company, 1999).*

Flexibility

The sit-and-reach test evaluates your level of flexibility. You need a yardstick and some tape for this test. Tape the yardstick to the floor at the 15-inch mark. Sit on the floor with the yardstick between your legs and your feet 12 inches apart and even with the 15-inch mark. With one hand over the other, gently lean forward as far as you can, and hold for 2 seconds. Write down your score. Repeat two more times, and use the best score to find your flexibility level for your gender in the following two tables. Log your score and your flexibility in your profile.

Male Norms for the Sit-and-Reach Test

Age (Years)	18–25	26–35	36–45	46–55	56–65	65+
Flexibility Level						
Excellent	22–28	21–28	21–28	19–26	17–24	17–24
Good	20–21	19	18–19	16–18	15–16	14–16

continues

Male Norms for the Sit-and-Reach Test (continued)

Age (Years)	18–25	26–35	36–45	46–55	56–65	65+
Above average	18–19	17	16–17	14–15	13	12–13
Average	16–17	15–16	15	12–13	11	10–11
Below average	14–15	13–14	13	10–11	9	8–9
Poor	12–13	11–12	9–11	8–9	6–8	6–7
Very poor	2–11	2–9	1–7	1–6	1–5	0–4

Source: Reprinted by permission from the YMCA of the USA, YMCA Fitness Testing and Assessment Manual, 4th ed. *Lawrence A. Golding, editor (Chicago).*

Female Norms for the Sit-and-Reach Test

Age (Years)	18–25	26–35	36–45	46–55	56–65	65+
Flexibility Level						
Excellent	24–29	23–28	22–28	21–27	20–26	20–26
Good	22	21–22	20–21	19–20	18–19	12–16
Above average	20–21	20	18–19	17–18	16–17	17
Average	19	18–19	17	16	15	15–16
Below average	17–18	16–17	15–16	14	13–14	13–14
Poor	16	14–15	13–14	12–13	10–12	10–12
Very poor	7–14	5–13	4–12	3–10	2–9	1–9

Source: Reprinted by permission from the YMCA of the USA, YMCA Fitness Testing and Assessment Manual, 4th ed. *Lawrence A. Golding, editor (Chicago).*

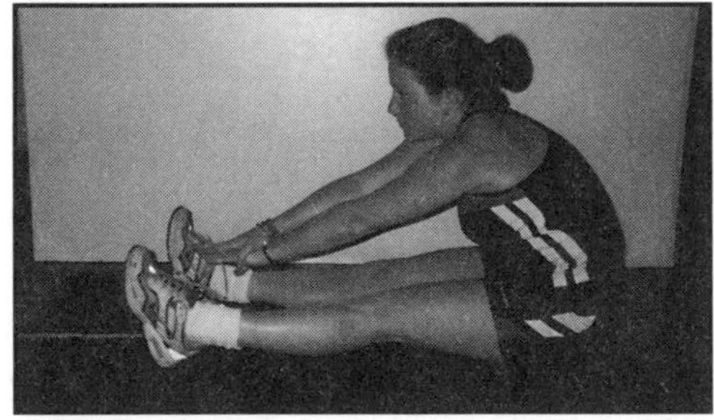

This shows the correct form for the Sit-and-Reach test.

Custom-Design Your Home Hard Body

With your home hard-body profile completed, it'll be easy to match your current level to one of my custom exercise routines. By training smart (not just hard), you'll soon be able to transform your fitness fixer-upper into a show-stopping physical palace.

The Least You Need to Know

- Use your health history as a guide for exercise choices and modifications.
- Work with your body type to create the shape you want with angular illusions.
- Doing the right workout for your fitness level will prevent injury and unnecessary soreness from doing too much too soon.
- Check your progress by doing follow-up assessments.

Chapter 3

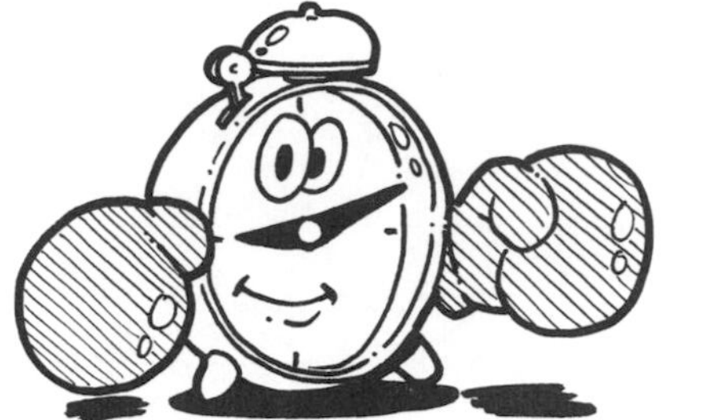

Punch the (Alarm) Clock

In This Chapter

- Getting your priorities straight
- Planning your work, and working your plan
- Discovering your workout time options
- Getting creative in finding time

Schedules fall into two categories: the friendly ones that organize your life so that your only decision is what to do with all your free time, and the straightjacket ones that make you feel like you're doing time.

Keeping your schedule simple will keep it user-friendly. Let your priorities decide the order of when things get done. Since you're reading this book, you already know that taking care of yourself should be at the top of your list. It doesn't take a rocket scientist to know that when you feel great, you do great.

Remember, the best-planned workouts won't do you any good if you don't do them. This will come in handy when picking your perfect hard-body workout time. If just thinking about 5 A.M. freaks you out, then it's probably not your best choice. Giving yourself room to breathe in your schedule is your insurance policy against missing an important appointment, such as your valuable hard-body workout, if you get caught in traffic or stuck in a doctor's waiting room because he's (big surprise) behind schedule.

Step 1: Get Your Priorities Straight

The first step to creating a schedule that will make you look forward to even Monday morning is to identify your priorities. Take a few minutes and write down the five most important things to your life in order of importance. I've taken the liberty of starting you off with number one.

My Priorities

1. Taking care of myself
2. ________________________________
3. ________________________________
4. ________________________________
5. ________________________________

Step 2: Where Does Your Time Now Go?

Saying that we will make time for something is an inaccurate statement because we can't *make* time. There are only so many set hours in a day, so if we really want to do something, we take the time away from another event that suddenly becomes less important.

If you've ever said, "If I only had more time" or "There aren't enough hours in a day," then chances are good that there might not be enough hours in your day for your current schedule. It's time to find out where you spend most of your time and to see if your priorities guide those time choices.

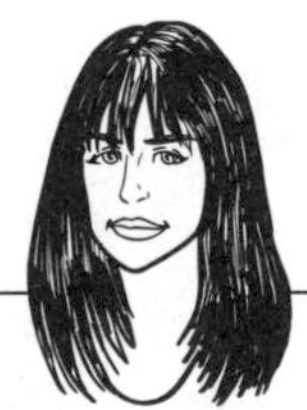

Jourdan's Gems

An event can be important, but if it's not fun, it could easily take a back seat when a fun opportunity comes along. To prevent this from happening, give yourself a fun reward (massage, new clothing) if you complete the important event by the appointed time (such as completing all scheduled hard-body workouts for the week).

Fill in the time table below with the average number of hours that you now spend on various activities. Then subtract the total hours from the starting hours to see if you actually have any time left over at the end of your day. Once completed, answer the following questions:

- Do I have time left over?
- Do I spend my time on my priorities?
- Does how I spend my time reflect a balance in my life?

If you answered "yes" to any or all of these, then you're on the right track or might have to make just a few adjustments. If you answered "no" to all three, then that explains why you might feel wiped out and overworked at the end of the day.

Go back over your time table and highlight the activities that could be rescheduled to another time, given less time, or eliminated if a better opportunity came along (such as getting your home hard body).

(Add Your Name)'s Current Time Table

	M	T	W	TH	F	S	S
Starting Hours	**24**	**24**	**24**	**24**	**24**	**24**	**24**
Sleep	______	______	______	______	______	______	______
Work	______	______	______	______	______	______	______
School	______	______	______	______	______	______	______
Time to get ready	______	______	______	______	______	______	______
Commute	______	______	______	______	______	______	______
Errands	______	______	______	______	______	______	______
Cooking	______	______	______	______	______	______	______
Laundry	______	______	______	______	______	______	______
Significant other	______	______	______	______	______	______	______
Childcare	______	______	______	______	______	______	______
Exercise	______	______	______	______	______	______	______
Fun time	______	______	______	______	______	______	______
Friends	______	______	______	______	______	______	______
Total Hours	______	______	______	______	______	______	______
Leftover Hours	______	______	______	______	______	______	______

Step 3: Taking Time

You are now going to start creating your new, friendly Hard-Body Training Schedule. It will be *friendly* because you are going to give yourself breathing space and will not try to do everything every day.

The first step is to block out the times for events that are pretty much set in stone, such as work or school hours. At the end of your week, make sure that you rope off a few hours or even a full day, and treat yourself to something special. It could be anything, just as long as it's fun for you. This time is your reward for all your hard-body hard work, and it is a mandatory requirement in your hard-body training program. (I've dedicated Chapter 16, "Return of the Couch Potato," to ways to pamper you.)

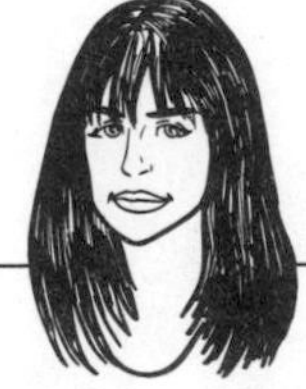

Jourdan's Gems

Time can easily slip away from you, so it's important to be really honest with your current time table. If you're not sure about a certain entry, try leaving it out of your new schedule and see if you actually miss it. The result might surprise you.

(Add Your Name)'s Current Time Table

	M	T	W	TH	F	S	S
5:00	____	____	____	____	____	____	____
5:30	____	____	____	____	____	____	____
6:00	____	____	____	____	____	____	____
6:30	____	____	____	____	____	____	____
7:00	____	____	____	____	____	____	____
7:30	____	____	____	____	____	____	____
8:00	____	____	____	____	____	____	____
8:30	____	____	____	____	____	____	____
9:00	____	____	____	____	____	____	____
9:30	____	____	____	____	____	____	____
10:00	____	____	____	____	____	____	____
10:30	____	____	____	____	____	____	____
11:00	____	____	____	____	____	____	____
11:30	____	____	____	____	____	____	____
12:00	____	____	____	____	____	____	____
12:30	____	____	____	____	____	____	____
1:00	____	____	____	____	____	____	____
1:30	____	____	____	____	____	____	____
2:00	____	____	____	____	____	____	____
2:30	____	____	____	____	____	____	____
3:00	____	____	____	____	____	____	____
3:30	____	____	____	____	____	____	____
4:00	____	____	____	____	____	____	____
4:30	____	____	____	____	____	____	____
5:00	____	____	____	____	____	____	____
5:30	____	____	____	____	____	____	____
6:00	____	____	____	____	____	____	____
6:30	____	____	____	____	____	____	____
7:00	____	____	____	____	____	____	____
7:30	____	____	____	____	____	____	____
8:00	____	____	____	____	____	____	____
8:30	____	____	____	____	____	____	____
9:00	____	____	____	____	____	____	____

Step 4: What Time Is Your Right Time?

Keeping your schedule's vacant time blocks in mind, it's time to look at the various hard-body workout time options and decide which one works best for you. You're already saving time by working out at home, so make sure that your workout time is realistic for you. When you know your final answer, block out your new hard-body workout times in your training schedule. Remember, these times now qualify as "set in stone," so make sure that you feel really comfortable about your choices.

Rise and Shine Renovations

One option is to get up an hour earlier and train your hard body before you start your day. The beautiful thing about training at home in the morning (besides not dragging all your stuff to the gym) is that you can roll out of bed and roll right into your workout room. Since you're the only member in this private club, there is no one to stop you from training in your pajamas, if you so desire. After you're done, you can get ready for work in the privacy of your own bathroom, with real towels. (Gyms aren't fooling anyone with those pint-size strips of sandpaper.)

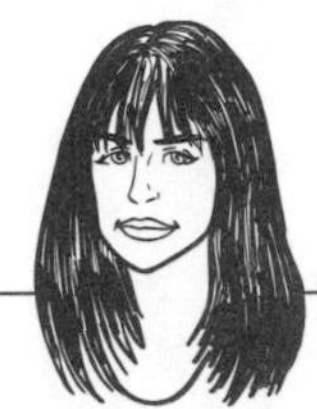

Jourdan's Gems

To make my schedule more fun to do and easier to read, I color-code regular events such as work, training, chill time, family time, and personal "all about me" time. An equal amount of each color means that my schedule is balanced.

Personally, I exercise in the morning and feel that if you can fit it in, morning training has the largest list of benefits. Some of the benefits of morning workouts include these:

- Working out in the morning jump-starts your metabolism and keeps it elevated for hours. This means that you'll burn more calories all day just because you exercised in the morning.
- Working out in the morning energizes you.
- Working out in the morning controls your appetite so that you eat less and eat better.
- Working out in the morning makes you sharper mentally.
- If you consistently wake up and work out at the same time each morning, your body's *endocrine system* adjusts to your new time schedule, making it easier to wake up alert and feel ready to exercise.
- Working out in the morning is one way to make sure that it gets done.

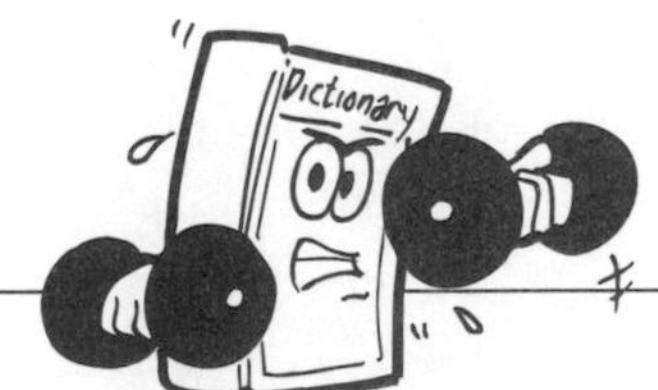

Workout Wisdom

The **endocrine system** is a group of organs and tissues of the body that release hormones. The endocrine glands and their hormones regulate the growth, development, and function of various tissues, and they coordinate many of the processes of metabolism.

High-Noon Hard Body

If you work far from home, then it's unrealistic to consider midday home workouts. If you work nights, by appointments only, or, best of all, at home, you have the option of training late mornings, noontime, or late afternoons. Exercising in the middle of the day is your best defense against the late-day lags. Benefits of midday workouts include these:

- Working out midday will supercharge you mentally and physically for the remainder of the day.
- Working out midday or late afternoon will mean stronger workouts because your body temperature has increased.
- Working out before your midday meal increases the amount of food that your body will use up for fuel before it starts to store it as fat.
- Working out late afternoon will make you more active in the evening and less likely to overeat at dinner.

Nighttime Transformation

Working out in the evening after you get home is an option if you don't regularly work late or meet clients after work. Even with the best intentions, not being able to break away at a set time will increase your chances of missing your workout. If being at home in the evening works for you, then the benefits of evening training include these:

- Working out in the evening will mean stronger workouts because your body temperature is higher and your lung airways are more open.
- Working out in the evening can be a great stress reliever from your day.
- Working out in the evening can become a creative way to spend time with your family.
- Working out in the evening will get you off the couch and help you avoid the temptation of nighttime snacking.

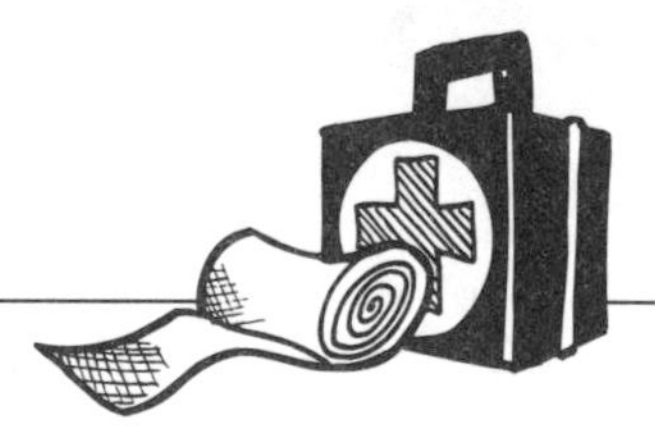

Safety Scoop

The increased adrenaline rush from weight training too close to bedtime can make it difficult to go to sleep right away. Give your body two to three hours to wind down after training before going to bed.

Split-Shift

Split training is dividing your workout into two separate sessions of lesser time, or adding a second workout session of equal time to your training day. Split training for beginners will maximize their results because it's easier to do two 30-minute intense workouts than it is to do one 60-minute intense workout.

Two ways that I split train are to weight train in the morning and then do cardio in the evening, or weight train one body part in the morning and weight train another body part in the evening. If your weight-training program consists of full-body workouts, then the second workout in your split shift shouldn't be another weight-training workout. In Chapter 9, "Custom Home Hard Bodies," I also break down split-training programs. Benefits of split training include these:

- Split training gives your metabolism two boosts for the day so that your body burns more calories.
- Split training first thing in the morning and last thing in the evening before meals will maximize your fat-burning potential.
- Split training with two longer sessions will maximize your muscle-building results because you will be working your muscles more often.
- Split training can help alleviate muscle soreness.
- Split training will build up your endurance for longer sessions.
- Split training for beginners allows them to maintain a higher level of workout intensity by doing two shorter workouts.
- Split training allows you to do more cardio sessions so that you lose body fat quicker.

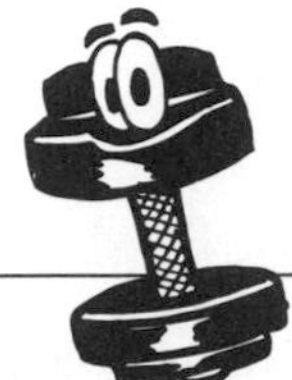

Hard-Body Headliners

You can help eliminate muscle soreness from an intense leg workout by split training later that day with a martial arts class, a yoga class, or a running session. Each of these will eliminate blood pooling in the lower body, increase circulation, and remove any remaining lactic acid that could cause muscle soreness.

Your New Hard-Body Success Schedule

After you've given your hard-body workout time a permanent address on your new schedule, you can add some of the activities that you highlighted in your time chart. If you start to feel the straightjacket coming on, then you know that you've added too much.

Leaving enough time between events will prevent unexpected time bandits from stealing time away from important events. Make it a point to have leftover hours at the end of each day so that you'll be able to enjoy the benefits from your labor any way you like.

After you've finished a schedule that you feel good about, make several copies of it, and place one in your Home Hard-Body Journal and one in your daily organizer. Post the remaining one somewhere visible, such as your refrigerator door or bulletin board.

Getting Creative and Getting Time

Finding ways to include fitness in your daily events is the gateway to getting more things done while maximizing your hard body results. Here are some ideas to get you started:

- Do an exercise video with your kids or spouse.
- Stretch or train with your mate, followed by an exchange of massages.
- Exercise while cleaning house (lunge while you vacuum).
- Exercise while playing with your baby (doing crunches while holding the baby on your chest).

Having a schedule will help you organize your life so you always have time for your hard-body workouts. Keeping your schedule simple so you can live with it will help you make sure your hard-body workouts become an important part of the rest of your life.

The Least You Need to Know

- Taking care of you should be your number-one priority because how you feel affects how you do.
- Creating a schedule that you look forward to following increases your chances of success.
- The right workout time should make it easy for you to work out.
- Finding creative ways to include exercise in your daily activities will increase your hard-body results, increase the amount of available time that you have, and create healthy alternatives that are fun for the whole family.

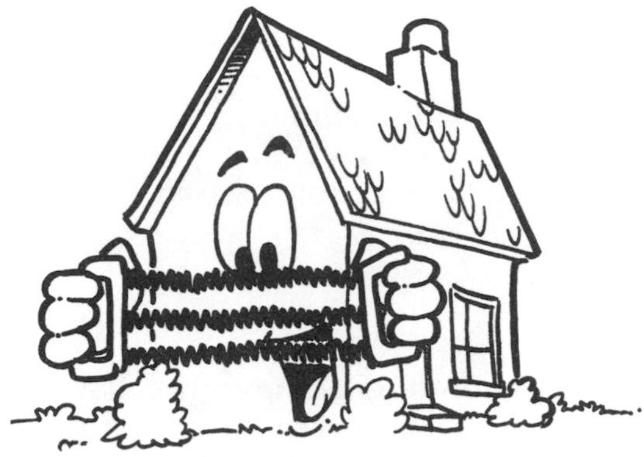

Chapter 4

Home Grown

In This Chapter

- What's your workout bag?
- Find the right strength and cardio gear
- Discover cool new gear options
- Hard-body accessories that maximize your workouts
- The hard-body workout wear is not just for working out

With all the testing behind you, it's time to pick out your cool new fitness toys. In your home hard-body program, you'll be doing strength training, cardio training, and flexibility training. The good news is that there are so many options to choose from in each category that you'll be sure to find something to suit your personality. It's important to pick a type of exercise equipment that's fun for you because even the best gear won't do you any good if it's moonlighting as a clothes hanger. I have several friends who have lost their lifecycles to their laundry. Oh, it's still there somewhere ....

After you've picked out your exercise gear, you need some fun clothes that'll get you excited to work out. If you think that cute workout clothes can't be comfortable, wait until you see the great clothes I've found. The cool thing about this gear is that you can exercise in it, hang out in it, and even go out in it. (How's that for major bang for your buck?)

If that isn't enough, I have also found the killer sport support bra that works without casting the "uniboob" spell on you. You know when you've been hexed. You have to stop in the middle of your sentence and say, "Oh by the way, I'd like you to meet ...

my breasts." I usually don't know whether to laugh (the look on their face is priceless) or to cry because I've just bought a $40 dust cloth.

It's not written anywhere in the home hard-body training manual that getting a hard body means you can't have fun along the way. Whoever thought up the saying "No pain no gain" missed the "happiness isn't supposed to hurt" boat. (He was probably too sore from squatting.)

Your Workout Options

To find what type of workout will get you psyched to sweat, look over the following list of exercises and their descriptions. Fill in the columns for each exercise with a 1 (not in this lifetime, buddy), 5 (maybe), or 10 (yes, bring it on). After you finish, total your scores—you should be able to get a good idea or maybe even a definite wakeup call to the type of activities that can take the work out of your hard-body workouts.

Exercise	It'll be fun.	I can do it.	It's convenient.	I can afford it.	Totals
Walking	______	______	______	______	______
Running	______	______	______	______	______
Elliptical machine	______	______	______	______	______
Exercise bike	______	______	______	______	______
Treadmill	______	______	______	______	______
Stair machine	______	______	______	______	______
Rowing machine	______	______	______	______	______
Weights	______	______	______	______	______
Yoga	______	______	______	______	______
Aerobic exercise	______	______	______	______	______
Dancing	______	______	______	______	______
Kickboxing	______	______	______	______	______
Boxing	____	______	______	______	______
Step work	______	______	______	______	______
Rebounding	______	______	______	______	______

Home Strength Gear

To do strength training, you're going to need some resistance to lift. Your options are store-bought or possibly homemade weights. Some possibilities for homemade weights could be water bottles (with the water in them) ranging from half-gallon containers down to 24 oz.-containers, or soup cans in various sizes. I've included some store-bought options that will do a great job and that won't cost you a fortune.

Dumbbells Do the Job

One of the most effective types of resistance that doesn't require a large living space is a set of dumbbells in various sizes or a straight bar with different size plates.

You can get a complete set of dumbbells in a neoprene finish (which look cool and won't scratch your floors), with a tiered rack to store them on, which makes it easy to switch weights during exercises without having to bend down to the floor to find them.

As your strength increases, so will the weight that you lift. At this time, you might think about adding a barbell set to your home hard-body gym. In addition to expanding your weight options, having a barbell set gives you more exercise options. If you have the room, I suggest getting a bench that has a barbell rack so that you have the option to upgrade.

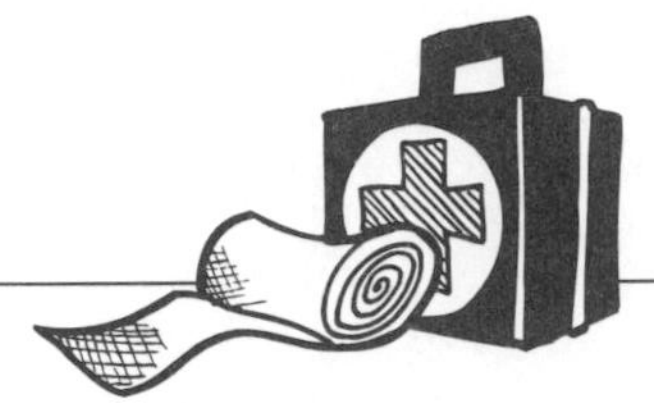

Safety Scoop

As you begin to lift heavier weight, it's important to really focus on your form. Having a spotter can help if you get stuck to either complete the rep or assist you in getting some extra reps. If you don't have a spotter, don't go for the extra reps, and please don't lift it up if you can't lift it off.

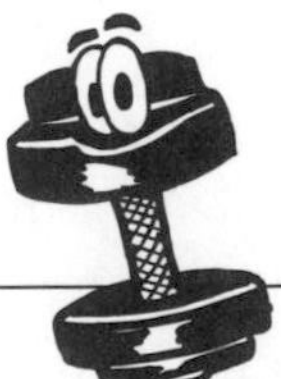

Hard-Body Headliners

Training with free weights (dumbbells) strengthens the muscles that stabilize and assist your main muscles so that they can act more efficiently. Machines direct your movement pattern so that these muscles don't have a chance to get stronger. Free weights also allow each side of your body to train independently of the other side so that you don't wind up with one side looking bigger then the other.

Raising the Bar

Bars come in different sizes and can be used for a variety of exercises that include squats, lunges, curls, presses, and rows. They can be easily stored in a closet or under a bed. Body bars start at around $27 for a 9-pound bar and go up to $50 for a 27-pound bar.

A weighted exercise bar can be used for a wide variety of exercise options.

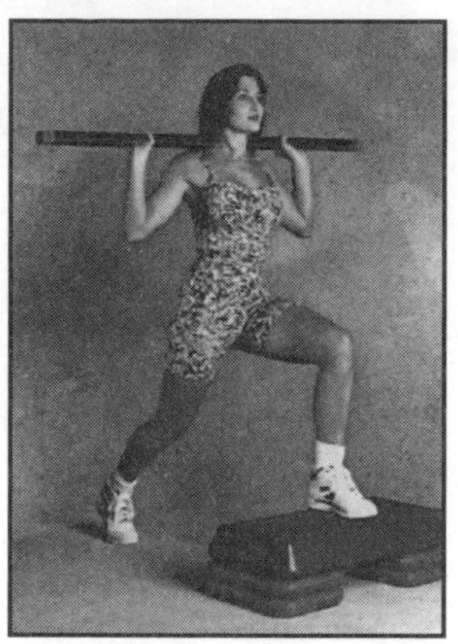

Have a Ball

Fitness balls, which have been used for years in rehabilitation, have found their way onto the home fitness front. They can be used for a variety of *core stabilizer* and other muscle group strengthening exercises. Used by people of all fitness levels, they are especially good for senior lifters or those who experience back pain because the back muscles are completely supported during the exercises.

Specifically, I have used the Resist-A-Ball's fitness ball because the ball makes it possible for me to work the abdominal muscles through their full range of motion. This is something that cannot be done with floor exercises. I use it for my video and "Move of the Month" column routines.

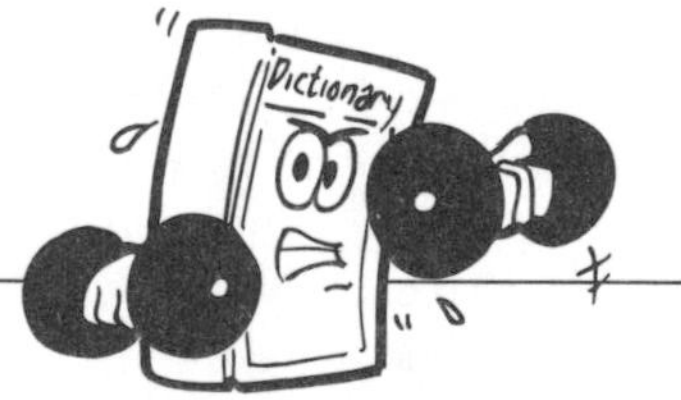

Workout Wisdom

The term **core stabilizers** refers to the abdominal muscles and the muscles of the lower back.

I recommend getting a ball pump with your Resist-A-Ball. (Blowing this thing up manually is never an option.)

The following are the suggested ball sizes based on height:

5 feet, 5 inches to 5 feet, 7 inches (55 cm)

5 feet, 8 inches to 6 feet, 2 inches (65 cm)

6 feet, 3 inches, to 6 feet, 9 inches (75 cm)

A pump will quickly inflate and deflate your fitness ball so you can store it in a small space and blow it up when it's time to use it.

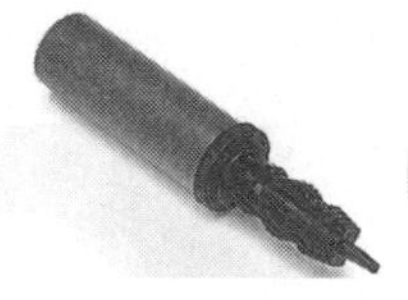

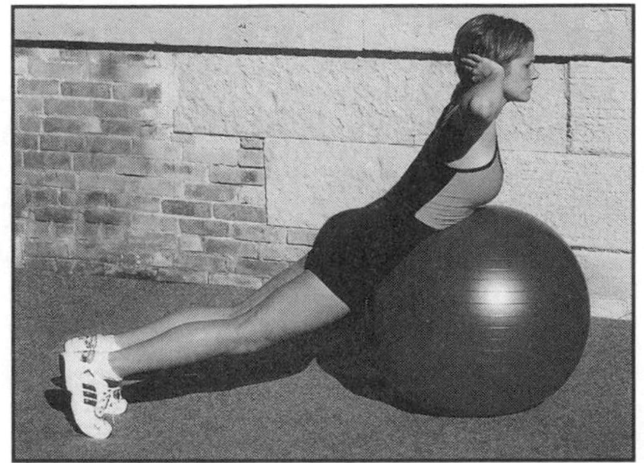

Fitness balls allow you to work your abdominals through their full range of motion.

Fitness Furniture

Exercises can be done on the fitness ball or a weight bench. An adjustable bench gives you more exercise options and gives you the ability to do *multiangular movements*.

Workout benches include the following options:

- Multipositioned back rest
- Barbell rack
- Squat rack
- Leg extension or leg curl attachment
- Roman chair
- Preacher curl attachment
- Pull-down bar attachment

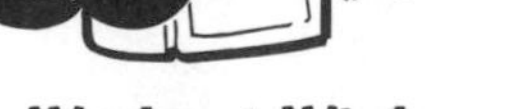

Workout Wisdom

Multiangular movements are exercises done in a variety of body angles. Doing makes you work harder because changing the angle allows a fresh muscle to pick up where the other left off. Working the angles also gives you muscles that are more rounded and defined in appearance.

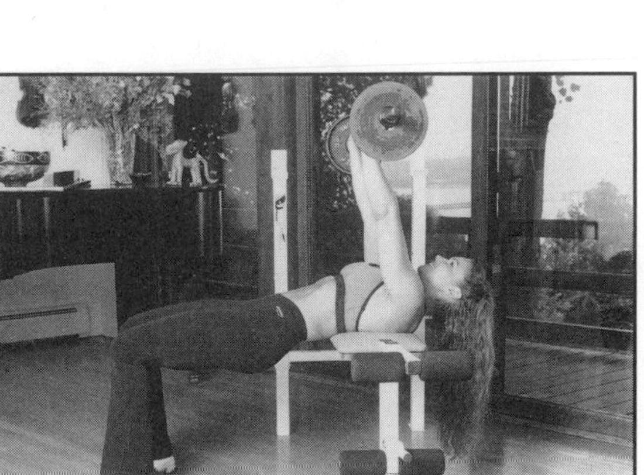

An adjustable weight bench will give you more exercise options.

Multistation Machines

If you have the room, you might think about adding a multistation machine to your home gym arsenal. Machines can offer exercise options that can't be done with dumbbells. A weight stack also allows you to lift more weight as your strength increases. The disadvantages, though, are that the bench doesn't adjust to different angles, and your range of motion is limited. If both aren't in your budget, then go with the bench and dumbbells, and add a barbell set when you're ready. A pull-up bar doesn't cost much and will fill any back exercise void.

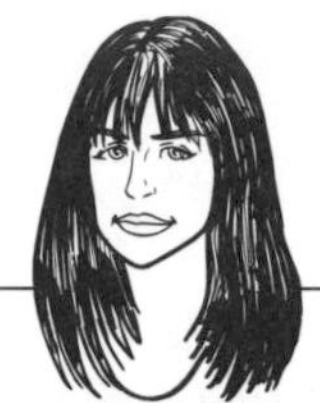

Jourdan's Gems

Machine pull-downs are great back exercises if you aren't strong enough to lift your own body weight, or even if you're so strong that your body weight poses no challenge.

A well-equipped multistation home gym includes the following features:

- Single or dual weight stacks
- Bench press for chest, arms, and shoulders
- Butterfly for inner chest
- High pulley for back, shoulders, and arms
- Military press for shoulders and arms
- Leg extension/curl for legs
- Squat station for lower body
- Ab pulley

Punch and Sweat

A training program that produces both explosive strength and marathon endurance has to be serious. That's why boxing has become a popular workout option. This is a workout in which the right gear is crucial. Over the years, I've seen too many people hurt their hands because they were hitting bags with gloves that looked more like oven mitts. (A complete breakdown of the right gear, along with the workouts that work best, can be found in Chapter 11, "Hard-Body Knockouts.")

Cool New Options

I recently discovered a piece of exercise equipment that strengthens my muscles and also gives me a good cardio workout. The Pro Fitter was initially developed to rehabilitate knee injuries and now has been used in many sports medicine and rehab centers for everything from ACL rehabilitation to strokes. Benefits include these:

- Improved cardiovascular endurance
- Improved upper-/lower-body strength
- Improved core strength and stability

- Improved balance and coordination
- Improved sports performance
- Reduced risk of sports-related injuries

If it's in your budget, the Pro Fitter is definitely one piece of equipment that won't be collecting much dust.

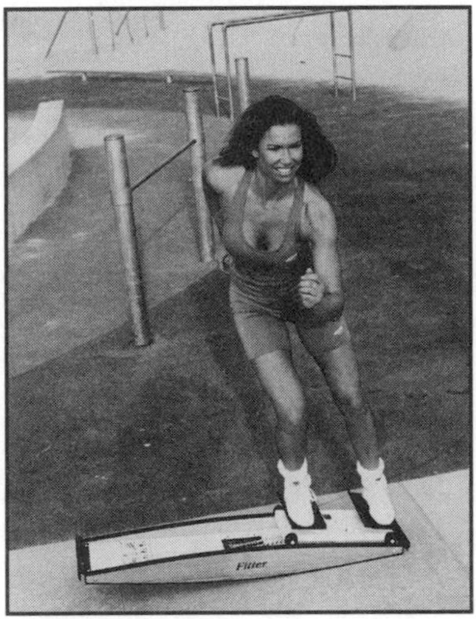

In addition to cardio benefits, the Pro Fitter gives you the feeling of slalom skiing, so it can be used in pre-ski season to get you ready for the slopes.

Home Cardio Gear

There are numerous options when it comes to doing cardio. I've included options for every preference and every budget in the next sections.

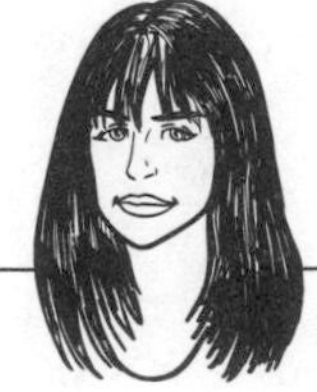

Jourdan's Gems

For a killer leg routine using a step, try my Triple Crown Leg Routine, discussed in Chapter 13, "Ten-Minute Ticket to Tone."

Step It Up

A step can give you a big sweat for a small price. Besides cardio benefits, you can also use your step in your strength-training routines. For home use, I recommend the Studio Step model. The only difference is length—the Studio Step is 28 inches long, and the Health Club model is 43 inches. To me, the extra length isn't worth the price difference.

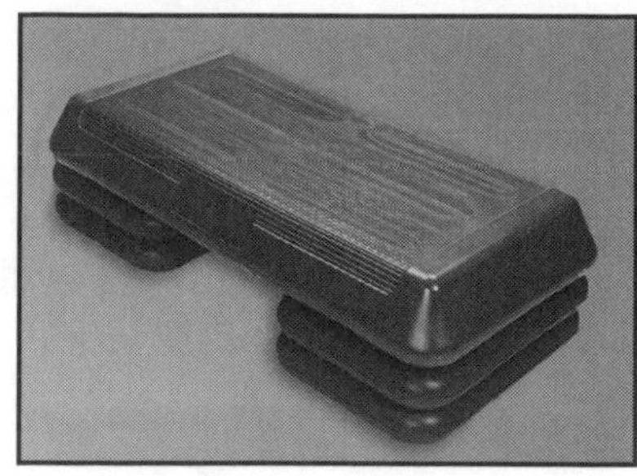

Because of its reduced size, the Studio Step is great for small spaces.

Bounce Your Butt Off

Urban rebounding is like doing a high-impact aerobic class without the high impact. By bouncing to the beat on your own mini trampoline instead of the floor, the stress is taken off your joints without diluting the exercises.

New Kid on the Cardio Block

One of the newest types of training is quickly becoming one of the most popular ways to get a phenomenal cardio workout. Elliptical trainers give you all the benefits of running without the impact that's hard on your joints. That means no more shin splints. Depending on your body weight, you can burn around 600 calories in 60 minutes.

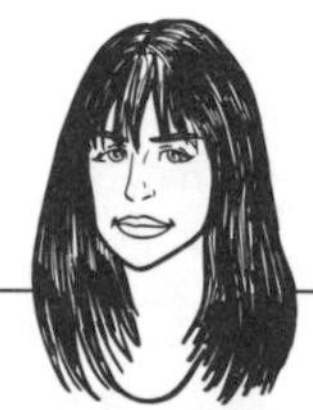

Jourdan's Gems

To up the intensity, get a better leg workout, and work on core stability, turn the tension high enough so that you don't have to hold on to the handles. Find a happy medium at which you can maintain your balance while training for a minimum of 30 minutes.

Because this item has a higher price tag, you need to try out several to see which is the best for you. Remember that you will be spending a lot of time together, so you want to make a love connection.

Questions to ask when considering an elliptical trainer include these:

- Does it feel sturdy when I ride it?
- Could I do this for an hour?
- Does it display time exercised and calories burned (and is it easy to read?)
- What are the options (rack for water bottle, magazine shelf)?
- Is it easy to pedal? Do my feet slip at all?
- What does the warranty cover? How long is it in effect?
- What is the repair process (local or long distance)?

Living Room Laps

If walking and running are your cardio exercises of choice, a treadmill is your best bet. This is another high-ticket item that is a very personal choice. My recommendation is that you spend the time to try out several before making your choice. That means you're on your own on this one. Remember that it might be better to bite the bullet and spend more for something you'll enjoy versus having the most expensive coat rack in town.

Questions to ask when considering a treadmill include these:

- Is the walking space long enough that I can make full strides?
- Is the tread wide enough that my feet have space from the edge?
- Does it feel smooth under my feet when I walk? When I run?
- Are the handles long enough (sturdy enough) if I need to jump off quickly?
- What are the options?
- What does the warranty cover? How long is it in effect?
- What is the repair process (local or long distance)?

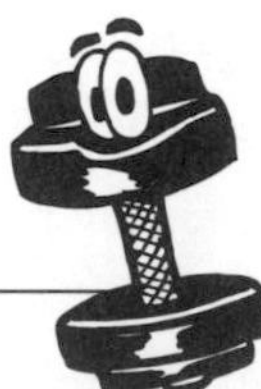

Hard-Body Headliners

Overweight women that use a treadmill at home as part of their exercise program can lose twice as much weight as those without this option, according to a study at Brown University. Of the 115 women ages 25–45 who were asked to do the same amount of brisk walking, one third were allowed to use a treadmill at home. Those who exercised at home lost an average of eight pounds more and maintained a higher level of exercise than those who didn't. (How's that for a home hard-body testimonial?)

Sit and Sweat

If you have lower-back pain, a recumbent bike might be the right cardio choice for you. This is another item that I wouldn't be too cheap on because it might literally wind up being a pain in your glutes. Comfort should be right up there with cost in the decision process, so take on some road tests, check out the options, and do some comparison shopping. The salesmen work on commission, so they will take the time to answer your questions.

Questions to ask when considering a fitness bike include these:

- Does the seat adjust?
- Could I sit on this for an hour?
- What are the options (rack for water bottle, magazine holder)?
- Is it easy to pedal? Do the straps adjust?
- What does the warranty cover? How long is it in effect?
- What is the repair process (local or long distance)?

Step Up and Sweat

If you're looking at steppers, my question to you is "Have you tried an elliptical trainer yet?" Elliptical trainers give you more exercise options and less joint stress than the stepper does. You want to be able to exercise for a long time, so the goal is to put the minimum amount of stress on the joints while getting the maximum exercise benefit. You will be the one doing the exercising, so test-ride both first and then decide. It took one session on an elliptical trainer to make a believer out of me.

Hard-Body Accessories

One hard-body cardio accessory that I find essential is a heart rate monitor. Knowing your heart rate at all times makes it easy to stay in the desired range for your fitness goal.

A perfect example for having a heart rate monitor is spinning. I know many dedicated spinners who never seem to lose any weight. I wore a heart rate monitor to a popular spin class and quickly solved the mystery. During the 60-minute class, I might have spent a total of 10 minutes in my fat-burning zone (warming up and cooling down). Since then, I always wear my heart rate monitor during my cardio sessions. I want to rest assured that when I want to burn fat, I'm actually burning fat.

Heart rate monitors range anywhere from $50 to $300, depending on the options. Some of the options include the following:

- Time of day
- Heart rate
- Target zone
- Calorie counter
- Time memory (exercise time and time zone)
- Stopwatch
- Calendar
- Face that lights up

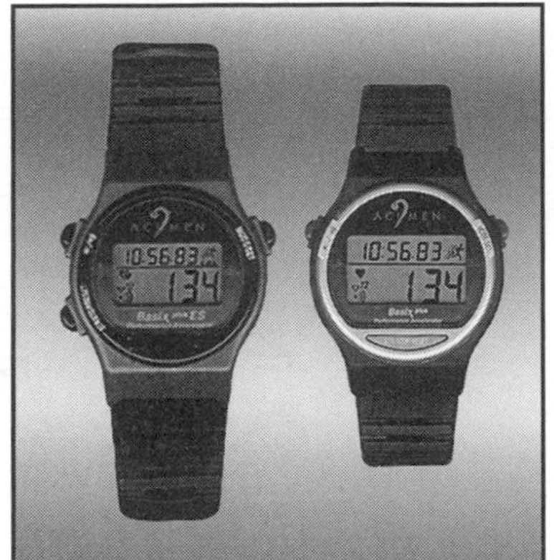

A heart rate monitor will make checking your heart rate during exercise extremely easy.

Watch Your Step

Another handy little gadget is a pedometer, which counts how many steps you take and how many calories you burn. This is ideal for walkers and joggers.

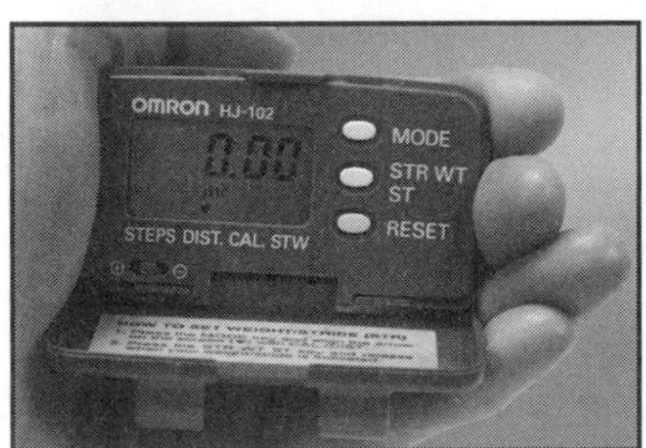

A pedometer is a great tool if walking or jogging is your cardio workout of choice.

Grip This

Using Progryp handgrips prevents rough bars from hurting your hands, weights from slipping out of your hands, and blisters from becoming a permanent part of your hands. I prefer using grips instead of gloves because they're easier to use and don't dye my hands. (Black leather gloves are notorious for this.)

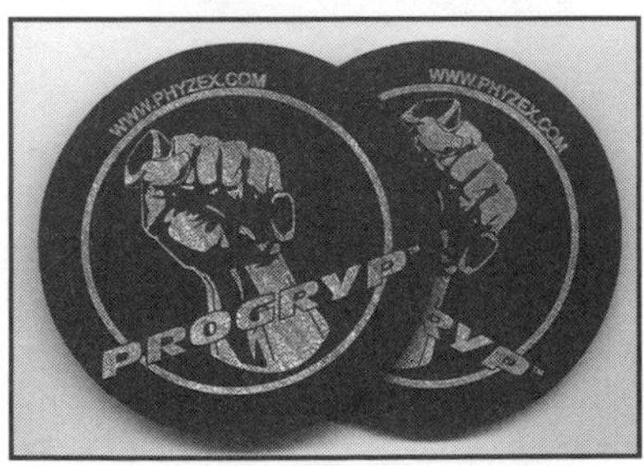

Progryp handgrips have become my grips of choice because of their small size, comfortable fit, and inexpensive price.

Women's Best Sport Support

Let's start with a quick lesson in ligaments. Cooper's ligaments are the only support system for women's breast tissue. Once these ligaments stretch, there isn't a press or curl that can make them retract. The only solution is to find a good support bra to hold you and your ligaments in.

Up until last year, I was the master of creative breast support. Wearing two or three sports bras when I boxed or taught my classes was common. Any bra that had promising support cast the "uniboob" spell on me. (That's when it looks like you have one big breast in the middle of your chest.) My clients, especially the larger-breasted, had the same problem.

Last year I was introduced to Nike Inner Actives, which has quickly become my favorite new sports bra. You can bounce all you want in it, and those breasts aren't moving. In addition to superior support, these bras are comfortable, keep moisture away, and make your breasts look like breasts. They're sized like bras, so the fit is perfect.

The most important thing about finding a good sports bra is comfort and support. You definitely don't want to feel like your breasts are having their own, separate workout routine going on! Make sure that whatever kind you use supports you enough to keep your breasts intact, without feeling uncomfortable or binding, and also one that allows your skin to breath while you work up a sweat.

Working Out Never Looked So Good

I would like to know who passed the law that a big white T-shirt and baggy, PE-type shorts is the official dress code for working out. Besides being unflattering, you can't see your muscles working. If the only one watching is you, there's no excuse to hide in Fruit of the Looms.

What's better than comfortable, great-looking workout wear? How about comfortable, great-looking workout wear that you can work out in, hang out in, go out in, and even sleep in? If you don't think it's possible, you might want to check out HotSkins Bodywear.

Jourdan's Gems

Seeing your muscles in action is great for motivating you and checking your form. Seeing your hard work get hard can make those last few reps a lot easier to do.

If the Shoe Fits ...

The bottom line on athletic shoes is that they have to be comfortable. If you are going to do a variety of workouts, a good cross-training shoe will work well. I recommend trying on several brands to see which feels the best. Get the best-fitting shoe even if it costs a little more—if your feet aren't happy, you won't be happy.

The Least You Need to Know

- ➤ Exercises have different personalities, so pick the one that's perfect for yours.
- ➤ Different-sized dumbbells and an adjustable bench should be first on your strength-training gear list.
- ➤ Take your cardio gear on a test ride before you buy. Buy the one that you (not your clothes) will use.
- ➤ A sports bra should be comfortable, should keep you dry, should not give you a uniboob, and, above all, should give you support.
- ➤ Pick workout clothes that make you want to get dressed to work out.

Part 2

Home Hard-Body Training Tricks

In this hard-body how-to section, I give you all the necessary information—my best exercise routines and my best-kept transformation secrets so that you can get maximum hard-body results in minimal time.

Chapter 5, "Warming Up!" gives you the details on warming up and cooling down so that your hard body can have a showroom shine that stands the test of time. To get you started, I've given you a complete warm-up and stretching routine.

Chapters 6, "Legs to Rock Your Hard-Body House"; 7, "Phenomenal Abdominals"; and 8, "Hard-Body Tower of Power," are your complete "Hard-Body Exercise Encyclopedias."

Chapter 9, "Custom Home Hard Bodies," is filled with my hard-body heavy-hitter programs that can turn a home body of any level into a hard-body homestead. With your exercise encyclopedia at your fingertips, these programs can change and grow as you do.

Getting the lowdown on cardio training in Chapter 10, "Home Is Where the Heart Gets Fit," makes it easy to keep your body fat level low so that you can show off all your hard-body hard work.

My 10-minute ticket to tone routines are fast and serious. They'll give your muscles that perfect pump when time isn't on your side. These timesaver gems can be used alone, put together for a full-body routine, added to your regular workout, or used as a split-training workout to help prevent soreness.

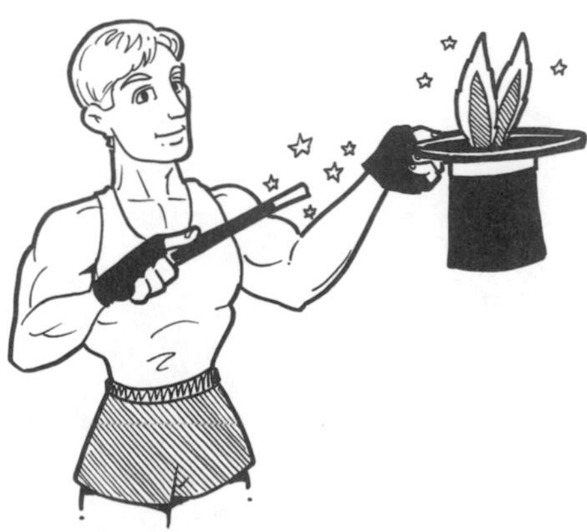

Chapter 5

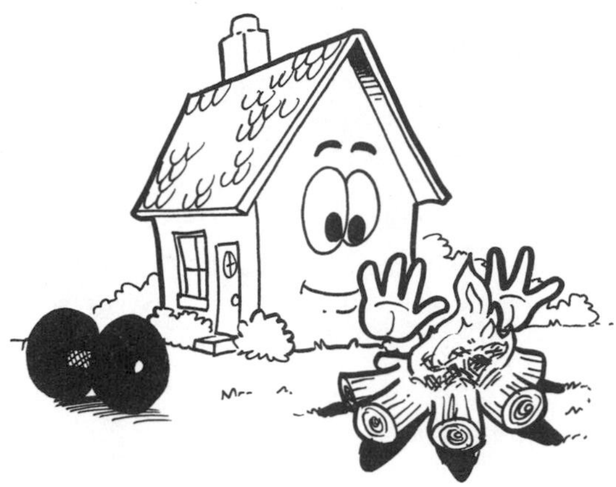

Warming Up!

In This Chapter

- Getting primed to pump
- Stopping soreness before it stops you
- Stretching 101
- Your "Home Stretch Exercise Encyclopedia"

When I started weight training, I knew it was something that I wanted to continue doing for the rest of my life. To me, this meant that I needed to learn how to train smart, not just hard. So, on the road to getting my hard body right, I put overtime into the small details that most people overlook or feel are unnecessary. Taking time and making the extra effort has paid off so far by giving me 10 injury-free and virtually pain-free years of weight training. So, at 37, I'm able to train as intensely as those in their early 20s.

Giving your home hard body a showroom shine means not skipping important details such as priming the surface before you paint. Applying a topcoat to seal the surface is the insurance that your hard-body shine can stand the test of time. Simply put, warming up primes your body for exercise, increases your level of performance, and prevents injury. Ending each workout session with a proper cool-down and stretching routine is your body's topcoat against injury and soreness.

If you want to create the Taj Mahal of home hard bodies, you have to stretch regularly. Stretching gives your muscles better development and gives your body incredible symmetry. My step-by-step routines and stretching encyclopedia give you the tools you need to create a hard body that only gets better with time.

Start Your Engines

I like to think of my body as a Formula One race car in the Fitness 500. To win the race and keep my million-dollar car in peak condition, I make sure that I warm up my engine gradually so that I'm ready when it's time to put the pedal to the metal and capture the checkered flag.

A proper warm-up that'll get your engines revved and race ready consists of three phases:

- General warm-up
- Light stretching
- Sport-specific activity

The purpose of the warm-up is to gradually raise your core body temperature and get the blood flowing to your muscles so that they are ready to exercise. Warming up also improves muscle performance and flexibility, and reduces the likelihood of injury.

Phase 1

It's important that you perform the general warm-up before you stretch. This consists of at least 5 minutes of light aerobic activity. Your muscles will stretch easily if they're warm. When muscles are cold, they are stiff and can be easily injured.

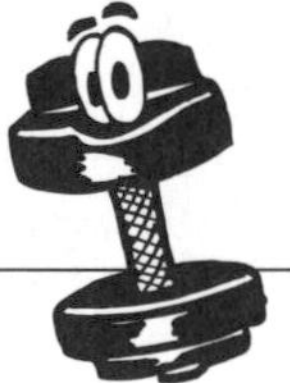

Hard-Body Headliners

Light cool-down exercise immediately following your workout will clear lactic acid from your blood better than resting will. If you're still sore the next day, doing a light warm-up routine will reduce lingering muscle tightness and soreness.

Phase 2

Light, static stretching follows the general warm-up. Static stretches for each muscle group are done in a slow and relaxed manner. If you don't have time to stretch all your muscles before your workout, you at least need to take the time to stretch all the muscles that will be heavily used during your workout.

Phase 3

The final phase of the warm-up is performing similar movements that will be used during the training phase at a reduced intensity level. In a weight-training session, this means doing one to two light sets of your first exercise before beginning your actual training sets. The warm-up sets are required only once at the beginning, unless you are doing a full-body workout. Then warm-up sets are needed before the upper-body and lower-body exercises.

Cooling Your Jets

After completing your workout, it's important to lower your heart rate slowly to about 100 beats per minute (bpm). Stopping suddenly without cooling down will put undue pressure on the heart because of the high amount of adrenaline that's still in the blood. Muscle soreness can be avoided by properly cooling down.

Cool Warm-Ups and Hot Cool-Downs

To start you off, I've included the following warm-up routine from my "Power Box" classes. My yoga cool-down routine, found in Chapter 12, "Have Floor, Will Lotus," is a combination of yoga moves and breathing techniques that's designed to restore your energy, release tension, and relax your body.

V-Steps

1. Start by placing an imaginary letter V in front of you, and stand with your feet together at the base of the V.
2. Using a four-count beat, step forward and to the right with your right foot, and extend your arms to the right. (1 count)

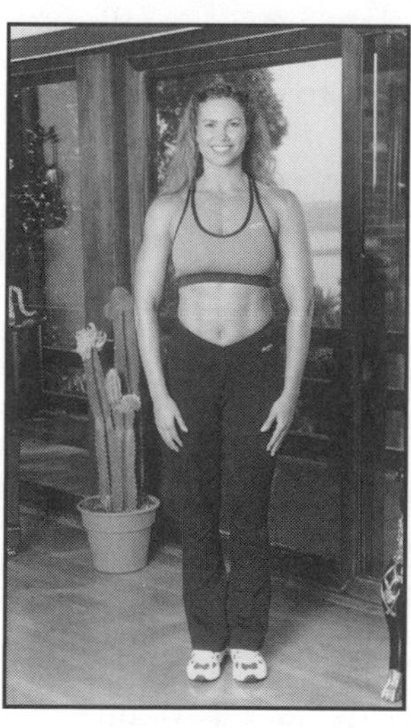

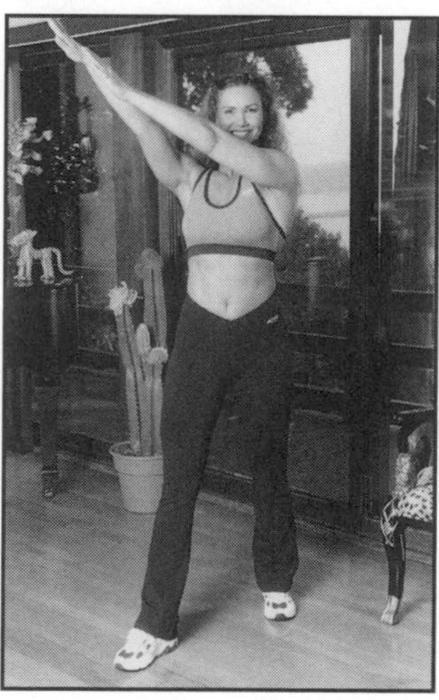

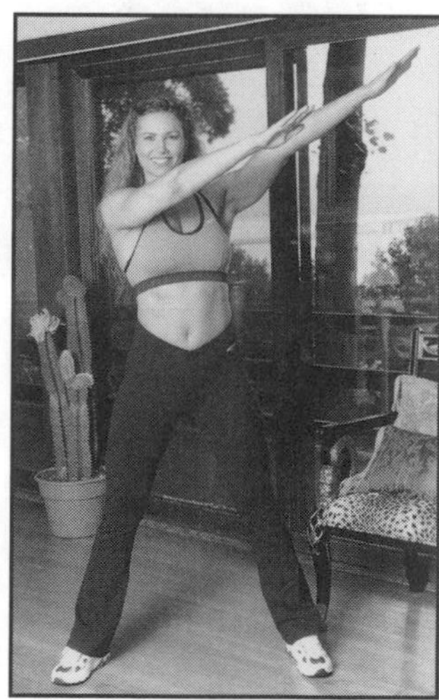

3. Then step left and forward with your left foot move your arms to the left. (1 count)
4. Finally, step back to the base, with your right foot first and then your left. (2 counts) You should be in the same position as in the first figure. Do four reps slowly on a double-time beat, and then pick up the tempo and do eight reps. Then go to jumping jacks.

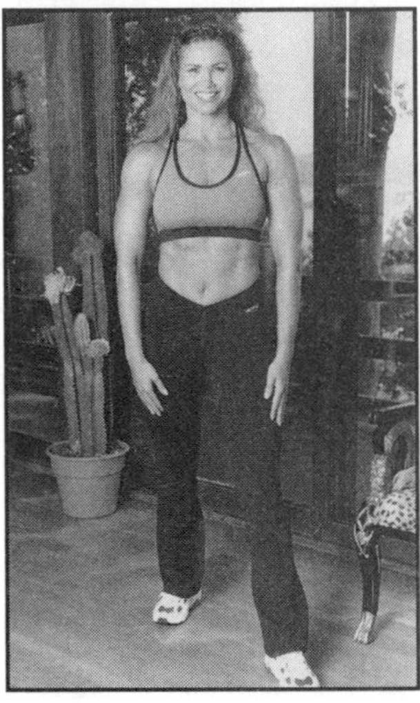

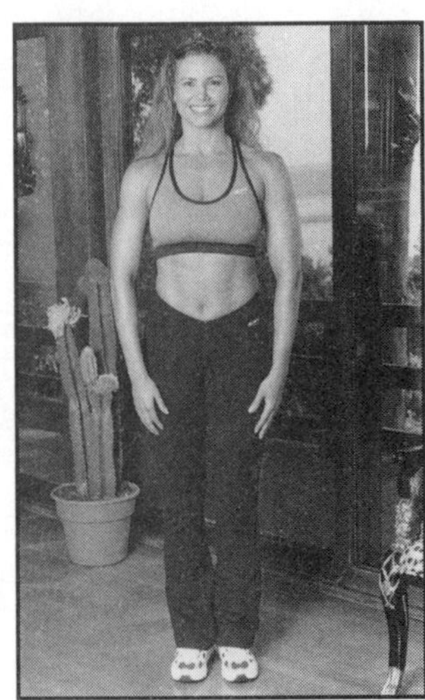

Jumping Jacks

Do jumping jacks for two sets, counting up to 10, and then back down to 1. Then go to the side step/knee up sequence.

Side Step/Knee Up Sequence

1. Step-touch side to side. Your arms go up when you step right with your right leg or left with your left leg.
2. Your arms go down when you bring your left foot to the right or your right foot to the left and touch-step. Do four touch-steps to the center.
3. Turn to your right, and reach out with your arms. Pull your arms in as you bring your left knee up. Do four knee-ups to the right.
4. Turn back to face the front and do four touch-steps.
5. Turn to your left and do four knee-ups to the left. Repeat steps 1 through 4 four times. Finish in the center, stepping side to side without your arms. Shorten your steps until your feet are together stepping in place. Come to a stop and go to the upper back/chest and shoulder stretch sequence.

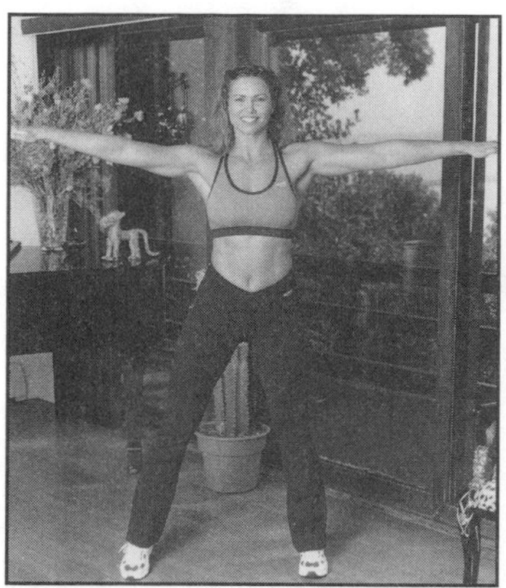

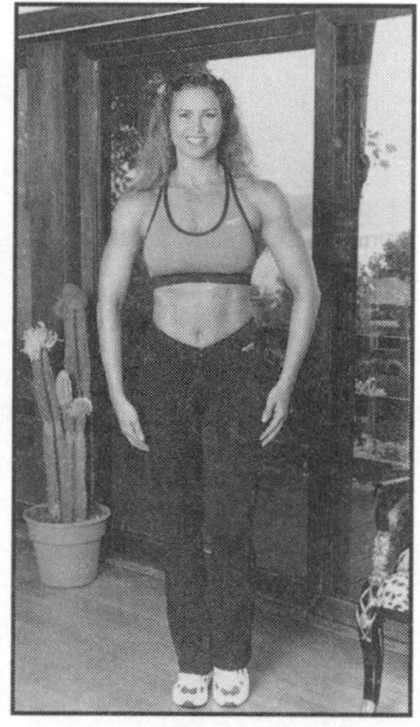

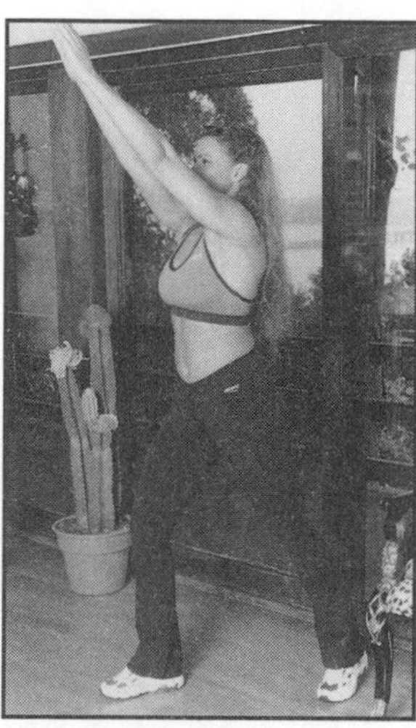

Upper Back/Chest and Shoulder Stretch Sequence

1. With your back straight, fingers interlocked, and arms extended overhead with your palms facing up, reach upward until you feel a good stretch—hold the stretch.
2. Now bring your arms forward and stop at shoulder height. Gently push your shoulders forward and around your back until you feel a stretch. Hold the stretch.
3. Release your hands and bring them behind your back. Interlock your fingers and push your shoulders back until you feel a good stretch—hold the stretch. Release and go to the hamstring/quadriceps stretch and balance sequence.

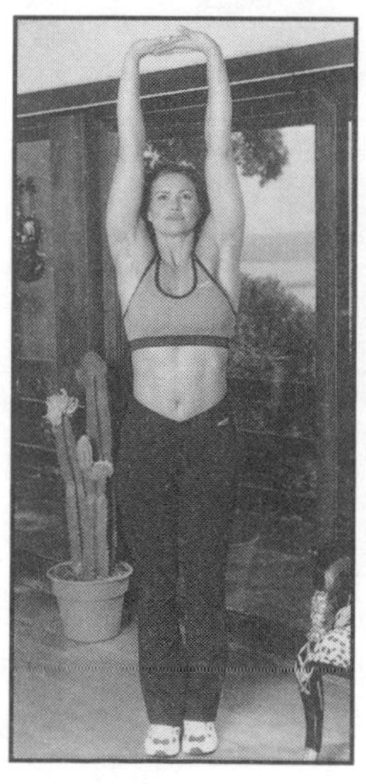

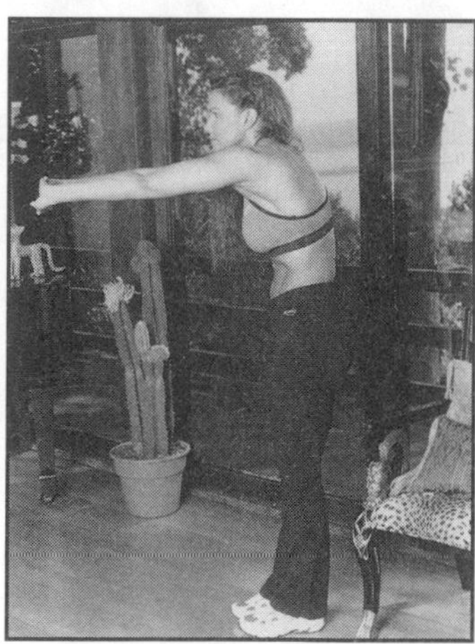

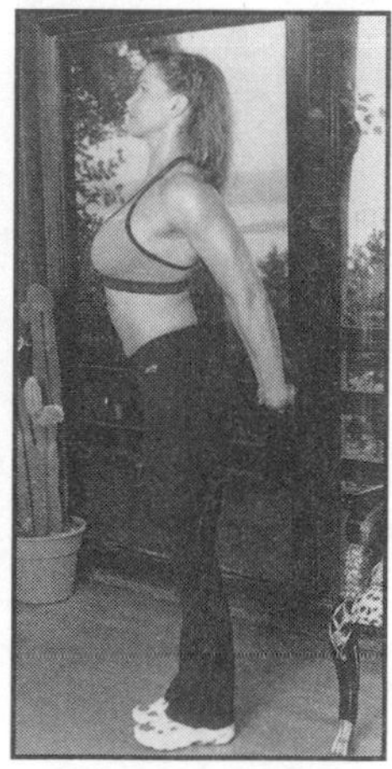

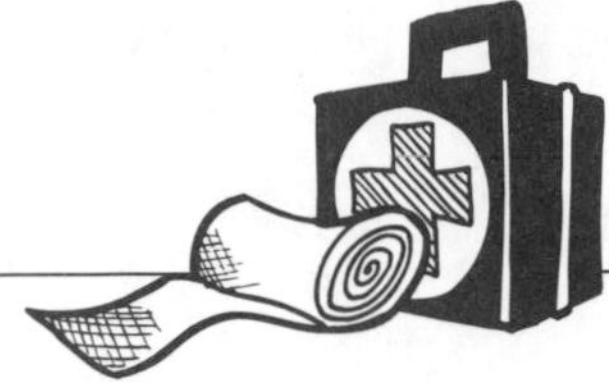

Safety Scoop

When placing your hand on your legs for support, always place them on your thighs instead of your knees. This will protect your knee joints from the pressure caused by the added weight.

Hamstring/Quadriceps Stretch and Balance Sequence

1. Start with your right leg forward, your foot flexed, and your left leg back. Straighten your front leg, and shift your weight to your back leg. Place your hands on your left thigh for support. Bend your left knee, and lean back until you feel a stretch in the right hamstring and calf. Hold the stretch.
2. To increase the stretch, reach down with your right hand and place it under the ball of your right foot; gently pull your foot back. Hold the stretch.

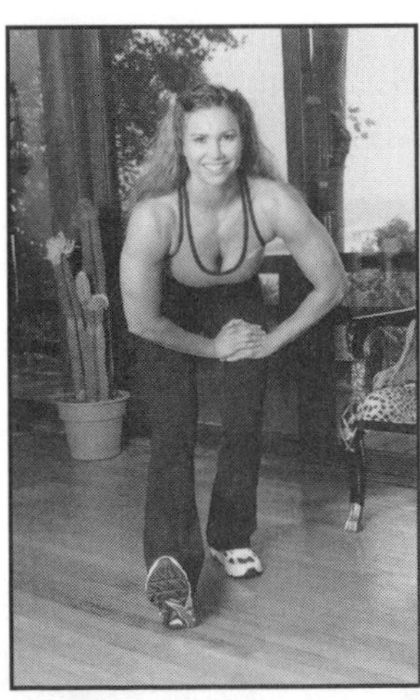

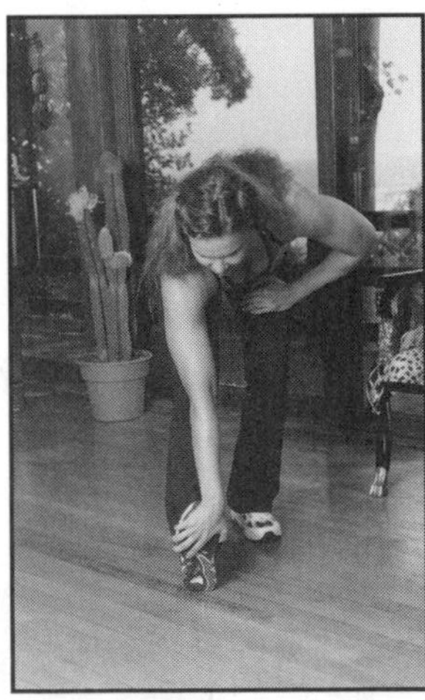

3. Press your foot into the palm of your hand, and raise your leg until it's parallel with the floor and at hip level. Hold this balance position.
4. Bend your right knee, and bring your right leg behind you slowly. With your knees together, gently pull back on your foot while pushing forward with your

hip until you feel a good stretch in the quadriceps of your right leg. Hold the stretch. Release. Repeat steps 1 through 4 through on your left side. Then go to the lunge stretch sequence.

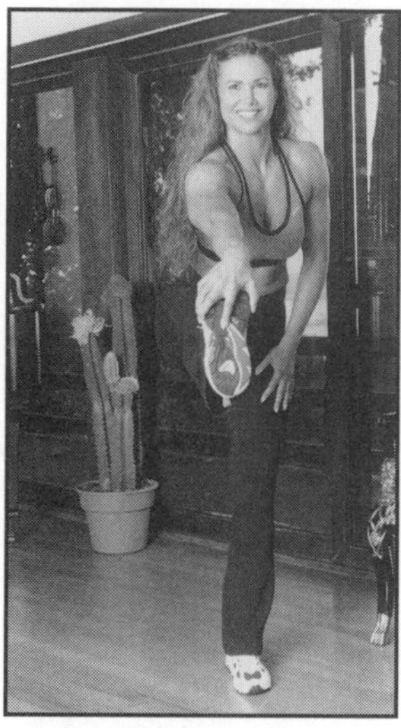

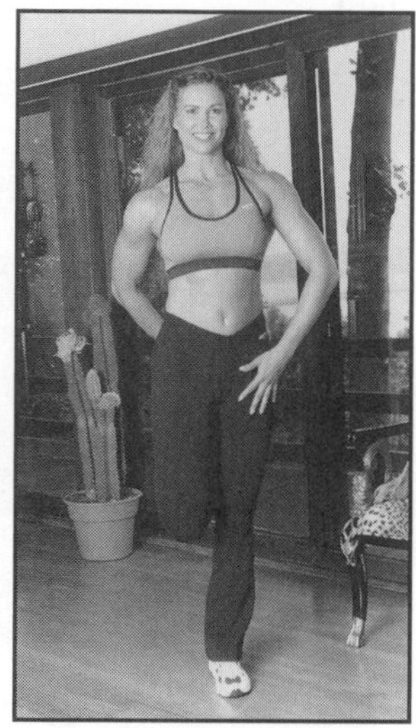

Lunge Stretch Sequence

1. Start this sequence facing forward in a wide stance.
2. Do a quarter turn to your right, and lunge back with your hands outside your feet and your front knee directly over your foot. Hold the stretch.

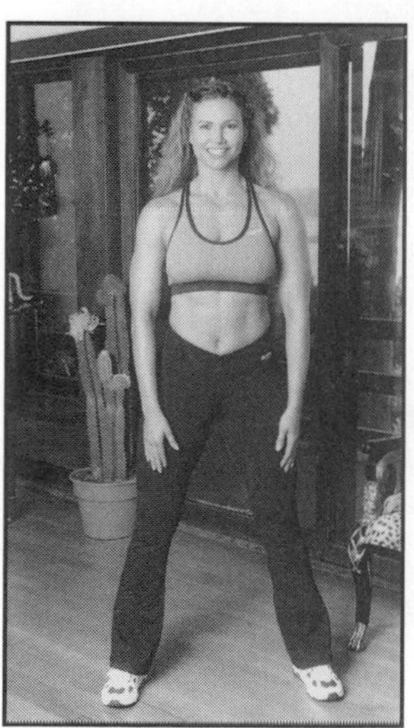

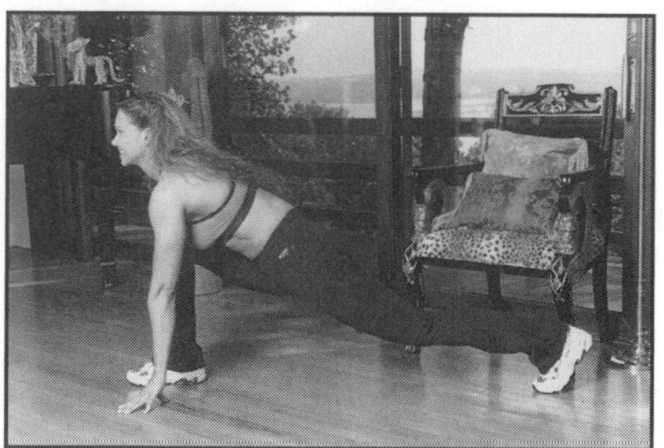

3. Straighten both legs, and bend forward from your waist, bringing your chest as close to your thighs as you can. Hold the stretch.
4. Lift your front foot up onto your heel, and hold. Make sure that both legs remain straight.

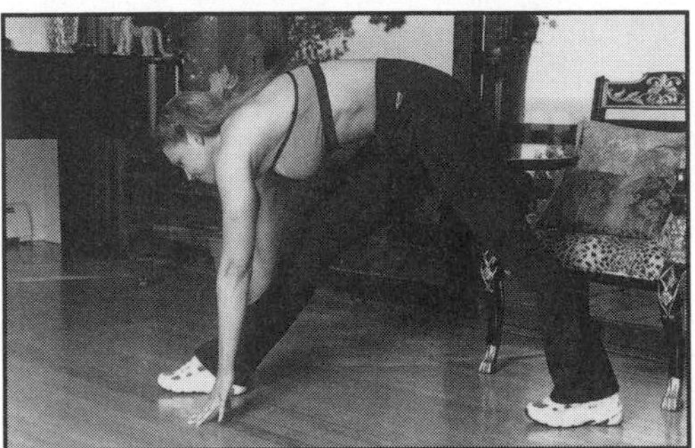

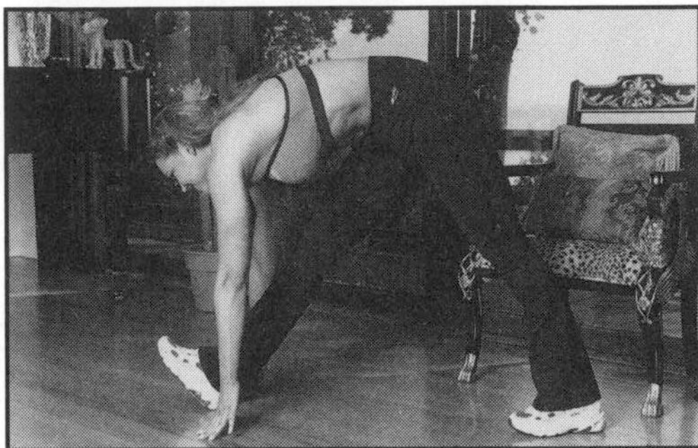

5. Lower your foot, do a quarter turn back to the center; assume the same position as in step 1. Bend forward from the waist and place your hands, forearms, or head on the floor in front of you. Hold the stretch. Release and return to standing. Repeat steps 2 through 5 without the forward bend on the left side. Then go to standing cat stretch.

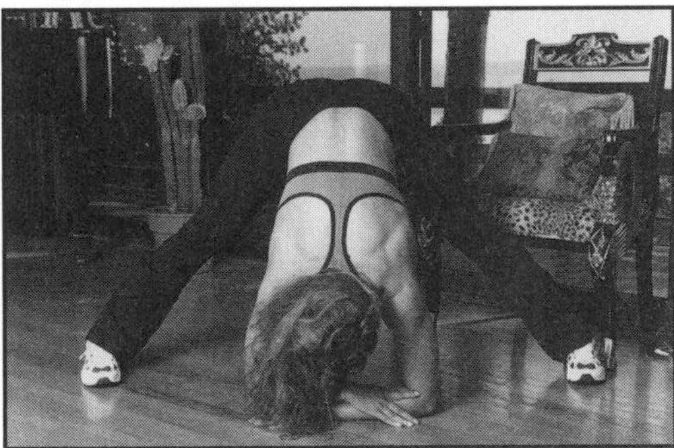

Standing Cat Stretch

1. Start this set in a wide stance, with your knees bent and hands on your thighs.
2. Inhale, arch your back up with your head down, and hold the stretch.
3. Exhale, let your back sink in with your head up, and hold the stretch. Repeat this two more times, and then go to the standing roll-up.

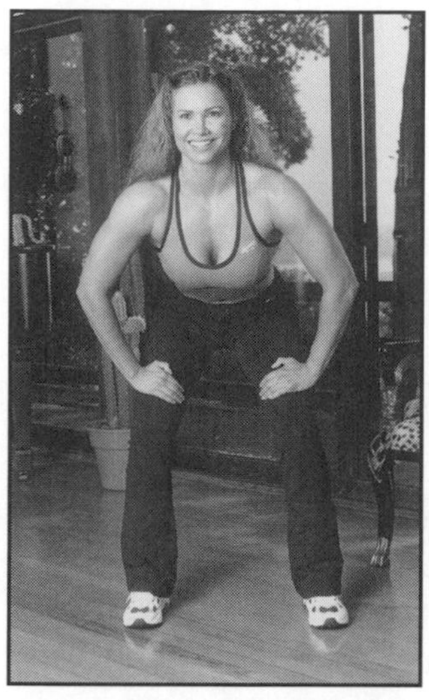
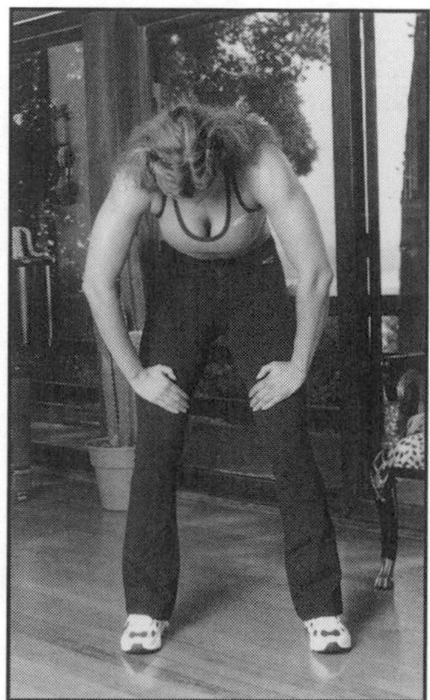
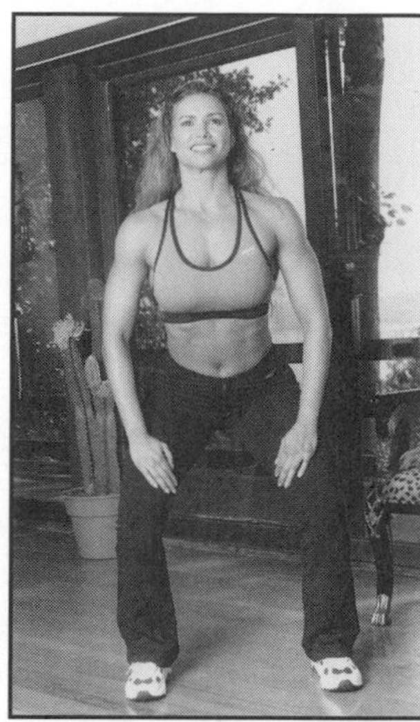

Standing Roll-Up

From position 3 of the cat stretch, inhale and arch back up with your head down. Continue rolling up one vertebra at a time, with the head being the last to come up, until you come to a standing position.

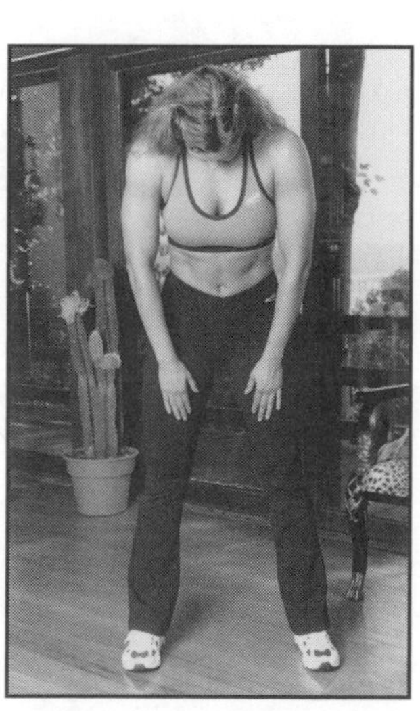
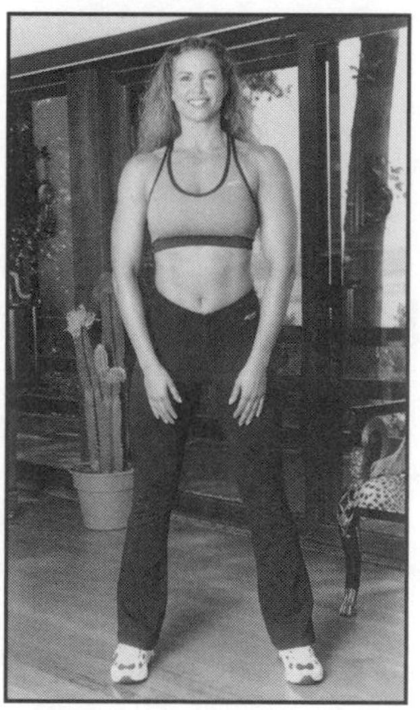

Your Flexibility Factor

Flexibility is defined as a joint's ability to move freely through a normal range of motion.

Benefits from flexibility training include these:

- Increased physical performance
- Injury prevention
- Increased blood supply to joints
- Improved circulation
- Improved balance and posture
- Reduced stress
- Decreased risk of lower-back pain

You can increase your level of flexibility by using a variety of stretching methods. Some of the most popular methods are these:

- Static stretching
- Ballistic stretching
- Isometric stretching
- Proprioceptive neuromuscular facilitation (PNF) stretching

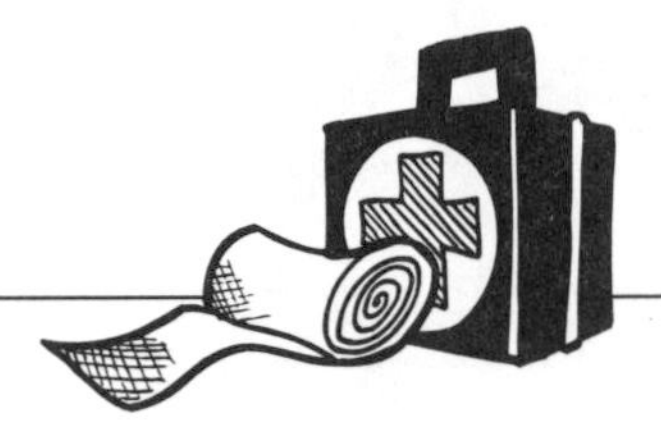

Safety Scoop

Because of its slow and controlled approach of elongation, static stretching is the least likely to cause injury. It is also the most widely recommended type of flexibility exercise for all fitness levels.

Static Stretching

Static stretching is a low-intensity, long-duration stretch technique. In static stretching, you slowly elongate the muscle through a full range of motion and then hold that position for 15 to 30 seconds.

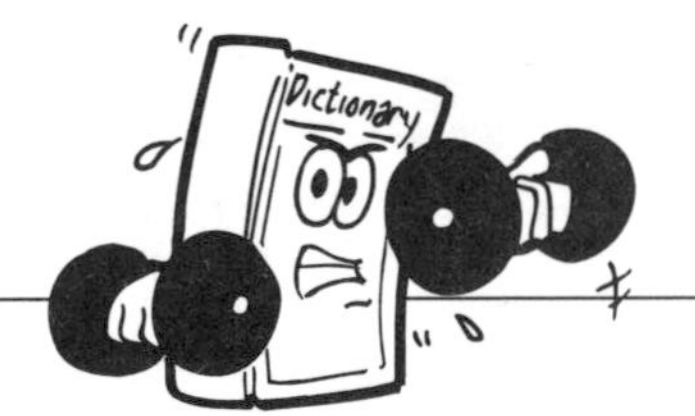

Workout Wisdom

Isometric contraction is a contraction in which a muscle exerts force but does not change in length because the muscular force is equal to the resistive force.

Ballistic Stretching

Ballistic stretching is a high-intensity, short-duration stretch technique that uses rapid, uncontrolled bouncing motions. Because of the high risk of injury, this technique should be avoided unless specifically used to prepare an athlete for a ballistic sports activity.

Isometric Stretching

Isometric stretching is a type of static stretching that involves the resistance of muscle groups through *isometric contractions* of the stretched muscles. In addition to increasing your flexibility level, isometric stretches also help develop strength in the "tensed" muscles.

The most common ways to provide the needed resistance for an isometric stretch are to apply resistance manually to your own muscles, to have a partner apply the resistance, or to use an apparatus such as a wall or the floor to provide resistance.

When doing an isometric stretch, you should first assume a static stretch position. Next, tense the stretched muscle for 10 seconds against a force that won't move, such as a wall. Finally, relax the muscle for at least 20 seconds.

PNF Stretching

Proprioceptive neuromuscular facilitation (PNF) stretching was initially developed and used to rehabilitate stroke victims. In PNF stretching, you stretch through a full range of motion and then apply an isometric contraction against maximum resistance for 10 seconds. You then relax the muscle and apply a slow, passive stretch to the point of limitation. The muscle is then relaxed for 20 seconds before doing another PNF technique. PNF stretching techniques are more effective with the assistance of a partner.

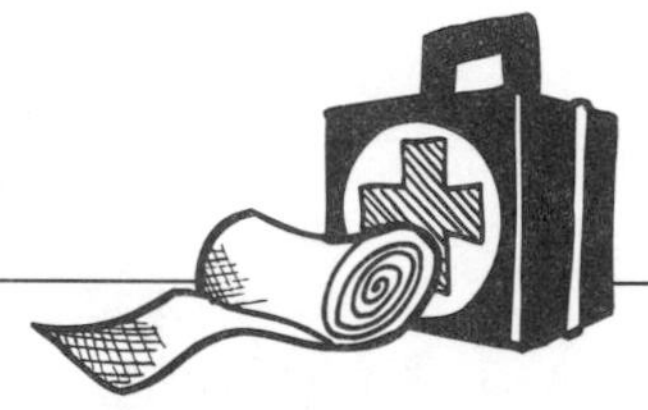

Safety Scoop

These exercises should be only done with a partner who is knowledgeable and experienced in PNF stretching. Communication between partners is critical to prevent injury from stretching a muscle beyond its limit.

Home Stretch Exercise Encyclopedia

In this section, you find a stretch for each muscle group. I've designed the order to go from top to bottom, and I've taken special care to make sure that each exercise easily flows from one to the next. So, the exercise encyclopedia is also a complete full-body stretch routine. (I always believe in getting more bang for your buck.)

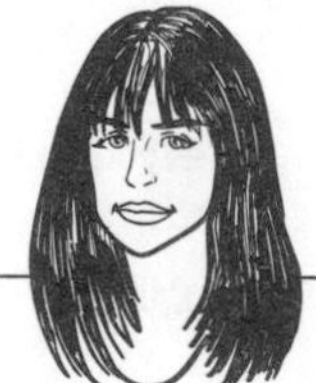

Jourdan's Gems

Stretching between exercise sets is key to better muscle development and definition. Regularly stretched muscles appear longer and give the body a more streamlined appearance.

Neck Stretches

The following neck stretches are for the neck regions and can be done separately at any time to increase flexibility and release muscle tension, or they can done together in the order shown as part of your stretching routine.

Neck Flexion/Extension

1. **Neck flexion.** Stretches muscles in the back of the neck. Relax your shoulders and slowly bend your head forward. To increase the stretch, place your hands, fingers laced, on the back of your head and gently press forward.
2. **Neck extension.** Stretches muscles in the front of the neck. Look up and stretch your neck by using your muscles to lift up and back.

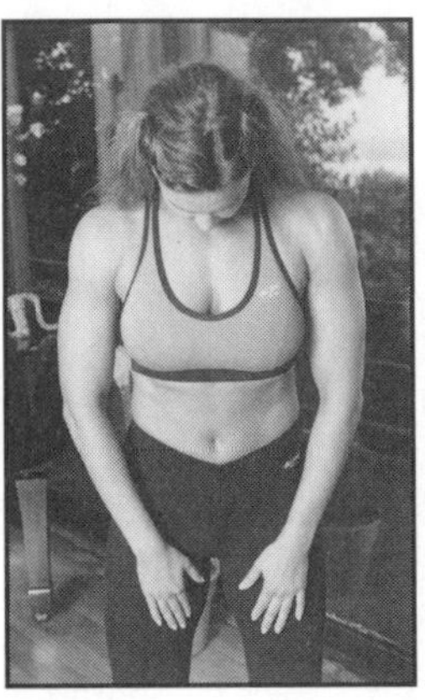
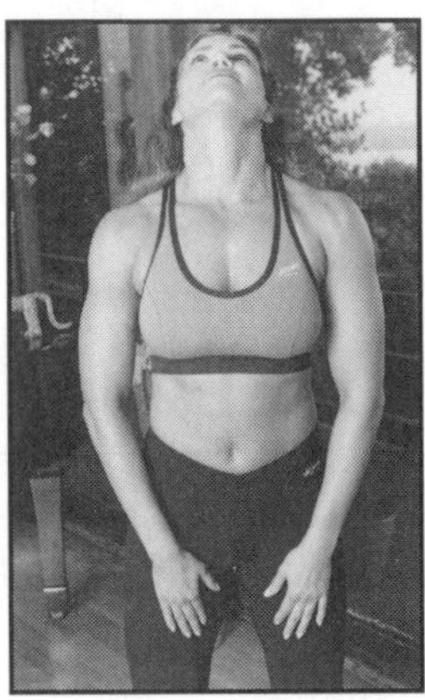

Neck Side Flexion/Rotation

1. **Neck side flexion.** Stretches the muscles on either side of the neck. Face forward, tilt your head to one side; hold the stretch. Release and repeat on the other side. Do not let your shoulders rise during the stretch.
2. **Neck rotation.** Start with your head and shoulders facing forward. While your shoulders remain forward, rotate your head as if looking over your shoulder; hold the stretch. Release and repeat on the other side.

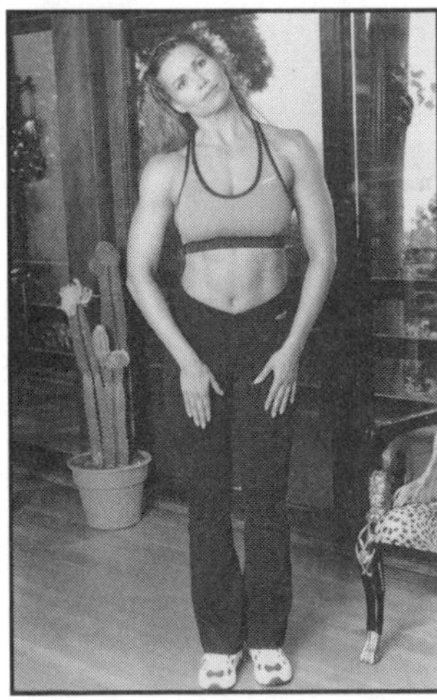
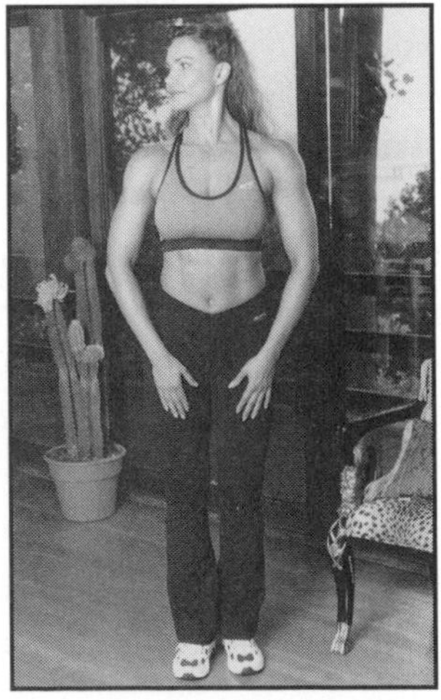

Pectoral and Deltoid Stretches

The following stretches are for the *pectoral* and *deltoid* regions and can be done separately at any time to increase flexibility and release muscle tension, or they can be done together in the order shown as part of your stretching routine.

Anterior Deltoid/Pectoral Wall Stretch

Stand and place your right palm against a wall or a doorway. Rotate your torso away from your hand until you feel a stretch, and then hold the position. Release and repeat on the other side.

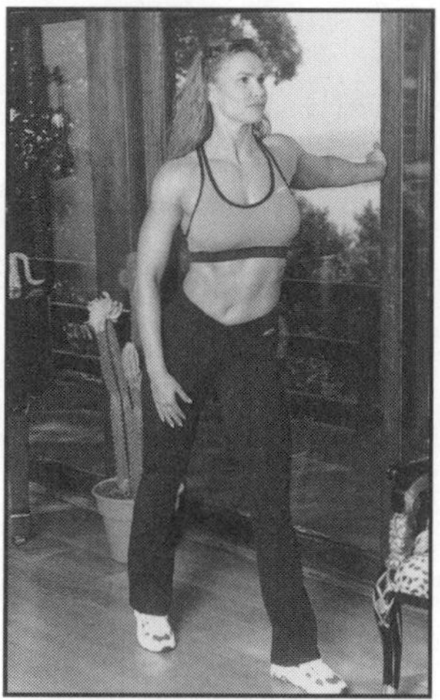

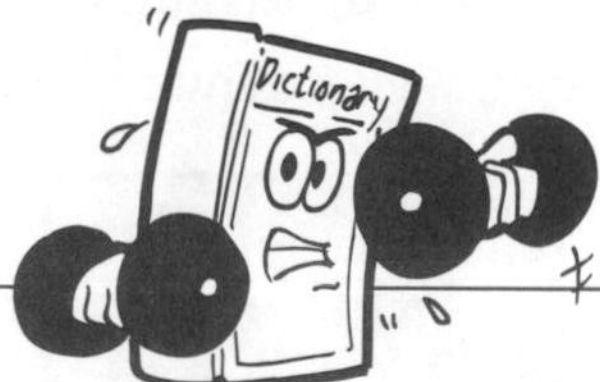

Workout Wisdom

The **anterior deltoid** is the group of muscles in the front part of the shoulder. The shoulder is divided into three sections (anterior, or front; medial, or side; and posterior, or back). To give your shoulders a well-rounded and defined appearance, exercises should be done for each section.

Pectoral muscles are the two muscles of the chest region (the pectoralis major and the pectoralis minor). The pectoralis major is the larger muscle and functions as a shoulder adductor and internal rotator.

Anterior Deltoid/Pectoral Standing Stretch

Start this by standing with your back straight. Interlock your fingers behind you, and then push your shoulders back until you feel a good stretch. Hold the stretch position.

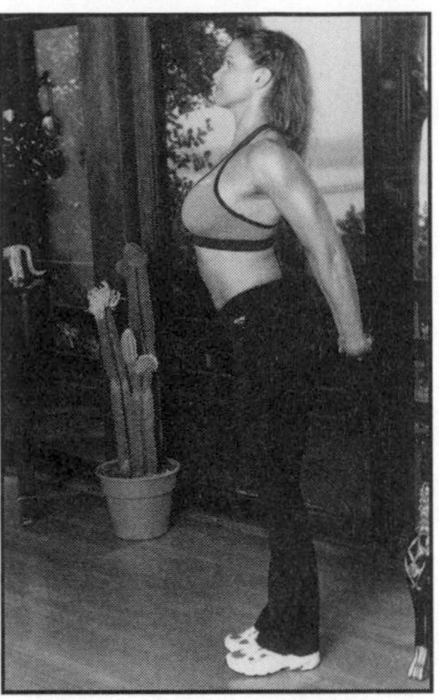

Posterior Deltoid Stretch

1. Start by standing with a straight back.
2. With your shoulders down and relaxed, bring your right arm across your chest. Place your left hand on your upper, arm and gently press toward your body.
3. Hold the stretch position. Release and repeat on the other side.

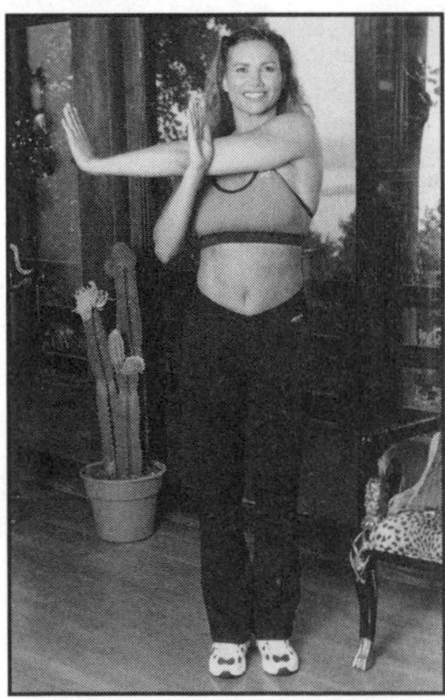

Upper Back Stretch

The following stretch is for the upper back region and can be done separately at any time to increase flexibility and release muscle tension, or it can be added to the other stretches as part of your stretching routine.

Standing Upper-Back Stretch

1. Start by standing with your back straight. Lace your fingers, and extend your arms overhead with your palms facing up.
2. Bring your arms forward, and stop at shoulder height. Gently push your shoulders forward until you feel a stretch.
3. Hold the stretch position.

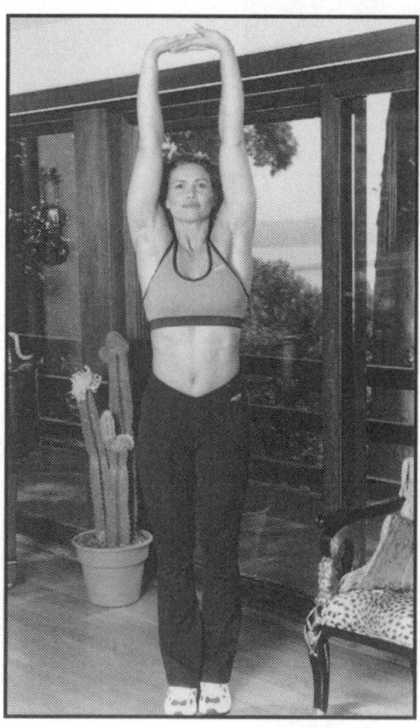

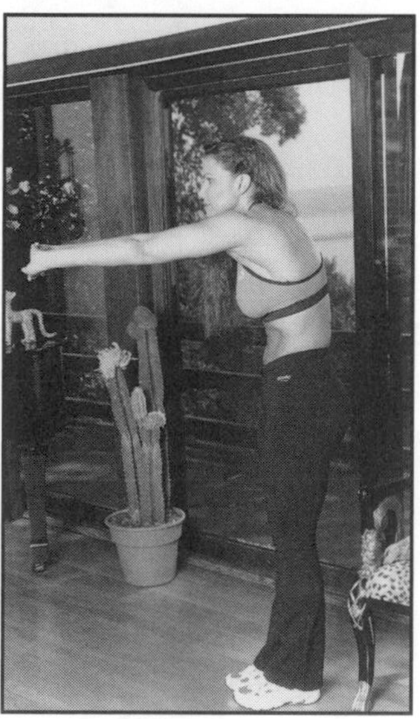

Arm Stretches

The following stretches are for the biceps and triceps and can be done separately at any time to increase flexibility and release muscle tension, or they can be done together in the order shown as part of your stretching routine.

Triceps Stretch

1. Bend your right elbow and place your left hand on your right upper arm below the elbow.
2. Bring your bent elbow behind your head until you feel a stretch on the outside of the upper arm. Hold the stretch position.
3. Repeat on the other side.

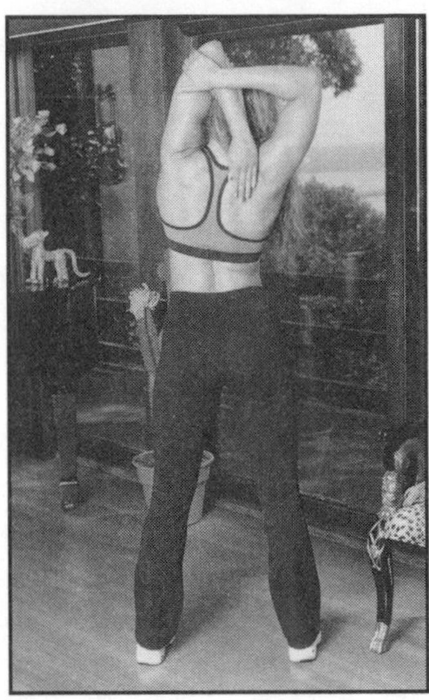

Biceps Stretch

1. Extend your arms out to the side at shoulder height.
2. Bend your hands back until you feel a stretch.
3. Hold the stretch position.

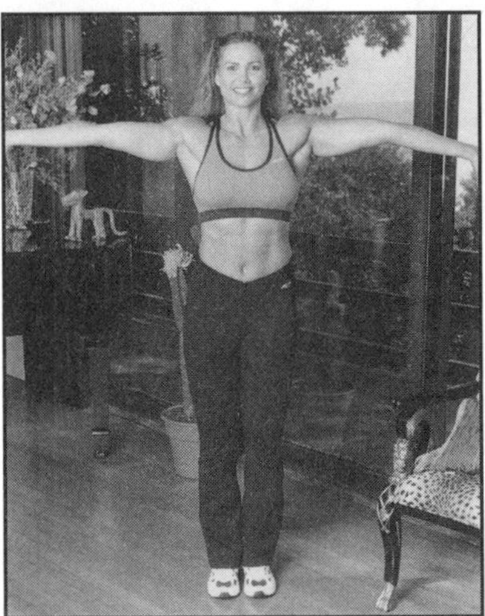

Lower Back/Abdominal Stretches

The following stretches are for the lower back and abdominal regions and can be done separately at any time to increase flexibility and release muscle tension, or they can be done together in the order shown as part of your stretching routine.

Lower-Back Stretch

1. **Lower-back stretch.** Start on your back. Lift both feet off the floor, and bring your knees toward your chest. Hold the stretch position and then relax.
2. **Single-leg variation.** This is done the same as the preceding stretch, except using one leg.

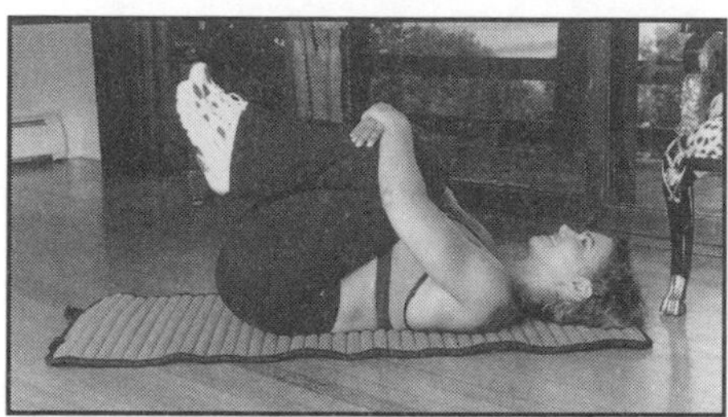
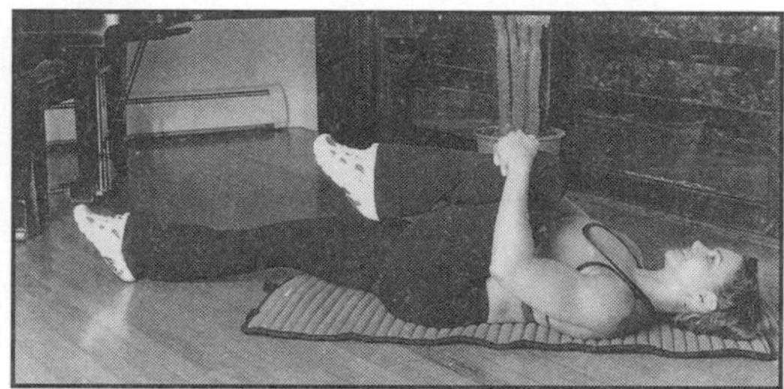

Kneeling Cat Stretch

1. Start on hands and knees. Inhale, arch back up with your head down, and hold stretch.
2. Exhale, let your back sink inward with your head up, and hold stretch.

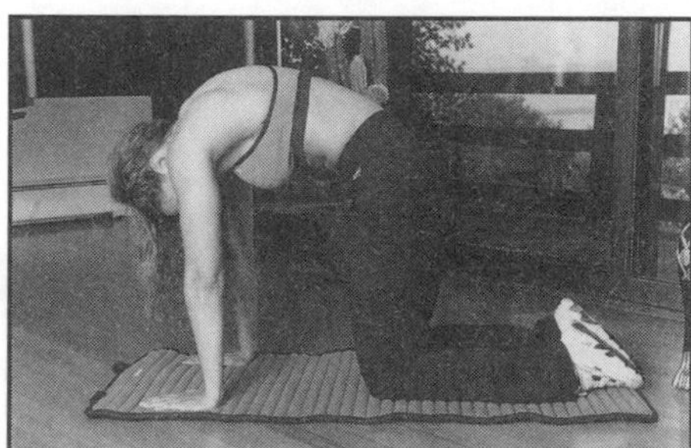
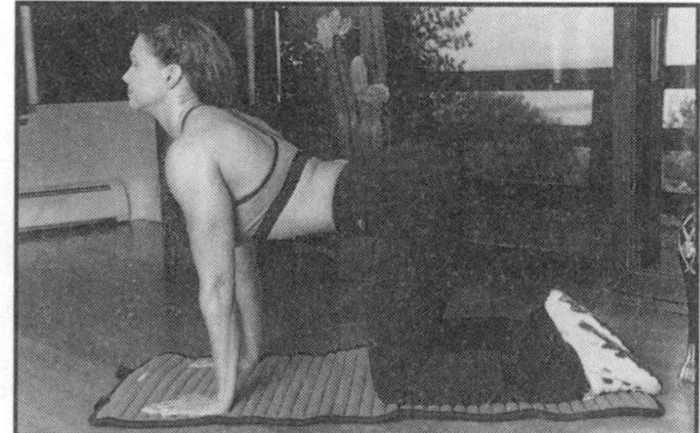

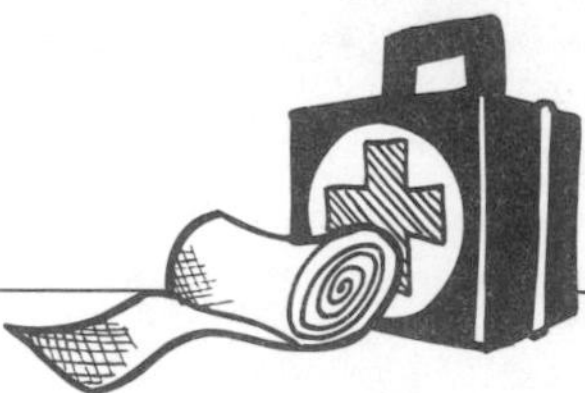

Safety Scoop

You should never feel pain during any of the lower or abdominal stretches. If you currently experience lower-back pain, do the kneeling cat stretch version, and do not let your back position drop below horizontal. Skip the torso stretch if you feel pain in your back when you lie face down on your stomach.

Lower-Back Release

1. From a hands and knees position, sit back on your heels, keeping your hands fixed in front of you, until you feel a stretch from your arms through your spine.
2. Hold the stretch position, and then relax.

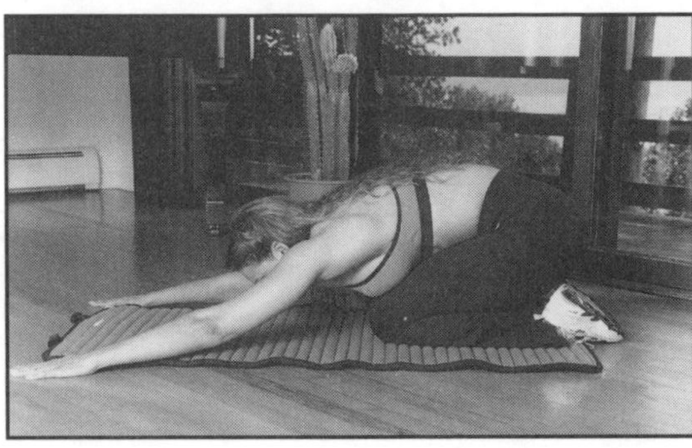

Torso Stretch

1. Start on your stomach with your hands at chest level, as if you're getting ready to do a push-up.
2. Exhale and lift your upper body while keeping your hips and lower body on the floor. Hold the stretch position.

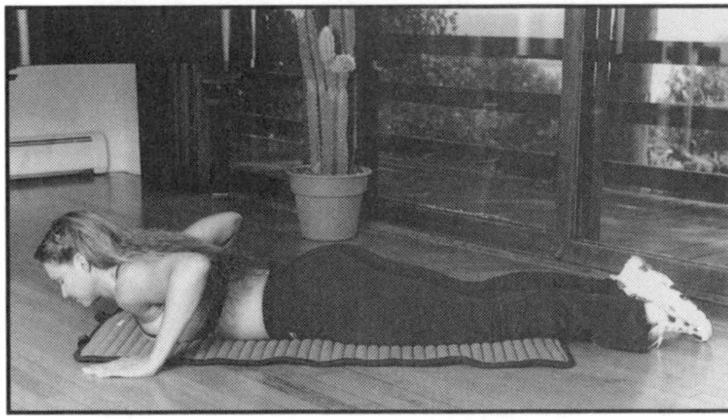

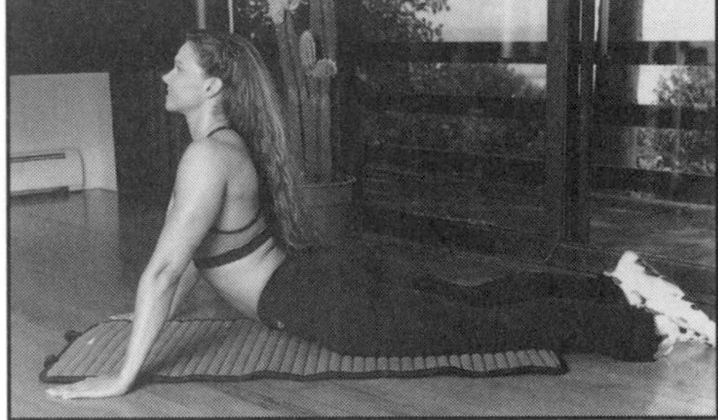

Lower-Body Stretches

The following stretches are for the lower body regions and can be done separately at any time to increase flexibility and release muscle tension, or they can be done together in the order shown as part of your stretching routine.

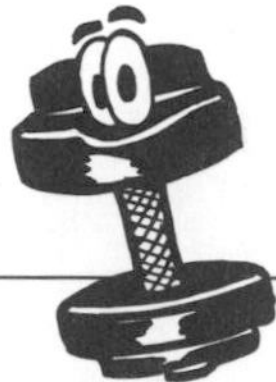

Hard-Body Headliners

You get better results from your hamstring exercises if you also stretch your quadriceps between sets. Increasing a muscle's range of motion increases the effectiveness of the exercise because more muscle mass is recruited during the exercise. Stretching the opposite muscle group (quadriceps) is one way to increase the range of motion because it reduces the muscle tension that can shorten the muscle.

Standing Quadriceps Stretch

1. Using a wall or a chair for support, reach back with your right hand and grasp your right foot.
2. Keeping your knees together, gently pull back on your foot as you push forward with your hip until you feel a good stretch. Hold the stretch position.
3. Release and repeat on the other side.

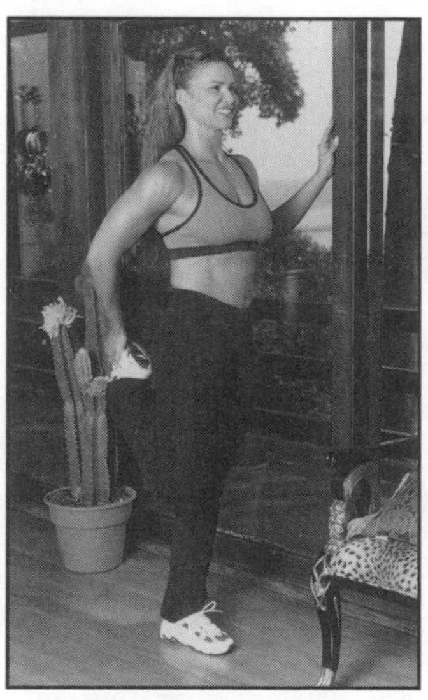

Standing Hamstring Stretch

1. Using a low bench or step, place your right heel on the bench, with your hands on your left thigh.
2. Lean forward and lower your back from the hips until you feel a stretch in the back of the leg.

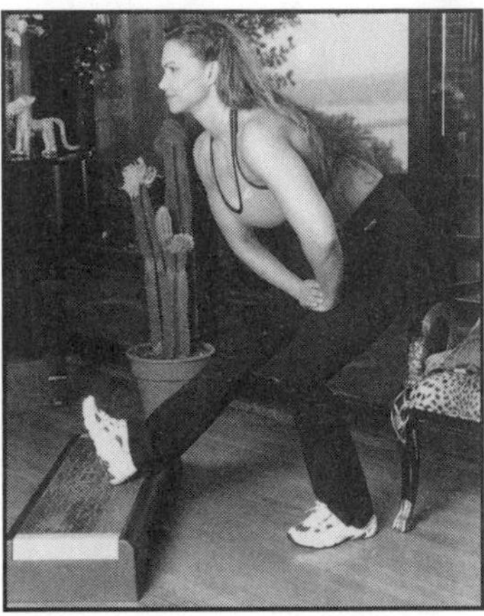

Lunge Stretch Sequence

1. Start this sequence by facing forward in a wide stance.
2. Do a quarter turn to the right, and lunge back with your left leg. Your hands should be outside your feet, and your front knee should be directly over your foot. Hold this stretch position.

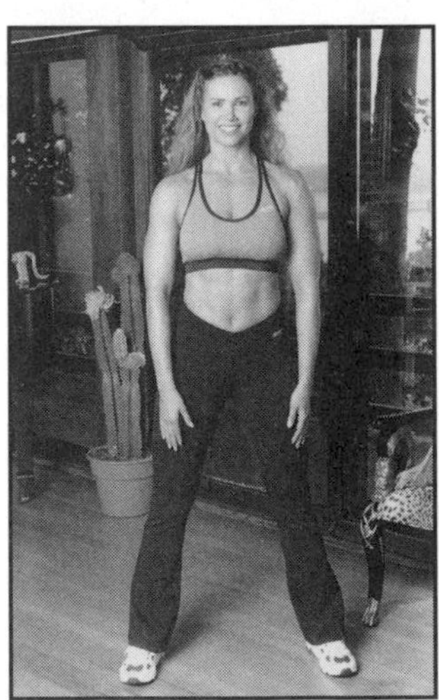

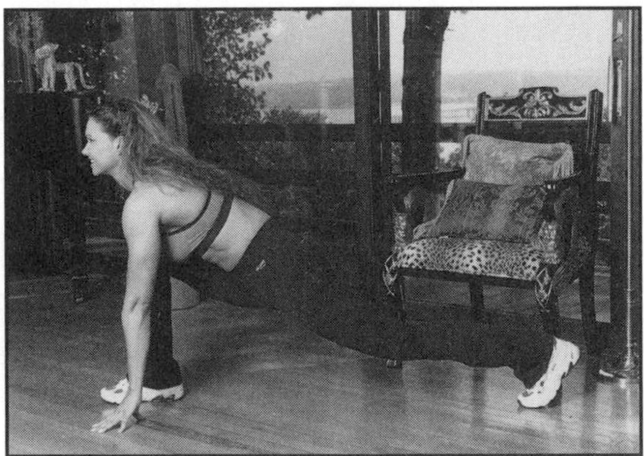

3. Straighten both legs, and bend forward from the waist, bringing your chest as close to your right thigh as you can. Hold this stretch position.
4. With both legs remaining straight, lift your front foot up onto your heel and hold. Lower your foot and do a quarter turn back to the center; assume same position as in step 1. Repeat stretch on other side.

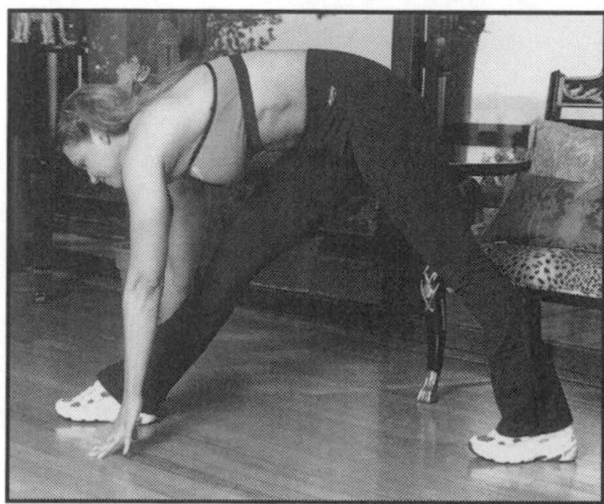
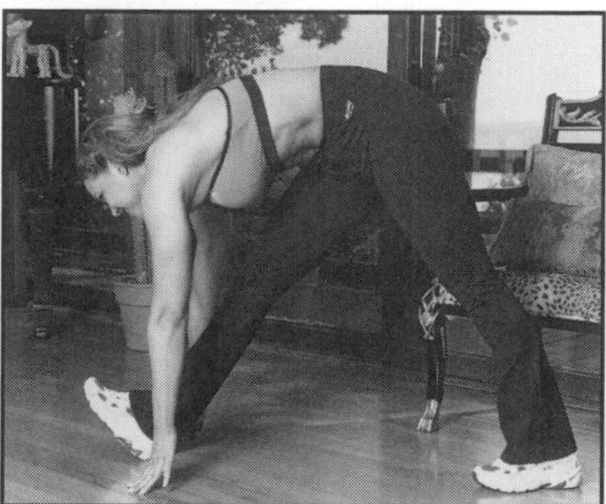

Outer Hip/Glute Stretch

1. Start on your back, and cross one ankle in front of a bent knee.
2. Put both hands around the bent leg, and gently pull your leg toward your chest until you feel a good stretch in the hip and butt area. Hold the stretch position.
3. Switch legs, and repeat this stretch on the other side.

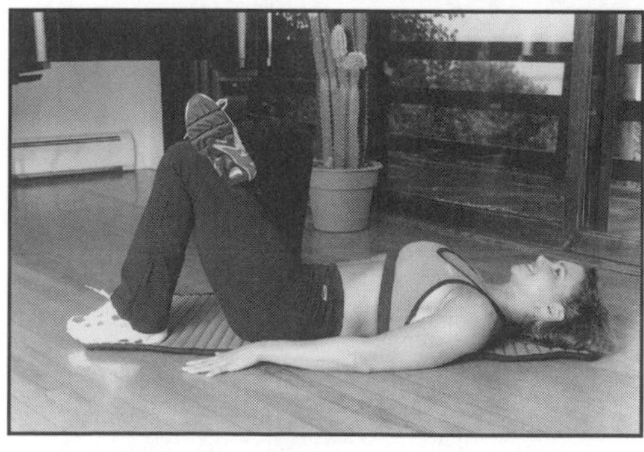
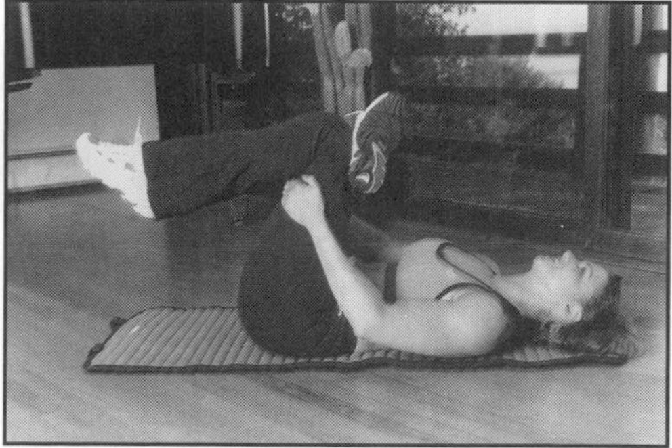

Butterfly Stretch

1. Sit tall with your back straight, shoulders back, and chest forward. Place your feet sole to sole.
2. With your knees out, gently pull your feet toward your groin, and press the inside of your knees toward the floor. Hold the stretch position.

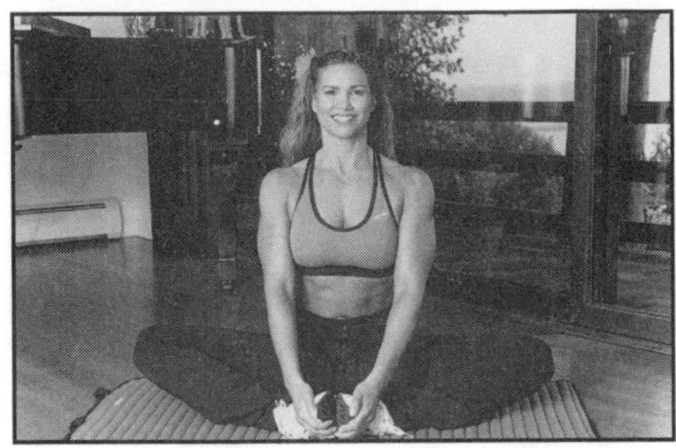

Calf Stretch

1. Using a wall or chair for support, place one foot in front of the other.
2. With your front knee slightly bent and your back knee straight and back heel down, lean your hips forward. Hold the stretch position.
3. Repeat the stretch on other side.

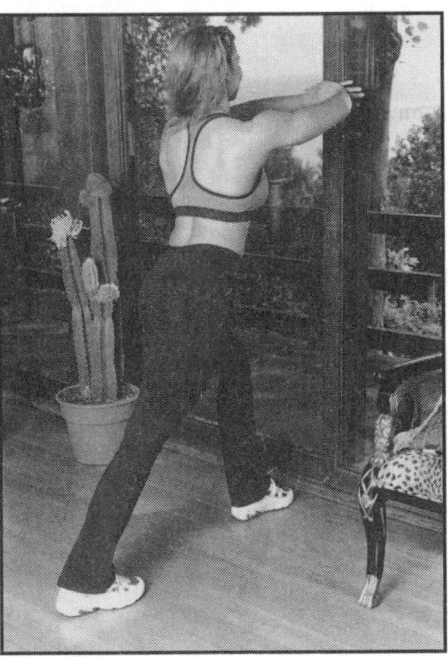

If you want to perform better and prevent injury, you have to warm up before you exercise. Doing a cool-down routine afterward will help you recover faster and experience less soreness. Stretching before, during, and after training is the key to creating muscles with an overall symmetrical appearance. Finally, whether you're doing a full body or specific muscle group workout, your stretch encyclopedia has you covered. Refer to it whenever you have a question about a specific stretch or need to check your form.

The Least You Need to Know

- Warming up will get your muscles ready to exercise, maximize your performance during exercise, and help prevent injury that could occur from exercising cold muscles.
- A proper cool-down will help prevent unnecessary soreness.
- Static stretching is the safest method of increasing your flexibility.
- If you don't have time to stretch all the muscles, you need to at least stretch the muscles that will be used in your training session.

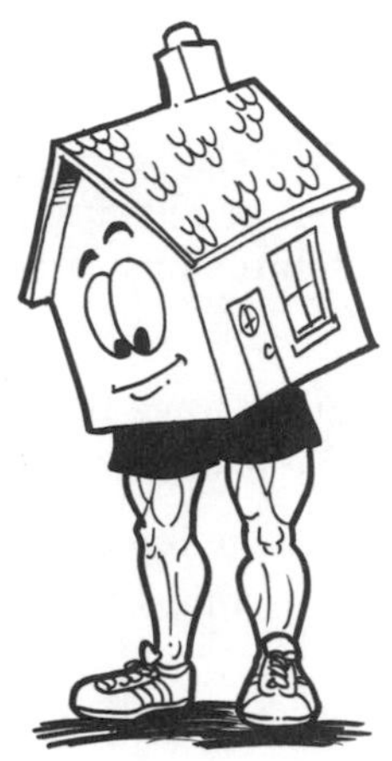

Chapter 6

Legs to Rock Your Hard-Body House

In This Chapter

- Muscles 101
- Your get hard home blue print
- Your home lower-body exercise encyclopedia

Before we break open your hard-body toolbox, it's back to the blackboard for Muscles 101. Understanding muscle makeup, function, and benefits will raise your desire to get them, dismiss all fear of "getting too big," and give you the confidence of knowing what does what and why. After your muscle introduction, you'll be briefed on your "Get Hard Guidelines," and then it's time to bring out your best hard-body building tools. To ensure that you become a "master builder," I've taken great care to fill your toolbox with only the best hard-body exercises.

Your lower-body exercise encyclopedia has what it takes to give you the legs that'll rock your hard-body house. You can select exercises for each muscle group to create your program, or you can use them as a reference for my custom programs in Chapter 9, "Custom Home Hard Bodies." If you're new to the building scene, it's best to follow one of my programs until you understand how to create your own muscle magic. During your apprentice period, pay special attention to how your body responds to each exercise. These responses will be your clues to creating your own hard-body muscle program.

Your Hard-Body Building Blocks

Each time you move, your muscles are called to action. Muscles respond to your request for movement by either contracting (getting shorter) or relaxing (getting longer). When a muscle contracts, it tenses and then attempts to shorten. Muscle contraction happens in one of three ways:

- **Isometric contraction.** This happens when the muscle force is equal to the resistive force. This results in no movement—an example is pushing against a wall.
- **Concentric contraction.** This happens when the muscle force is greater than the resistive force. The result is that the muscle shortens—an example is the lifting phase of a dumbbell curl.
- **Eccentric contraction.** This happens when the muscle force is less than the resistive force. The result is that the muscle lengthens—an example is the lowering phase of a dumbbell curl.

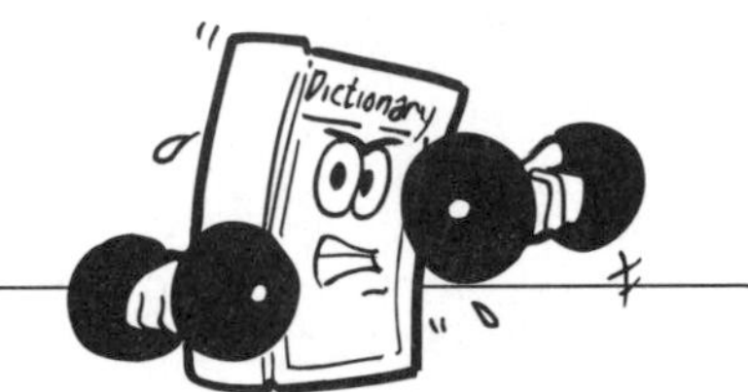

Workout Wisdom

The term **muscle fiber** refers to a muscle cell. These cells are made up of myofibrils and sarcomeres, and are the basic units of muscle contraction.

The intensity and duration of the muscle force is determined by the *muscle fiber*. Each muscle is made up of thousands of threadlike fibers that fall into one of two categories:

- **Slow-twitch fibers.** These are smaller and produce low levels of force for a longer period of time. These fibers are better for aerobic (with oxygen) energy use.
- **Fast-twitch fibers.** These produce high levels of force for shorter periods of time. These fibers are better for anaerobic (without oxygen) energy use.

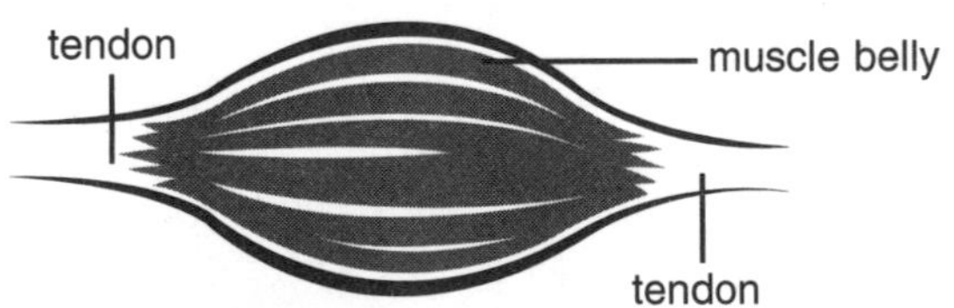

Muscle fiber diagram.

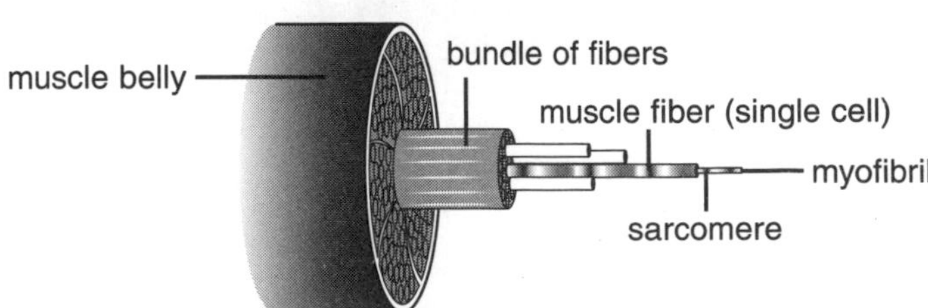

Muscle fiber cut away.

Building Better Blocks

Strength training is how you turn your muscle sticks to muscle bricks. Exercising with progressively heavier weights will increase the following:

- ➤ Muscle fiber size
- ➤ Muscle strength
- ➤ Bone strength
- ➤ Tendon strength
- ➤ Ligament strength

The presence of more lean muscle in your body will have a direct effect on your work capacity, physical appearance, metabolism, and likelihood of injuries.

- ➤ Muscle size and strength increases, so for the same amount of energy as before, you now are able to work harder and longer.
- ➤ Your body appears leaner and more defined with more muscle and less fat, even if body weight is increased. (Muscles weigh more than fat.)
- ➤ The metabolism is elevated by the presence of more muscle because it takes more energy (calories) to rebuild and maintain muscle than it does for fat.
- ➤ Overuse injuries can be prevented by maintaining a balanced level of strength between *opposite muscle groups*. Muscles are your body's shock absorbers against injuries.

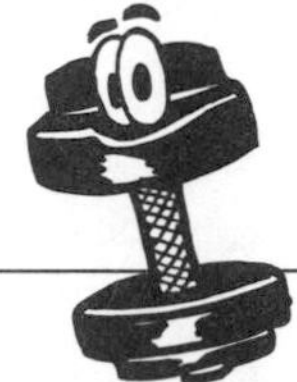

Hard-Body Headliners

People who strength-train for the first time gain about 2 to 4 pounds of muscle and 40 to 60 percent more strength after the first two months of regular strength training.

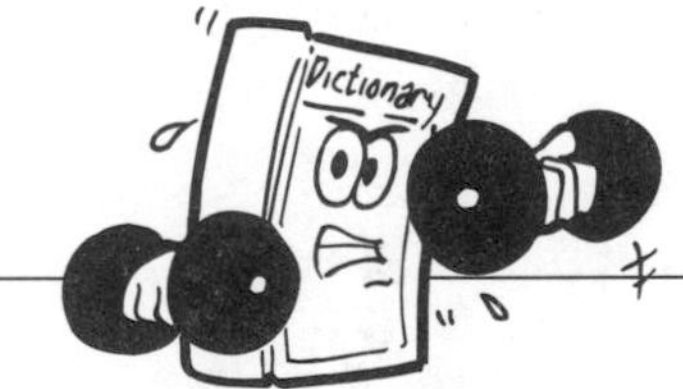

Workout Wisdom

Most muscles of the trunk and limbs are arranged in **opposite muscle groups.** When one muscle is contracting, its opposite muscle is being stretched. Examples of opposite muscle groups are these:

- ➤ Abs and lower back
- ➤ Quadriceps and hamstrings
- ➤ Pectorals and upper back
- ➤ Biceps and triceps

Home Hard-Body Training Guidelines

The following guidelines will ensure that you get your home hard body in the safest and most effective way.

- ➤ **Exercise selection.** Pick at least one exercise for each major muscle group to balance muscle strength and prevent injury.

- **Exercise sequence.** When doing a series of exercises, start with the largest muscle group and work down to the smallest. Doing this lets you do the hardest work first when you're not so tired.
- **Exercise speed.** Lifting too fast uses momentum to do most of the work and increases the risk of injury by placing extra stress on the muscles and connective tissue. Lifting at a slow pace uses more muscle strength throughout the movement. A good tempo is to lift on the count of 1 second and lower on the count of 3–4 seconds.
- **Exercise sets.** This refers to the number of reps done in a row without rest. Work up to three sets for each exercise.
- **Exercise resistance and reps.** Working between 70 and 80 percent of maximum resistance with 8–12 reps is safe and effective.
- **Exercise range.** Do each exercise through a full range of motion, with an emphasis on the contracted position. This will increase muscle strength and joint flexibility.
- **Exercise progression.** As your strength increases, you need to gradually raise the weight. Above all, never sacrifice perfect form to lift more weight.
- **Exercise frequency.** An intense workout may produce microscopic tears in the muscle fibers, so it's important to rest about 48 hours between same-muscle workouts to give the muscles time to recover and rebuild. The rule is, if it's still sore, it needs more time to recover.

Lower-Body Anatomy

Your lower body is made up of four major muscle groups: the quadriceps, the hamstrings, the gastrocnemius and soleus, and the tibialis anterior. The quadriceps, the largest group, are made up of four individual muscles: the vastus lateralis, vastus medialis, vastus intermedius, and rectus femoris. These muscles are responsible for extending your leg. The vastus lateralis and medialis are also known as the outer sweep and teardrop muscles. They are located on either side of the thigh. The vastus intermedius lies in between and extends upward below the rectus femoris.

The hamstring muscles are the quadriceps' opposite muscle group and are made up of three individual muscles: the biceps femoris, the semitendinosus, and the semimembranosus. The biceps femoris has two heads: the long head and the short head. The long head crosses the hip and the knee joint, and is involved in extending the hip and flexing the knee. The short head crosses only the knee joint, so it's involved in only flexing the knee. The semitendinosus and the semimembranosus cross the hip and knee joint, and are involved in extending the hip and flexing the knee.

The gluteus maximus (your butt) is the large muscle at the rear of your pelvic girdle, which is also involved in extending the hip. The gluteus medius is a smaller muscle that lies beneath the gluteus maximus. You use your "glutes" when you climb stairs and walk up an inclined plane.

The gastrocnemius and the soleus are the two major muscles that make up your calf. The tibialis anterior is located at the front of your lower leg and is commonly known as your shin muscle—or even more painfully as your "shin splints" muscle.

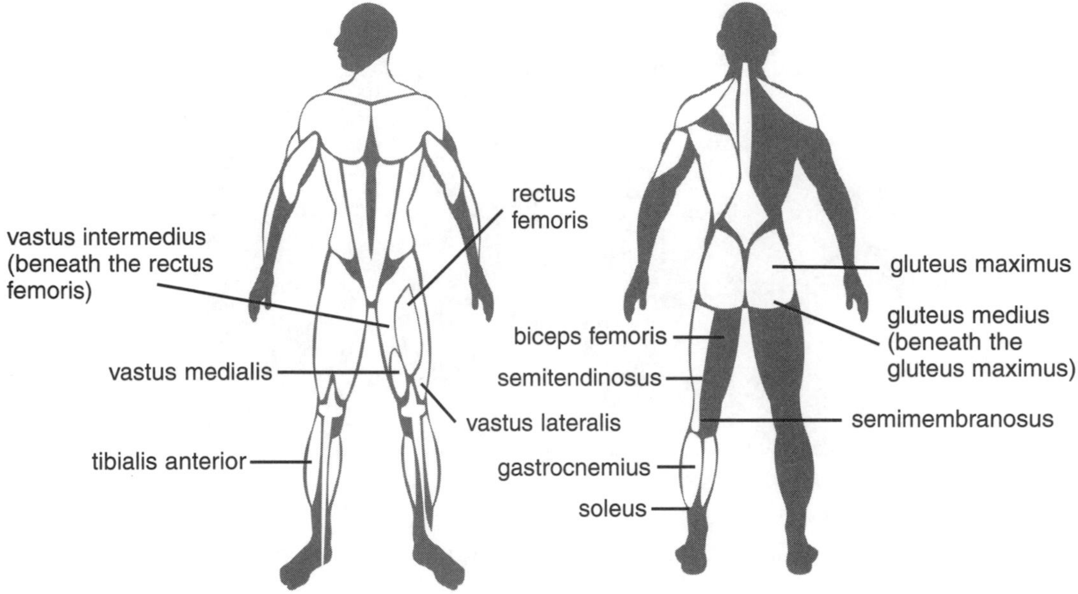

Lower-body muscles—front and rear view.

Your Hard-Body Exercise Encyclopedia

The most common workout mistake is usually incorrect exercise form. This can lead to poor muscle development and injury. To avoid even this possibility, I've created your "Hard-Body Exercise Encyclopedia." The exercises are categorized by muscle groups and are broken down step by step both in text and photos. These exercises can be used to create your own routines or can serve as a reference for my custom programs in Chapter 9.

Free Bar Squats

Squatting is the best overall lower body exercise for leg and glute development. No other exercise works as many major muscle groups as intensely and burns as many calories as squatting. Squatting with a free bar increases the intensity because your muscles also have to work as stabilizers. The bottom line is that if you want a great butt, you've got to squat.

This exercise works the quadriceps, hamstrings, and glutes.

1. Start standing with your feet hip-width apart, your shoulders back, and your chest forward. Keep a shoulder-width grip on a straight bar resting across your upper back.

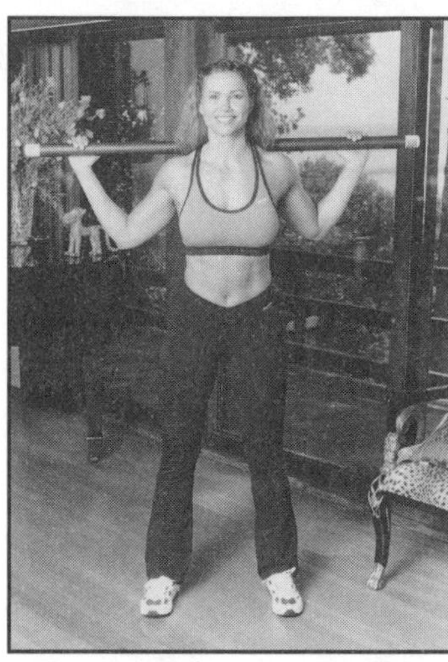

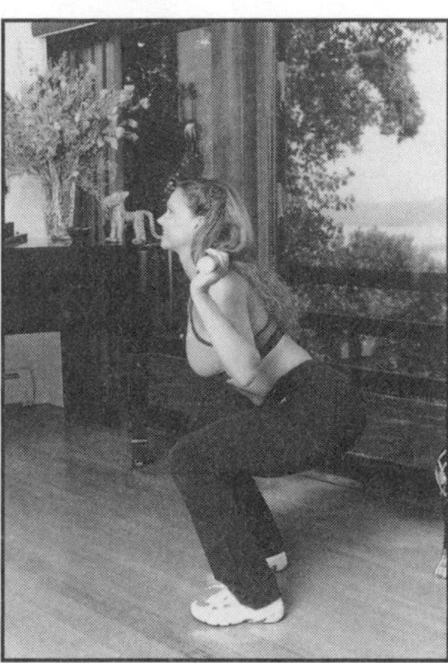

2. Look slightly up, inhale, and squat back, as if sitting on a stool, until your thighs are parallel to the floor. Exhale and rise up on a count of 1. Repeat for desired reps.

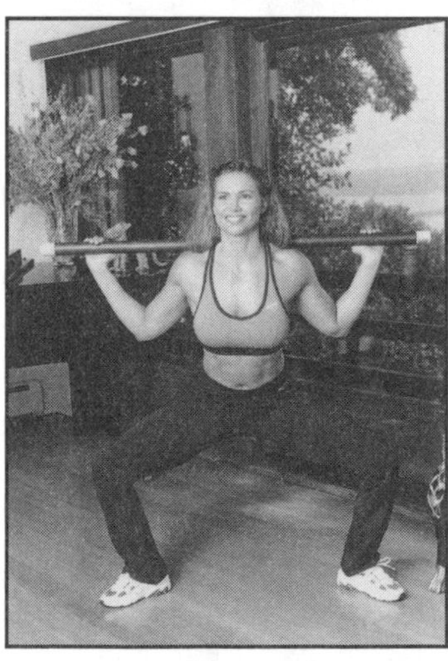

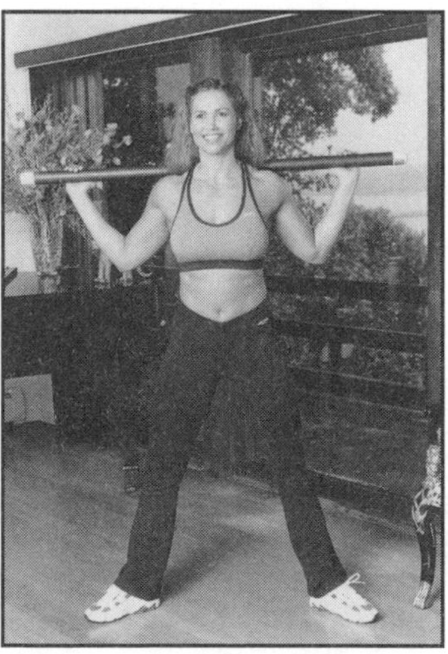

You can also squat from a wide stance to place more emphasis on the adductor muscles. In this position, toes are pointed out to a 10 o'clock and 2 o'clock position.

Front Squats

By going straight down instead of back, your quadriceps get extra work.

This exercise works the quadriceps (emphasized in this variation), hamstrings, and glutes.

1. Start standing with your feet hip-width apart, your shoulders back, and your chest forward. Hold the bar on your upper chest.
2. Squat down instead of back until you feel a stretch in your quadriceps, and rise up on a count of 1. Repeat for desired reps.

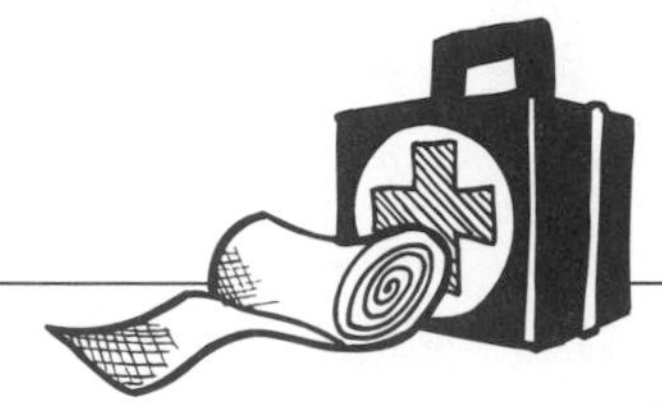

Safety Scoop

Front squats put extra tension on the quadriceps and the knee joints. If you have any knee problems, work on strengthening the joints first with single-leg squats.

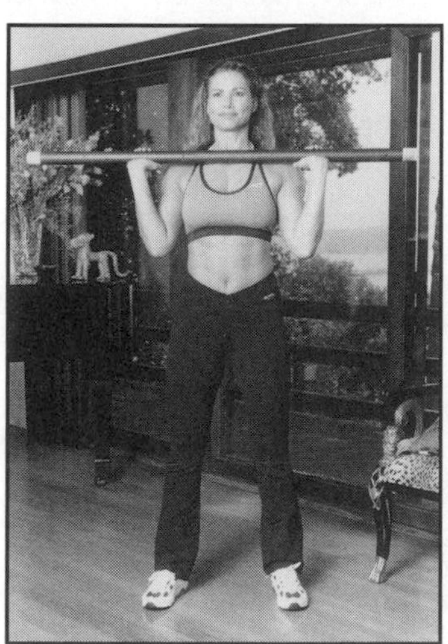

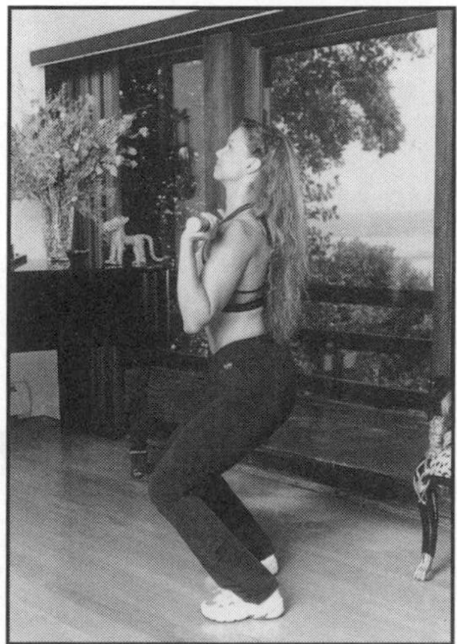

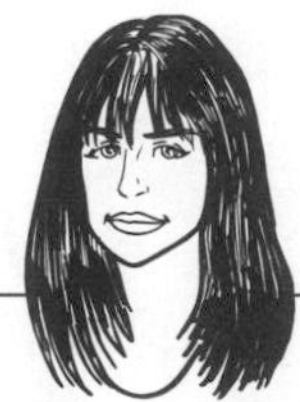

Jourdan's Gems

Flexibility is the secret to great side squats. Increasing your flexibility will increase your range of motion on the side squats so that you fully work the muscle from end to end.

Side Squats

The side squat is a variation that I created to really work the inner thighs.

This exercise works the quadriceps, hamstrings, glutes, adductors, and abductors.

1. Start by standing with a weighted bar on your upper back, with a grip slightly wider than shoulder width. Your feet should be in a wide stance, with the toes pointing forward.
2. With your left leg straight, squat to the right and back until your thigh is at a 90° angle to your knee, or as far as your range of motion allows. (Imagine sitting on a stool to your far right side.) Your shoulders should be in line with your knees, and your lower back should be slightly arched.
3. Rise up halfway, and go back down. Repeat for desired reps. (You should feel a good stretch in your adductor muscles in the squat position.) Switch sides, and do reps on other side.

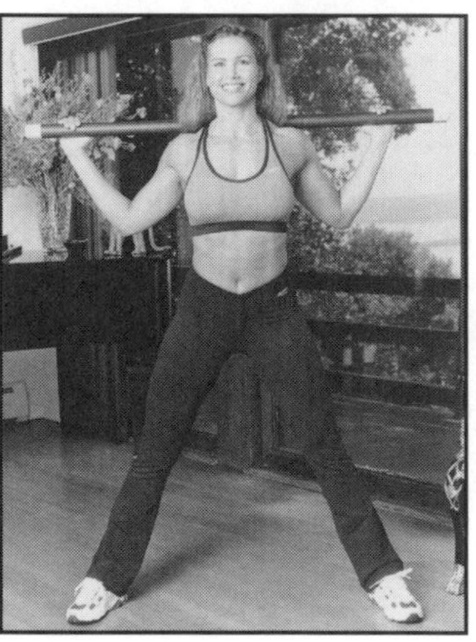

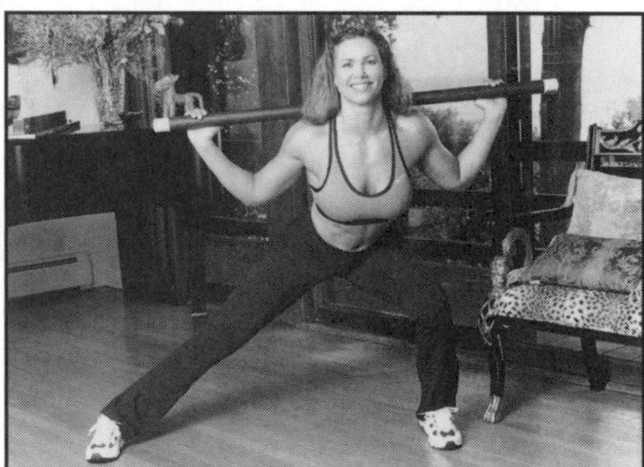

Single-Leg Squats

I primarily use this variation to strengthen the knee joints and surrounding muscles. (This also makes a great warm-up exercise for your leg workout.)

1. Keep your shoulders back, chest forward, and abs tight throughout this exercise. With your hands on your hips (or a chair for support), shift your weight to your right foot, and extend the left foot forward, with your foot flexed.
2. Slowly lower yourself up and down on your right leg. Make sure that your knee stays directly over your foot and doesn't sway from side to side. Repeat for desired reps.
3. Switch legs and do reps on your other side. As your strength increases, you will be able to go lower. At that time, you can stand on a step to increase the height.

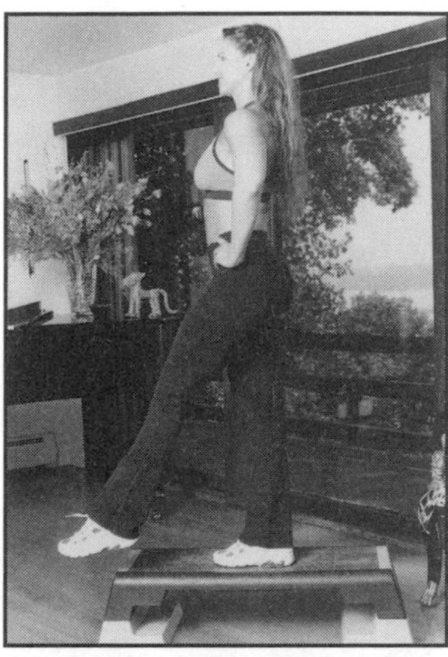

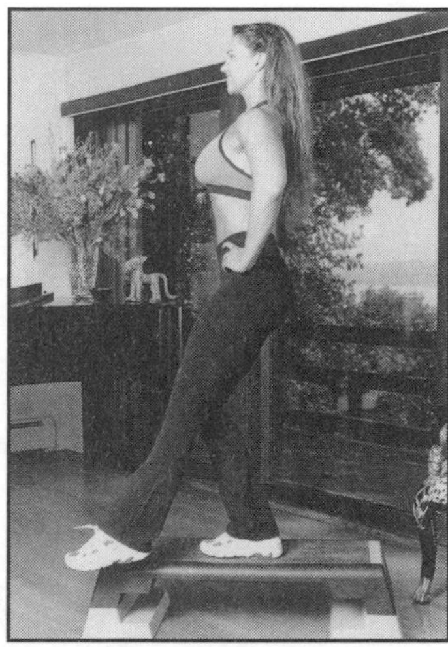

Walking Lunges

Next to squatting, the next-best leg exercise is walking lunges. You'll really feel this in your glutes.

This exercise works the quadriceps, hamstrings, and glutes.

1. Start standing, holding dumbbells at your sides.
2. With a straight back, your shoulders back, and your chest forward, step forward with your right foot and lunge down by bending your left knee. Your right knee should be directly over your foot.
3. Now pull your left leg through, and take a step forward. Lunge on the right side. Repeat stepping and lunging without stopping until you reach the desired distance.
4. Turn around and go back to complete the set.

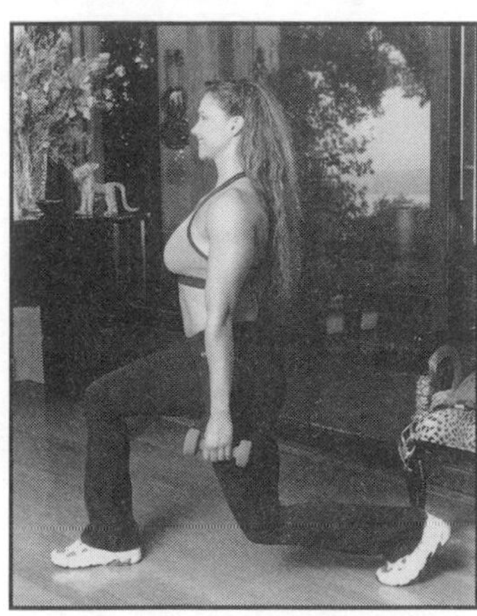

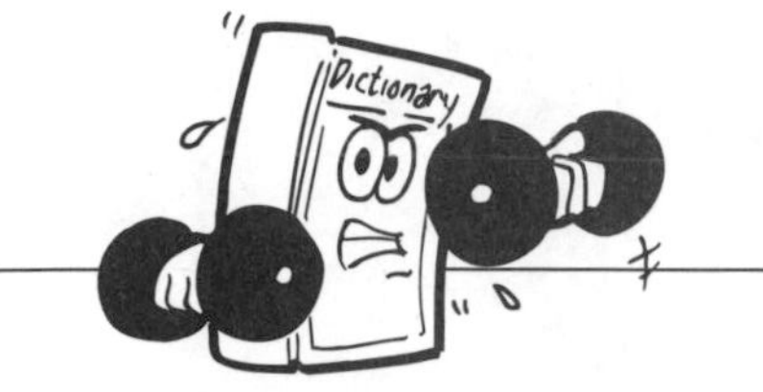

Workout Wisdom

In an **open-chain exercise** (**OCE**), a muscle or muscle group is isolated to function alone.

Leg Extensions

This *open-chain exercise* is a great isolation exercise to finish your leg workout. Leg extensions are done on a weight bench with an extension attachment.

This exercise works the quadriceps.

1. With your back straight and the roller above your ankles, extend your legs and squeeze your quadriceps at the top of the movement. Lower your leg slowly for a count of 3 seconds. Repeat for desired reps.

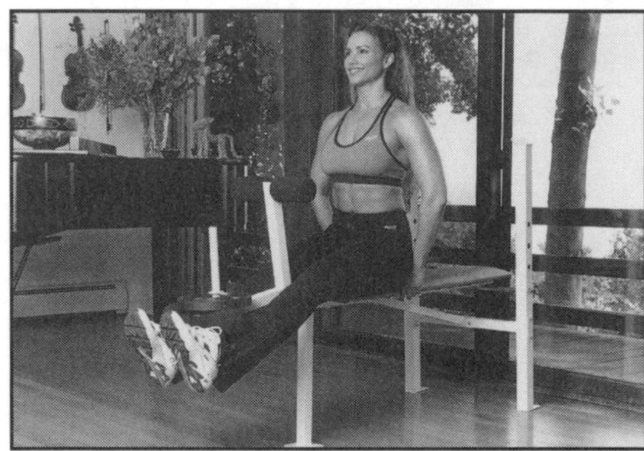

2. Turn your toes slightly in for a variation that focuses on a different angle.
3. Turn your toes slightly out for another variation.

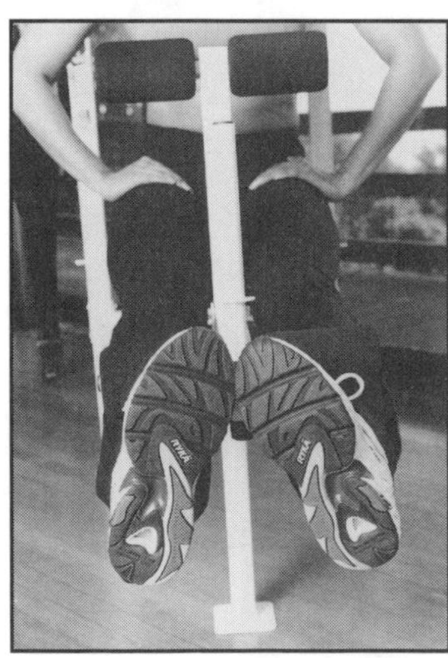

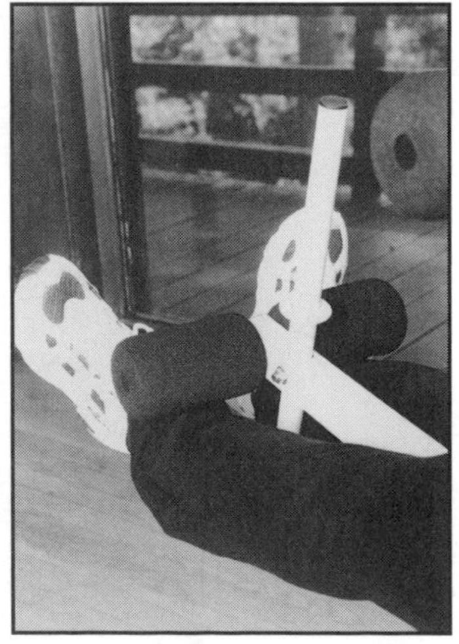

Leg Curls

I have added my own twist to leg curls to increase the level of muscle contraction and work the glutes better.

This exercise works the hamstrings.

1. Lay flat on your stomach. Keep your hips pressed into the bench throughout the movement to support your lower back from arching.
2. Curl the weight up toward your glutes, and contract your hamstrings.
3. Now lift your knees a couple of inches off the bench, and really squeeze your glutes.
4. Lower your knees to the bench, and then lower the weight to the starting position.
5. Repeat for desired reps.

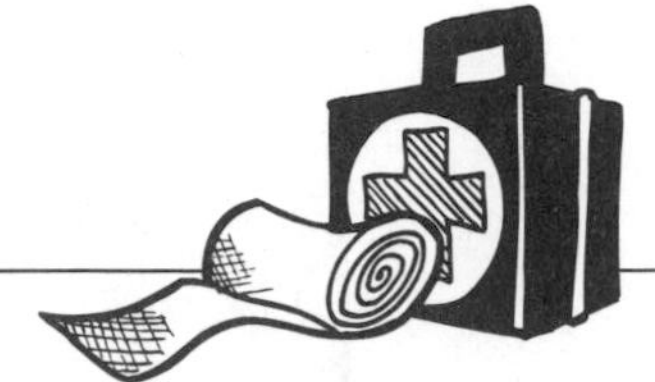

Safety Scoop

Leg extensions can put a lot of stress on the knees if you lift really heavy weights. To avoid this, I up the intensity by drop setting or super setting with another exercise, such as leg curls.

Stiff-Legged Dead Lifts

This exercise works the hamstrings and glutes.

1. Stand with your feet hip-width apart, with your legs straight, your back perfectly flat, and your hands gripping the bar outside your hips.
2. While looking forward, bend from the waist and lower the bar for a count of 3 seconds until you feel a stretch in your hamstrings.
3. Rise up on a count of 1. Repeat for desired reps. Keep the bar close to your legs as you lower and raise. The most important thing is to keep your back strong and straight.

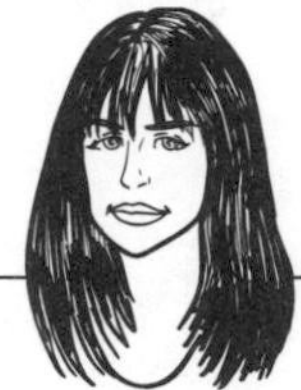

Jourdan's Gems

The secret to stiff-legged dead lifts is in the form. Many people round their back as they lower the bar. Doing this makes your lower back do a lot of the work. You know this is true if your lower back is sore the next day. The key to making this more of a hamstring and glute exercise is to keep your back flat during the entire movement.

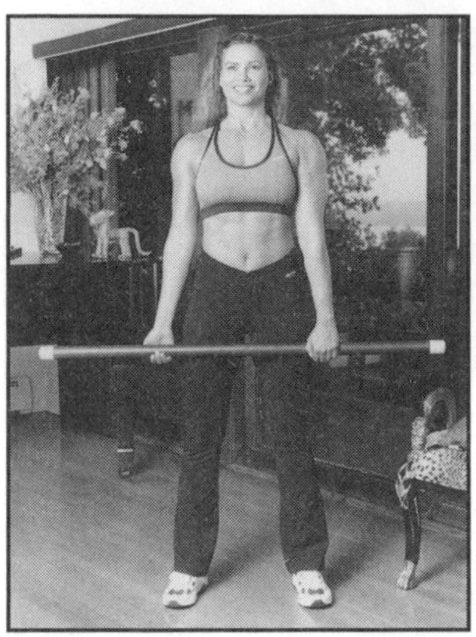

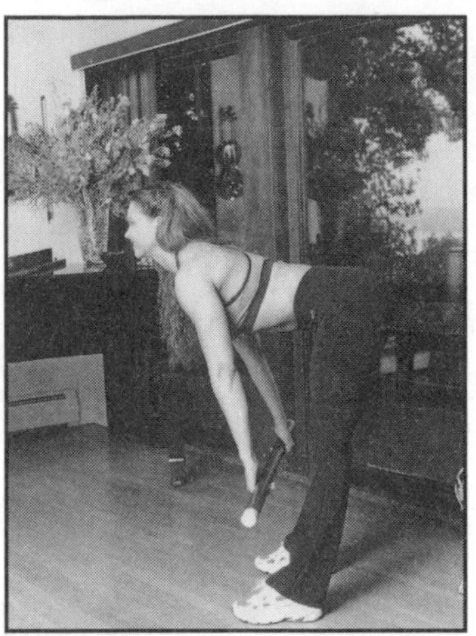

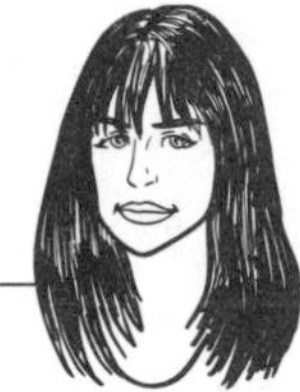

Jourdan's Gems

Because your hamstrings are mostly made up of fast-twitch muscle fibers, they respond better to high-weight, low-rep training. Increase the amount of sets that you do, and don't let the reps go over 10. I sometimes start my leg routine with hamstrings so that I can get the most out of the exercises. After my warm-up set, I do two hamstring exercises for four sets each. My reps descend from 10 down to 6 for the last set.

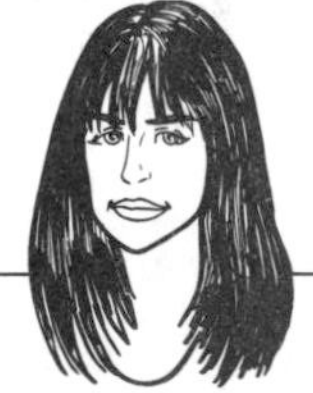

Jourdan's Gems

Taking stairs two-at-a-time is a great glute exercise that you can do anytime you see a set of stairs (unless you're in a dress).

Step-Ups

This exercise works the hamstrings and glutes.

1. Place your right foot on the step, and lift your left knee up, as if you were climbing stairs. (Raising your knee higher will give your butt a workout.)
2. Curl your right arm when your left knee goes up, and curl your left arm when your right knee goes up.
3. Lower back and lunge down. Repeat for desired reps.

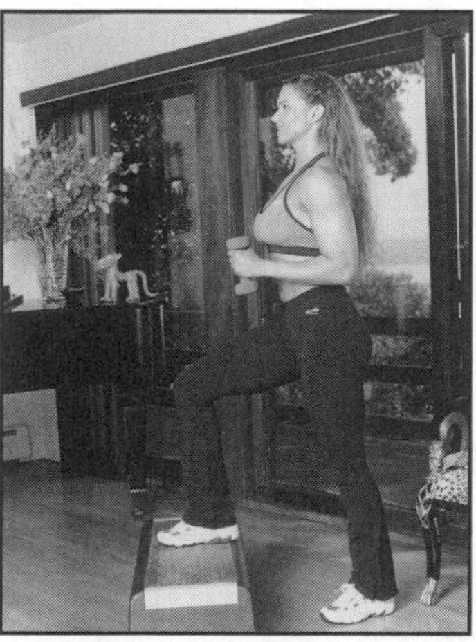

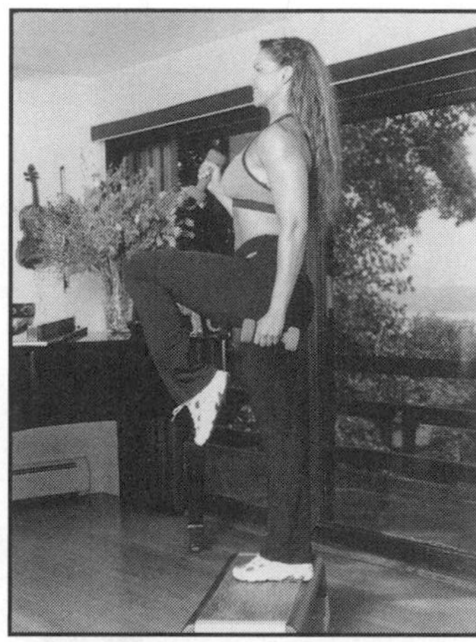

Hamstring Lean

Then rise up to the starting position. Repeat for desired reps.

1. Start on knees and extend your arms forward as you lean back as far as you can.

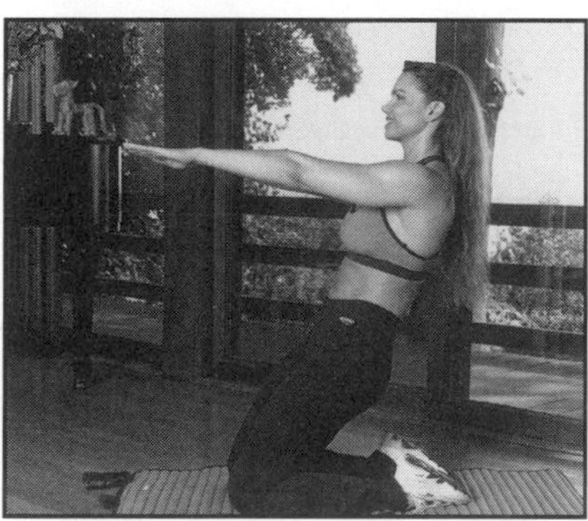

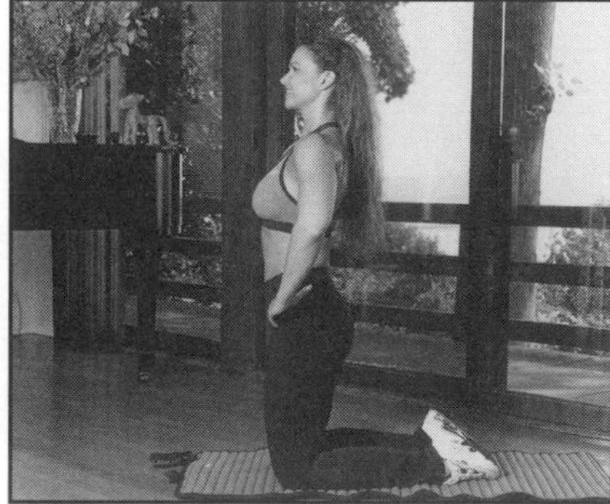

Calf Raises

As the name suggests, this exercise works the calves.

1. Using a step on a staircase works great for this exercise. Holding a dumbbell in one hand and the staircase for support, lower up and down on one leg.
2. Lower your foot below the step until you feel a good stretch. Contract the calf as hard as you can at the top position.
3. Switch sides, and repeat for desired reps.

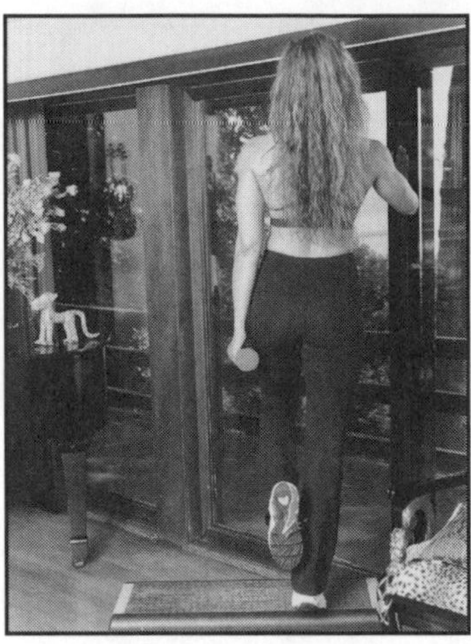

Knowing how to train right will give you the confidence that your home body fixer-upper is well on its way to becoming your best hard body. Keeping your Lower Body Exercise Encyclopedia handy when it's time to update your routine or when you need answers about a specific exercise will help you continue to rock your hard-body house.

The Least You Need to Know

- Strength training increases muscle fiber size, muscle strength, bone strength, tendon strength, and ligament strength.
- Having more muscle mass will increase your work capacity, enhance your physical appearance, raise your metabolism, and help prevent injury.
- The most common training mistake is using incorrect exercise form.
- Squatting works more major muscle groups and burns more calories than any other weight-training exercise.
- Hamstrings are made up of mostly fast-twitch muscle fibers and respond better to high-weight, low-rep training.

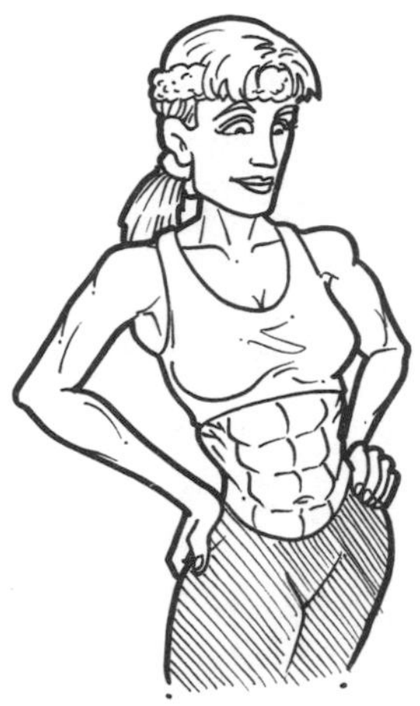

Chapter 7

Phenomenal Abdominals

In This Chapter

- Your hard body's power generator
- The lower-back link
- Your hard-core training guide
- Your core exercise encyclopedia

Abdominal training is another one of those details that many people let slip through the cracks. If you want proof, just start checking out midsections and compare the ratio of six-packs to gallon jugs. I don't know who came up with the name "love handles" because there is nothing to love about being able to grab a whole bunch of fat that's attached to you.

Training your core muscles is like the gift that keeps on giving. Increasing your core strength will also strengthen every other muscle in your body, improve your posture, and increase your spine's support so that you can kiss lower-back pain goodbye.

If you're doing 100 crunches a day 5 days a week and still look like the Pillsbury doughboy, then you're doing the thing wrong or doing the wrong thing. Your hard-core training guide gives you the pieces you need to put your phenomenal abdominals together once and for all.

The volume of your "Hard-Body Exercise Encyclopedia" contained in this chapter is dedicated to your core muscles. Exercises for each core region are given in full detail, so you'll soon be able to trade in your mediocre midsection for a show-stopping six-pack.

Your Hard-Body Power Generator

Let's start by listing your hard-body core credentials:

- All power that's generated by your upper- or lower-body muscles either started, passed through, or was stabilized by your core.
- If you strengthen your core muscles, you will be strengthening every muscle in your body.
- Strengthening your core muscles can straighten out shrimp posture, take the sway out of your back, and pull in that protruding abdomen.

I don't know how you feel about it, but those are some pretty serious credentials to substantiate putting core training high on your priority list. Just the possibility of getting posture that resembles a shrimp should be enough to make commercial crunch breaks a nightly ritual.

Your Lower Back Link

The strongest link in your hard-body chain should be your core link. Strong core muscles are your direct link to having good posture. Having your spine supported takes pressure off your lower back and prevents future problems that range from nagging pain to the posterior or anterior tilt of your pelvis.

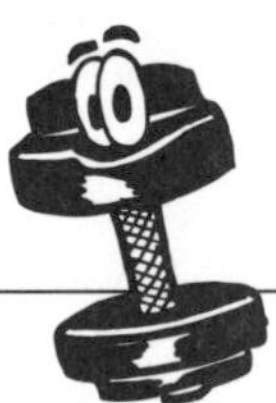

Hard-Body Headliners

Lower-back pain is often muscle-related and can be prevented by strengthening your core muscles.

Anterior or forward pelvic tilt is due to muscle strength imbalance between the quadriceps and the hamstrings. The stronger quads pull the pelvis forward, resulting in a protruding abdomen and lower-back pain. The swayback look is caused by a posterior or backward pelvic tilt.

Core strength is also a direct link to lower-back stabilization and overall balance. Having control over balance and stability will increase your performance and endurance level.

Your Hard-Core Training Guide

The following guidelines will maximize your core strength and development in the safest and most effective way:

- Train the weaker core regions first. Upper abs assist both lower and oblique regions during exercises and should be trained last so as not to decrease their productivity.

- Train your abs in the following order:
  1. Obliques
  2. Lower abs
  3. Upper abs
- Train opposite muscle groups (abs/lower back) evenly to prevent muscle imbalances.
- Limit the range of motion to 45° or less, to prevent the psoas and hip flexor muscles from becoming the *prime mover muscles*.
- Keep your knees bent and unsecured during ab exercises, to minimize hip flexor involvement.

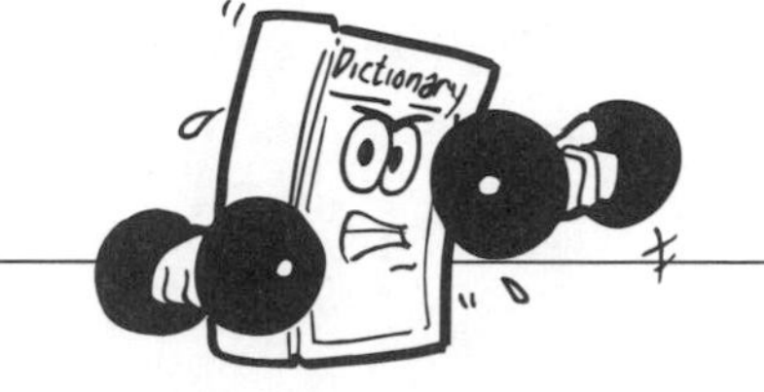

Workout Wisdom

A **prime mover muscle** is the muscle that contracts concentrically to accomplish the movement in any given joint.

- Avoid exercises that arch or severely hyperextend the lower back.
- Vary exercise direction, angle, and order for maximum development.
- Keep the abs contracted during the entire set.
- Exhale during the lifting phase of exercise.
- Increased sets with low reps and high resistance maximize abdominal development since the abdominal muscles are mostly made up of fast twitch muscle fibers. Keep exercise reps less than 20 in the beginning sets and less than 10 reps for the last few sets.
- Oblique exercises should follow a high-rep, low-resistance training program because overdeveloped obliques make you appear wider and heavier.

Core Muscle Anatomy

You have four paired muscles in the front and side abdominal wall:

- Internal oblique
- External oblique
- Transverse abdominis
- Rectus abdominis

Together these muscles flex the spine forward and sideways, rotate the lower and upper body, and compress the abdomen.

Three major muscles are responsible for movement of the vertebral column:

- Iliocostalis
- Longissimus
- Spinalis

Together these muscles are known as the erector spinae and are found on either side of the spine.

Abdominal muscles.

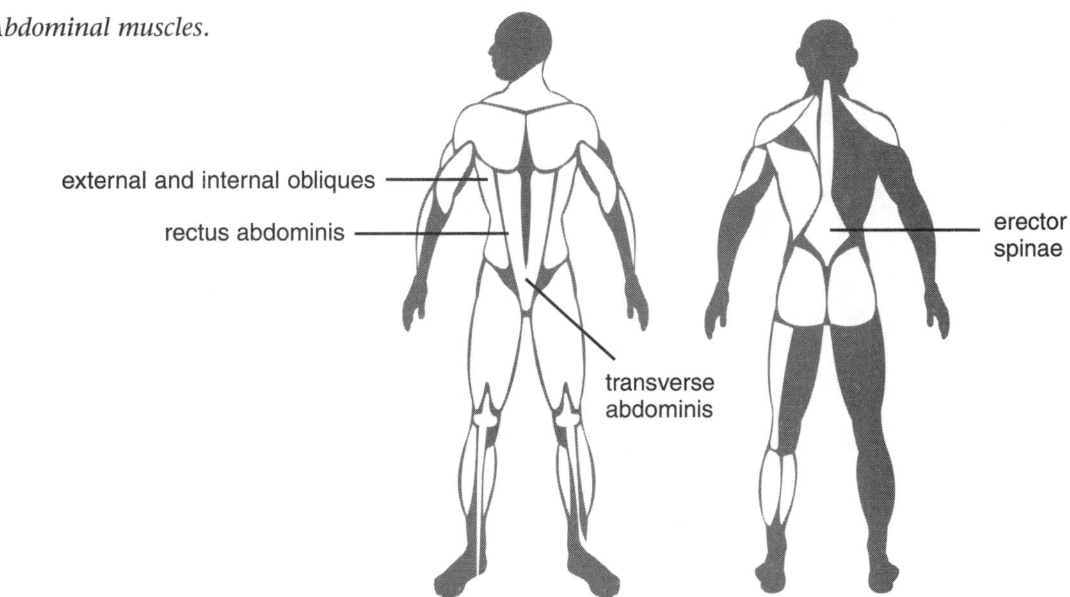

Core Exercise Encyclopedia

Core exercises are usually named after or classified by core regions, as follows:

- **Oblique exercises.** Internal and external obliques.
- **Lower ab exercises.** Lower portion of your rectus abdominis and transverse abdominis.
- **Upper ab exercises.** Upper portion of your rectus abdominis.
- **Lower-back exercises.** Entire lower-back region.

Weighted Crunch Variations

This exercise works the upper abs.

1. Start with your back on the floor, your knees bent, and your heels up; hold a dumbbell on your upper chest.

2. Exhale and lift up, using your abs while you simultaneously press into the ground with your heels. Hold for 1 second and lower down. Repeat for desired reps.

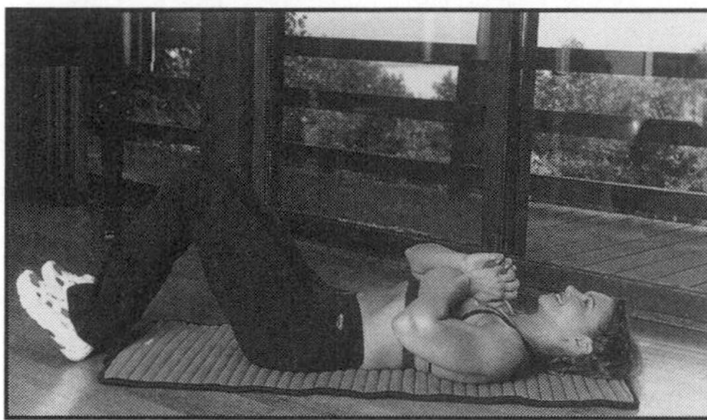

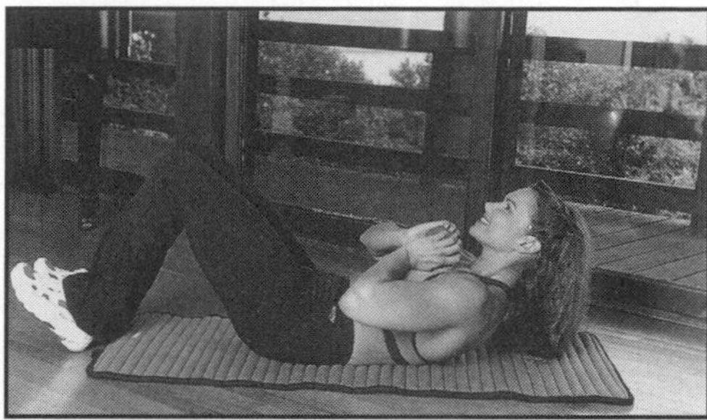

3. The movement is the same as in step 1, except that you are lying on the fit ball. The difference is that you now can stretch your abs through their full range of motion. Your lower back is fully supported throughout the movement by the fit ball.

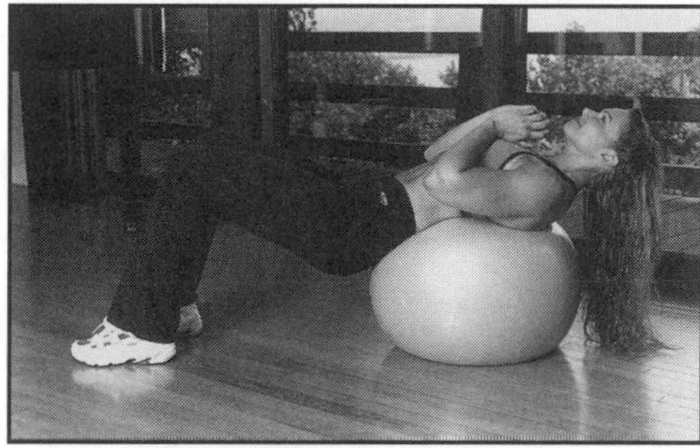

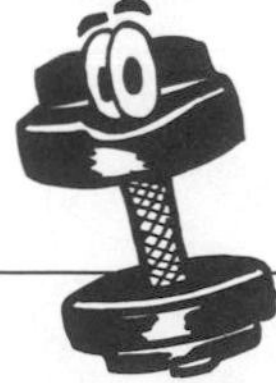

Hard-Body Headliners

Floor exercises are great for working the abs only through the first 30° of motion. Abdominal training should include exercises that also allow your abs to bend backwards the additional 15°. This will ensure that your abs learn how to properly contract when you bend backward.

Weighted Oblique Reach

This exercise works the upper abs and the obliques.

1. Start with your back on the floor, your legs extended straight up, and your arms extended up reaching for your toes, holding dumbbells.

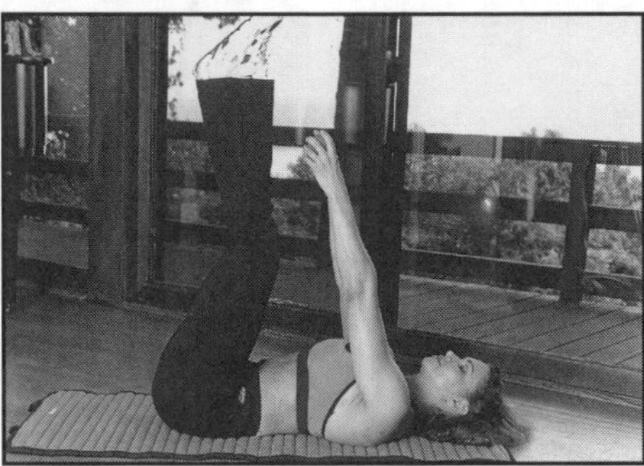

2. Using your abdominal muscles, lift your upper body off the ground toward your feet. Lower down and repeat for 10 reps.

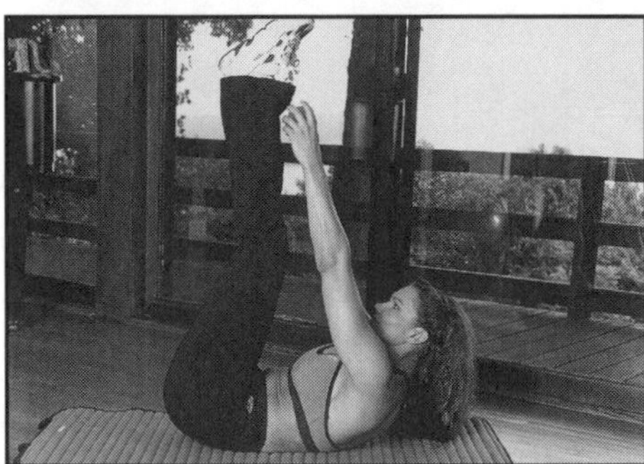

3. Now reach for your right little toe with the dumbbell. Contract your obliques on the way up, and then lower down. Repeat for 10 reps and switch sides. Finally, go back to center and do 10 reps to finish the set.

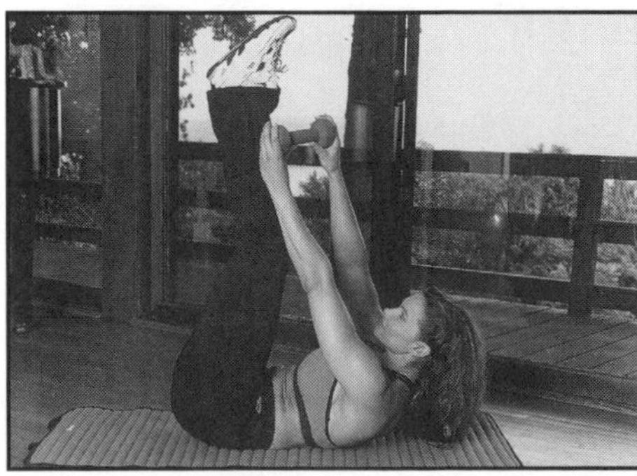

Leg Lift Variations

This exercise works the lower abs and the obliques.

1. Lie flat on your back with your arms by your sides and your palms down. Your legs should be extended up, toes pointed.

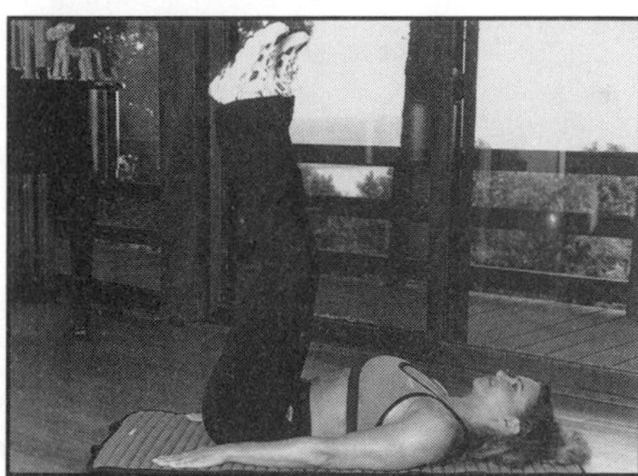

2. Using your ab muscles, lift your lower body a couple of inches off the ground, hold for 1 second, and then lower down. Repeat for desired reps. Go to step 3.

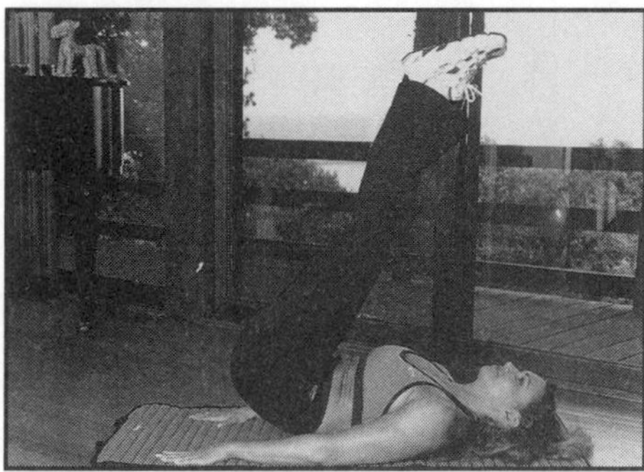

3. Now lift and twist to the right side. Hold for 1 second, untwist, and lower down for 10 reps. Repeat on the other side for 10 reps.

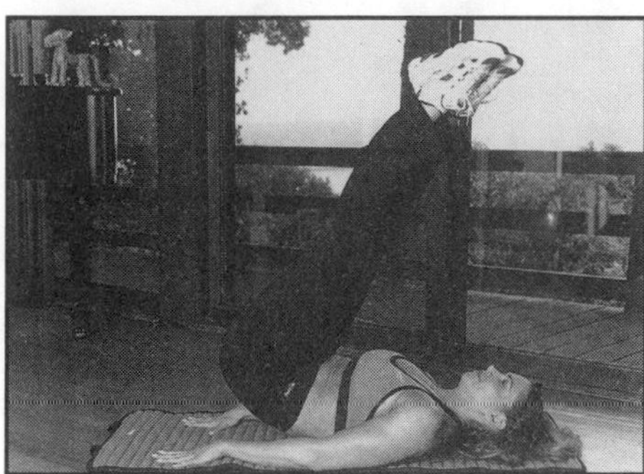

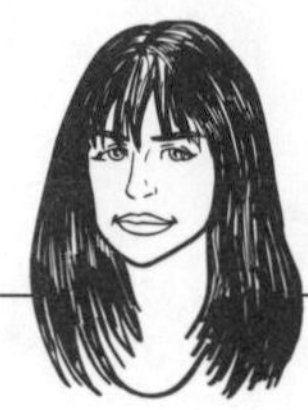

Jourdan's Gems

Your core muscles work together to give you strength and power in a multitude of directions and angles. To increase your overall power and strength, exercises should be done in various directions and angles.

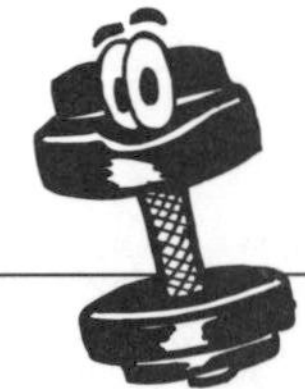

Hard-Body Headliners

All the training in the world won't give you a ripped set of abs. The only way you'll see your six-pack is to lose the excess body fat that's covering the muscles.

Upper/Lower Combined Crunch

This exercise works the upper and lower abs.

1. Start with your feet extended up and your toes pointed. Your hands can be on the sides of your head or holding a dumbbell on your upper chest to raise the intensity. You should be looking up with a fist-width distance between your chin and your chest. (This will prevent neck pain that results from having your circulation cut off.)
2. Exhale and curl up from your abs, while simultaneously lifting your glutes off the floor a few inches by using your lower abs. Hold in the center position for 1 second, and release. Repeat for desired reps.

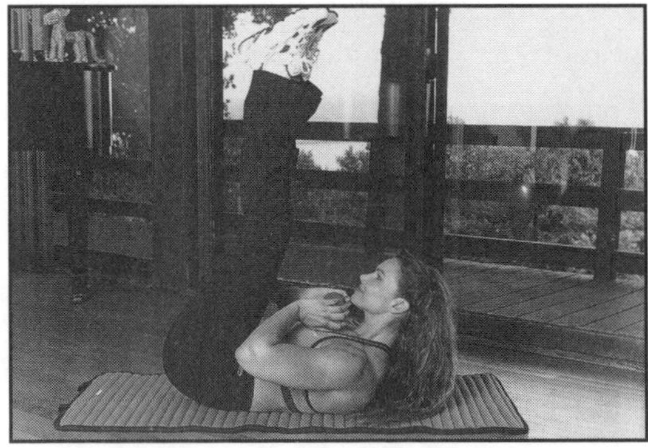

Knee-Ups

This exercise works the lower abs.

1. Start by sitting on the floor with your hands behind you, with your fingers pointing forward and your elbows flexed to stabilize the upper body. Your legs should be together, knees bent.
2. Bring your legs toward your chest while your upper body simultaneously crunches toward your knees.

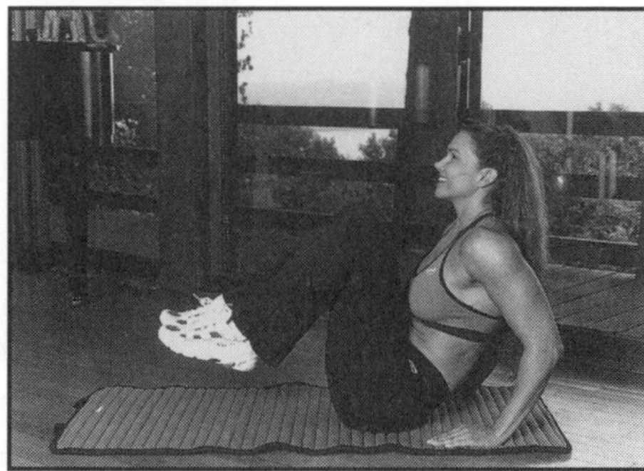

3. Exhale and extend your legs out to a 45° angle to your upper body. Repeat for desired reps.

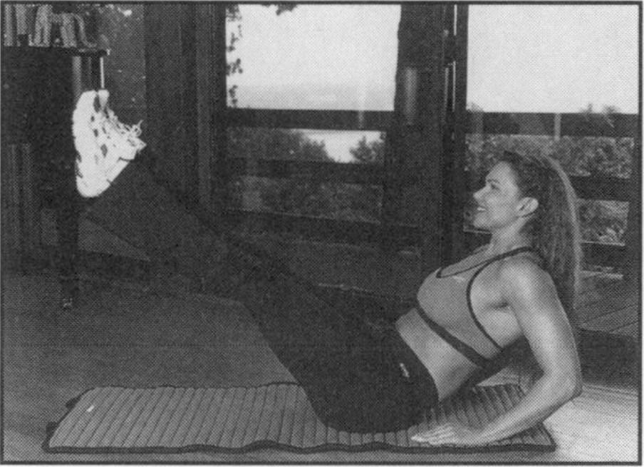

Lower-Back Lift

As its name suggests, this exercise works the lower back.

1. Lie on the floor, facing down, with your arms extended overhead.
2. Contract your lower back and glute muscles. Lift your upper and lower body three to four inches off the floor, and hold for two seconds. Release and repeat for desired reps.

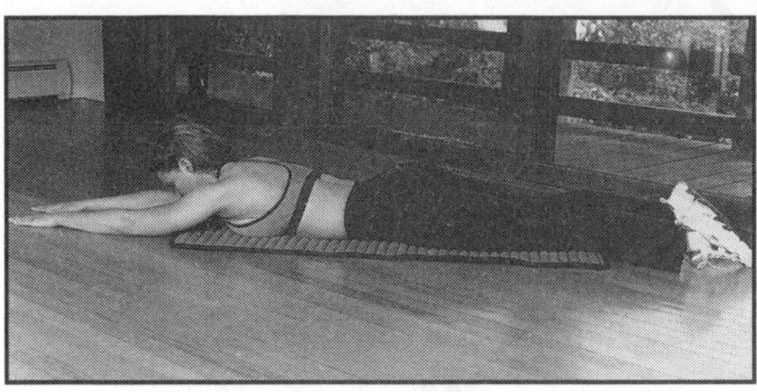

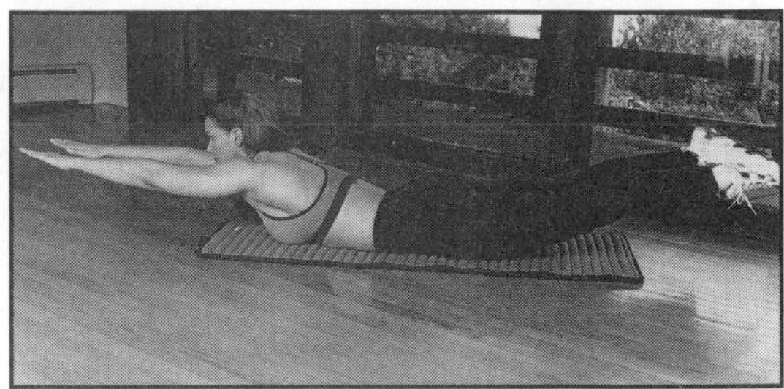

Fit Ball Extensions

This exercise works your core stabilization.

1. Lie on the floor, with your spine in contact with the floor and your arms by your sides. Flex your knees and hips to 90°, and place your heels on top of the ball.
2. Slowly extend yourself with both legs so that the ball rolls. Keep your abs and lower back tight throughout the movement. Hold for 5–10 seconds, and then slowly return to the starting position. Repeat for desired reps.

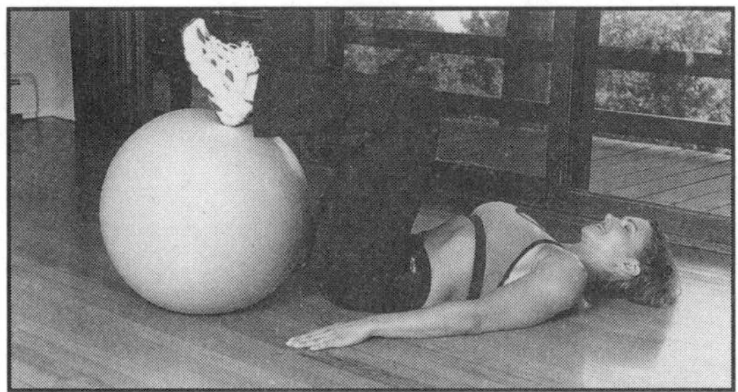

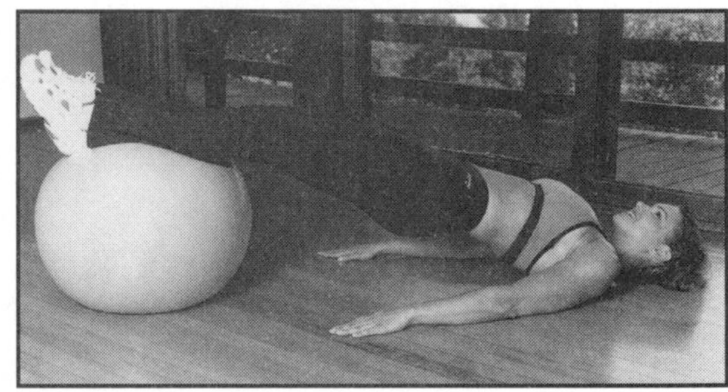

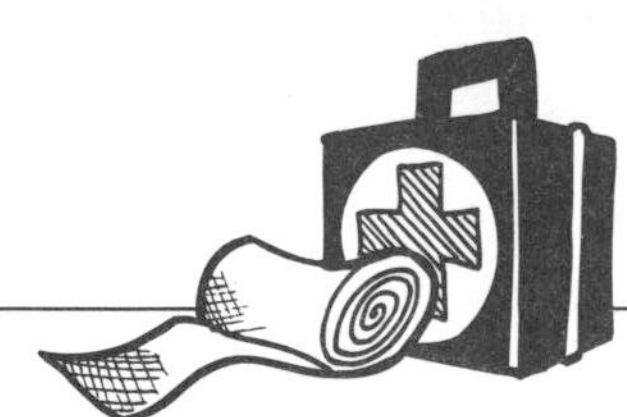

Safety Scoop

Do fit ball hypers on a surface that allows your hands to grip the floor. This will prevent you from slipping forward.

Fit Ball Hypers

This exercise works the lower back, the hamstrings, and the glutes.

1. Lie on the fit ball with your hands shoulder-width apart in a push-up position. The ball should be directly under your stomach, and your weight should be shifted forward. Extend your legs back.
2. Exhale and lift straight legs with toes pointed up as far as your range of motion allows for a count of one second. Lower slowly for a count of five seconds. Repeat for desired reps.

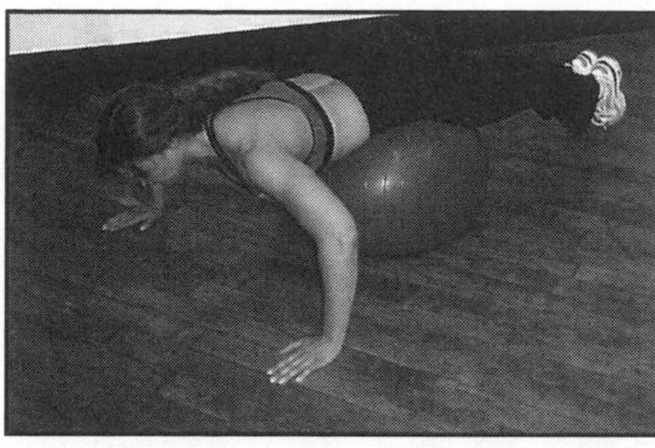

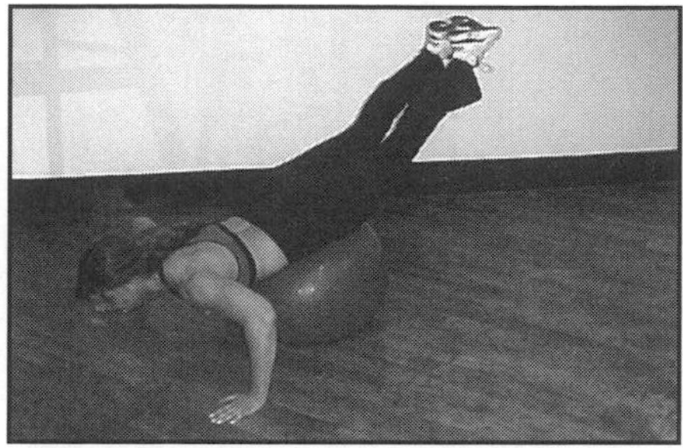

Core training should take priority in your workout because increasing your core strength automatically strengthens all the muscles in your body and improves your athletic performance. The health benefits include eliminating lower-back pain. The visual benefits include increased height (because of posture improvement) and a head-turning midsection.

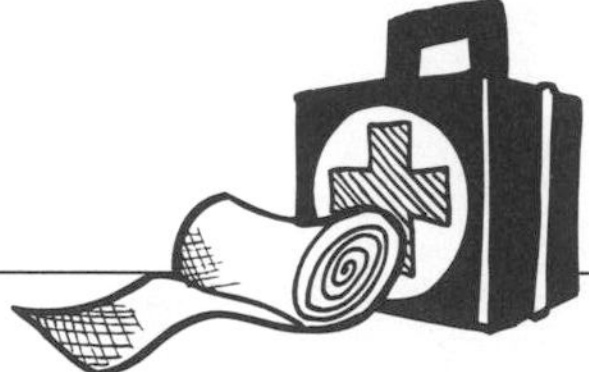

Safety Scoop

Do fit ball hypers on a surface that allows your hands to grip the floor. This will prevent you from slipping forward.

The Least You Need to Know

- ➤ All power that's generated by your upper- and lower-body muscles either started, passed through, or was stabilized by your core muscles.
- ➤ Lower-back pain is often muscle-related and can be prevented by strengthening your core.
- ➤ To minimize hip flexor involvement during ab exercises, keep your knees bent and unsecured.
- ➤ Abdominal muscles are made up of mostly fast-twitch muscle fibers and respond better to high-weight, low-rep training.
- ➤ The only way you'll see ripped abs is to lose the excess body fat that's covering them.

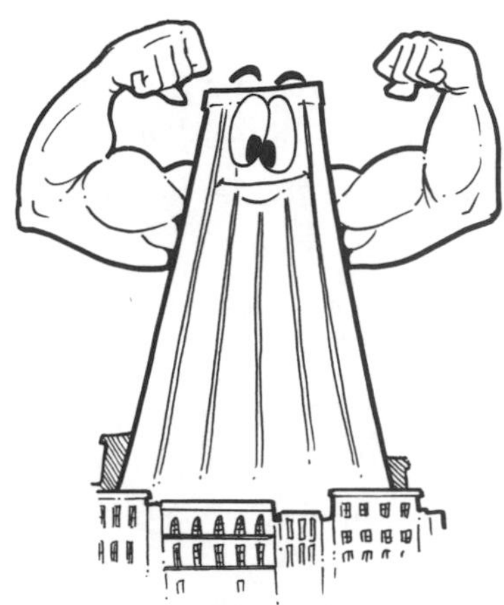

Chapter 8

Hard-Body Tower of Power

In This Chapter

- Learn how to create an amazing upper body
- Discover the big difference small muscles can make
- Your home upper-body exercise encyclopedia

It's time to create the angles and lines that dramatically change the shape of your body. When you learn the transformation tricks, such as increasing the width of your back and medial delts to dramatically decrease the width of your waist, you'll be ready to take your top level to the next level.

In hard-body training, sometimes little things can make a big difference. The added 10 minutes of training time makes this one a "no brainer."

The final volume of your "Hard-Body Exercise Encyclopedia" in this chapter defines each piece of your upper-body puzzle and contains all the right moves to turn you into a Home Hard-Body Houdini.

Top-Level Transformations

If we're only as strong as our weakest link, then the goal is to have no weakest link. A perfect example of unbalanced links is when someone is known as the one with the "great legs" or "great arms." You know that you've reached the pinnacle of home hard bodies when you're known as the one with the "great body."

In my experience, men seem to have better upper halves and women better lower halves. That's because most guys spend the majority of their training time benching and curling, and most women are busy busting a sweat in search of a better butt.

The following keys unlock the door so that you can take your top level to the hard-body max level:

- Training your muscle groups separately (split training) enables you to give each muscle group the amount of training attention at the required intensity level needed to change the shape of your body.
- Further separating similar muscle groups maximizes their development by allowing them to be trained more often (for example, separating chest and delt training, or separating back and biceps training).
- Depending on your goals, using techniques such as super setting and drop setting maximizes your results.
- If a muscle group has several sections, be sure that you include exercises that train the whole group or each section individually, or incorporate exercises that do both in your training session.
- Maintaining perfect form ensures that your body develops in the most desirable and safest way.

The Forgotten Little Muscles

With all the focus on your major hard-body muscles, some smaller but just as important muscles might not get the spotlight they deserve. I'm talking about your external rotators, in particular. These are the muscles that rotate your shoulder when you raise your hand to say hello. The two most important rotators are the *teres minor* and the *infraspinatus*. These muscles help prevent injury by stabilizing your shoulder.

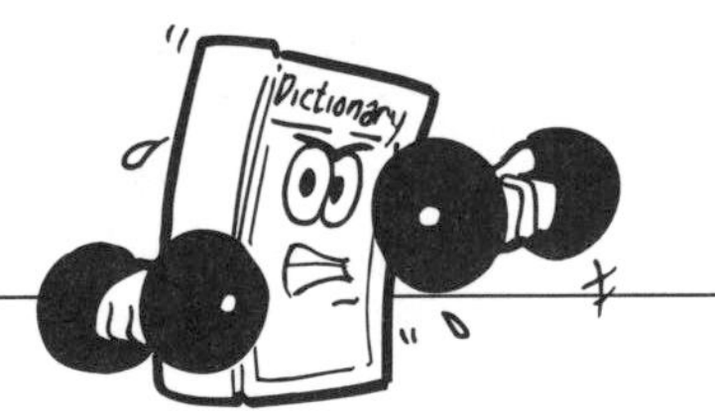

Workout Wisdom

Teres minor and **infraspinatus** are two of the four muscles that make up your rotator cuff. Their primary function is to externally rotate and stabilize the shoulder.

Besides injury prevention, the rotators also affect your posture and muscular physique. If you sit hunched over at a desk for long hours, strong external rotators are your best defense against developing rounded shoulders. Developed rotators also give your back better definition by creating deeper cuts between the muscles.

Rotate Right

The following guidelines maximize your results and ensure that you're rotating correctly:

- Rotate through a full range of motion.
- Do higher reps with lower weight (10–20 reps).

- Stretch your chest and back between sets (internal rotators).
- Use a slower exercise tempo.
- Start with your nondominant side to determine the amount of reps for a set.

Upper-Body Muscle Anatomy

Your pectorals, or "pecs," make up your chest muscles. Your pectorals consist of these components:

- **Pectoralis major** is the larger of the two and is involved in shoulder adduction and internal rotation.
- **Pectoralis minor** lifts the chest when your scapular retractors are stabilized, or tilts it forward and down when they're not. This affects your posture.

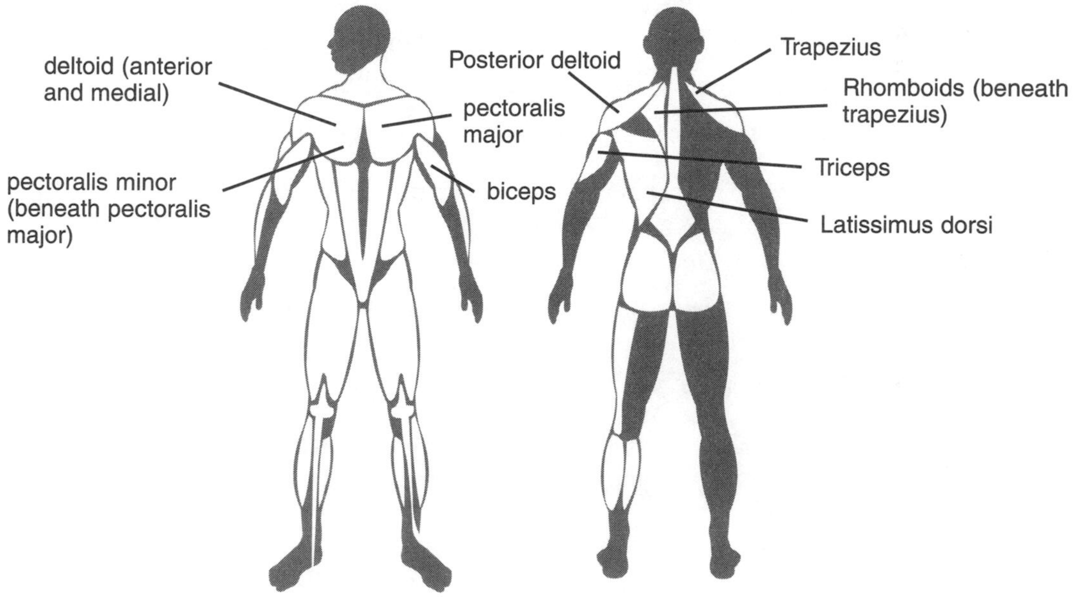

Upper-body muscles—front and back view.

Anytime you push something, throw something, or hug someone, you're using your pecs.

The *serratus anterior* is the muscle that connects the chest and back muscles. When defined visually, you will see diagonal lines on either side of your chest that point toward the center of your waist.

On the flip side you'll find the back muscles. Your back is made up of the following four major muscle groups:

- ***Latissimus dorsi (lats, for short).*** This is the largest back muscle. The lats are what give your body symmetry the V-shape. Anytime you pull something, you're using your lats.
- ***Trapezius (traps for short).*** Located right above your lats, these are used when you shrug your shoulders.
- ***Rhomboids (major and minor).*** Located beneath your middle and upper trapezius and between your spine and shoulder blades, these muscles are used when you try to touch your shoulder blades together.
- ***Erector spinae.*** These are the muscles of your lower back. (See Chapter 7, "Phenomenal Abdominals," for more on these muscles.)

The deltoids, or "delts," are your shoulder muscles. During chest training, your delts are the secondary muscles worked. You use your delts when you push things. The deltoids are divided into the following three sections, or heads:

- ***Anterior deltoid.*** The front part that raises your arm up and forward.
- ***Medial deltoid.*** The side part that raises your arm up from the side.
- ***Posterior deltoid.*** The back part that brings your arm back.

The biceps make up the front part of your upper arm. Their primary function is to bend your arm and pull things. As the name implies, the biceps are divided into two sections:

- ***Biceps brachii.*** The large muscle that's visible when you flex your arm. It flexes the elbow and assists in shoulder abduction.
- ***Brachiallis.*** The prime mover for all positions when your forearm is *pronated.*

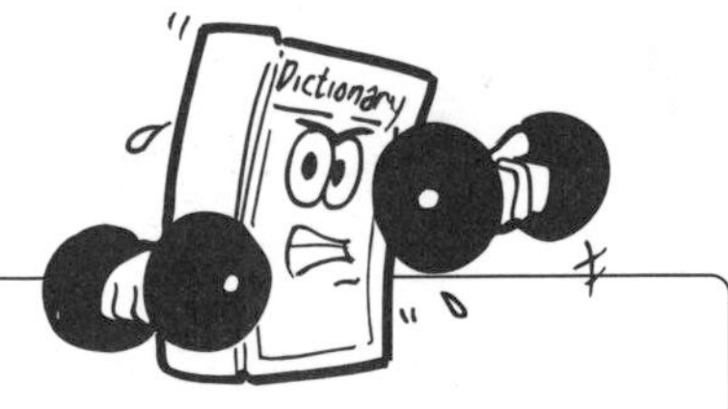

Workout Wisdom

Pronation is the position of the forearm with the palm facing down or back. Pronation is the opposite of supination, in which your palm is facing forward or up.

On the flip side of your arms you'll find the triceps bracchi. The triceps are the secondary muscles used in chest and shoulder training. Their function is to straighten the arm and to push things. The triceps are divided into (you guessed it) three heads:

- Long head
- Medial head
- Lateral head

The muscles of the rotator cuff are located on the scapula and function as stabilizers and movers. These muscles, also known as the SITS muscles, are made up of four muscles:

- ***Supraspinatus.*** Helps abduct and stabilize the head of the humerus in the socket.
- ***Infraspinatus.*** Externally rotates the shoulder.
- ***Teres minor.*** Externally rotates the shoulder.
- ***Subscapularis.*** Internally rotates the shoulder.

Upper-Body Exercise Encyclopedia

The following sections detail some upper-body exercises.

Multiangle Chest Press

This exercise works the pectorals, the anterior deltoids, and the triceps.

1. Start on an incline or a flat bench, with the back of your shoulders touching the bench behind you and with your chest elevated. (Keep your feet on the floor and your butt in the seat throughout the movement.) Arms are extended over your chest, holding dumbbells end to end so that they almost touch in the center.
2. Lower the dumbbells out to the side until you feel a stretch in your chest muscles. Exhale and raise the dumbbells up until your arms are straight, yet unlocked, and the dumbbells almost touch in the center. Contract your chest muscles. Repeat for desired reps.

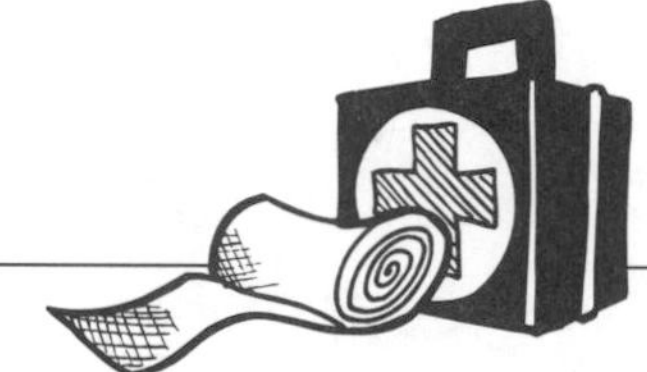

Safety Scoop

Because of the position your muscles are placed in during flyes, lifting too much weight could possibly strain or tear your pectoral muscles.

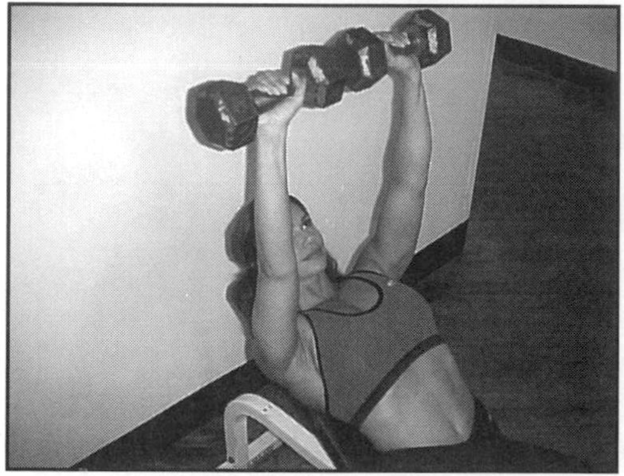

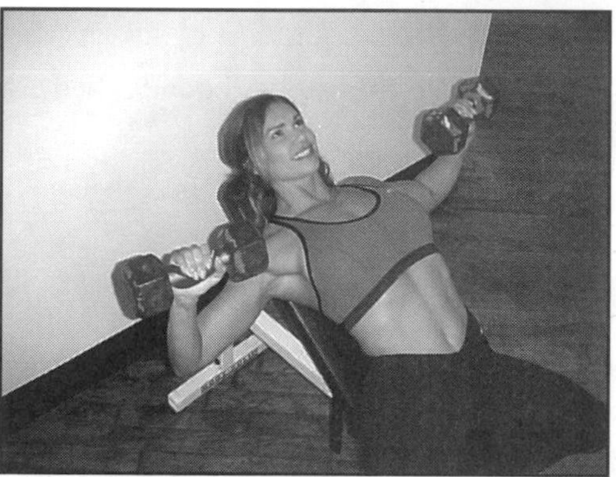

Multiangle Chest Flye

This exercise works the pectorals, the anterior deltoids, and the triceps.

1. Start on a flat or incline bench, with the back of your shoulders touching the bench and your chest elevated. Arms are directly over your chest, with elbows bent and palms facing each other, holding the dumbbells.
2. Extend your arms out to the side until you feel a stretch in your chest muscles. Exhale and bring the weights together, and contract your chest muscles when the weights almost touch. Repeat for desired reps.

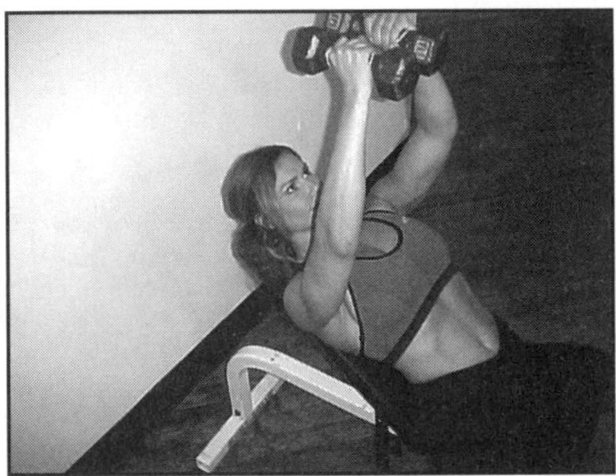

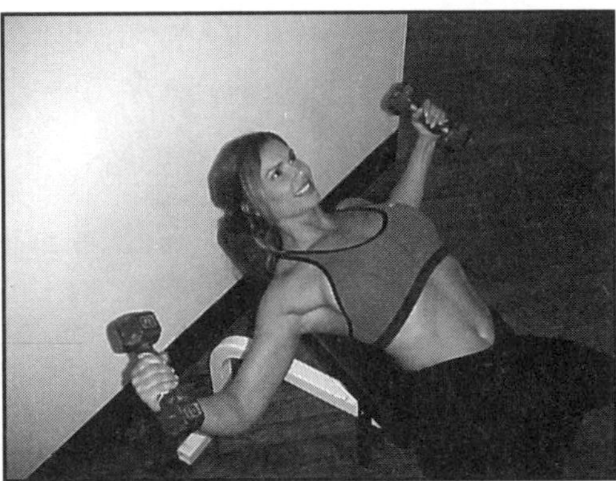

Push-Up Variations

This exercise works the pectorals, the anterior deltoids, and the triceps.

Regular Push-Up

1. Start with your arms shoulder-width apart, your abs tight, and your body in line from shoulders to ankles (or knees, if doing knee push-ups).
2. Lower your upper body by bending your elbows. Exhale and press up. Repeat for desired reps.

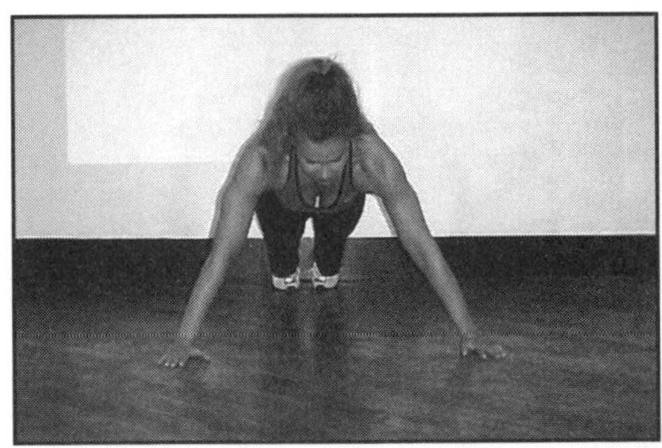

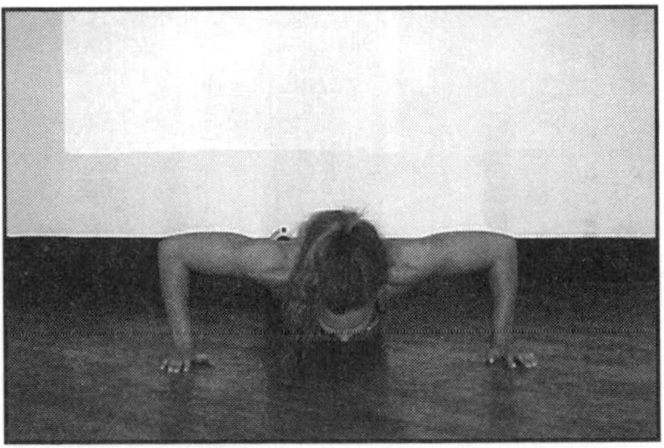

One-Arm Push-Up (Assist)

1. I developed this push-up to get you ready to do one-arm push-ups. Start with your feet in a wide V stance (bottom of a triangle). Place your left hand directly overhead at 12 o'clock. Place right hand at 3 o'clock.
2. With your body in a straight line and parallel to the floor, lower your body until your chest almost touches the floor. Press up and repeat for desired reps. (Keep the abs and the lower back strong during the entire movement.)
3. As your strength increases, you will be able to raise the 3 o'clock hand on its fingertips. Before you know it, you will be able to place that arm behind your back and lower yourself with one arm.

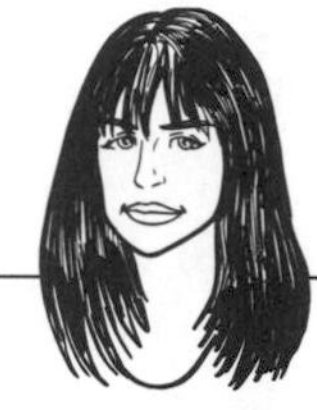

Jourdan's Gems

The secret to doing one-arm push-ups is even weight distribution between all points while keeping your body tight and parallel to the floor.

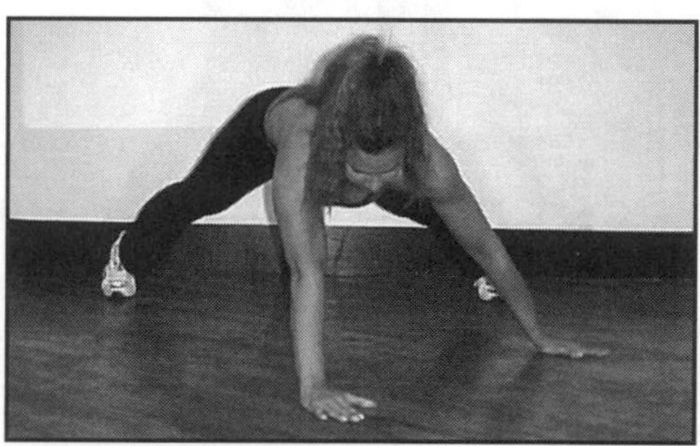

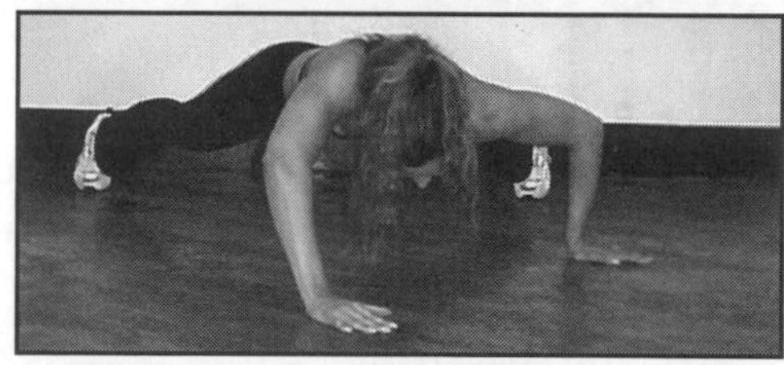

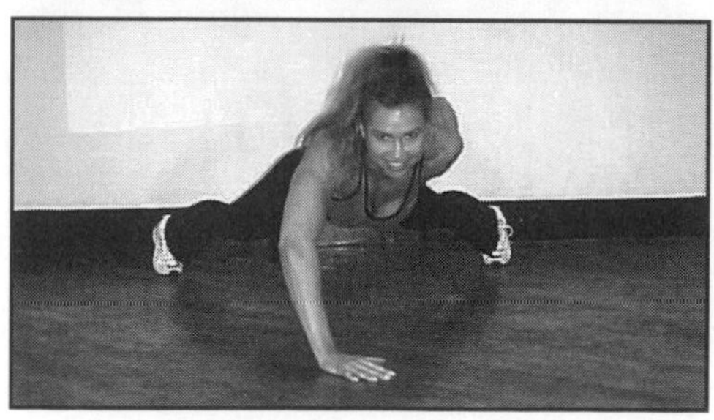

Forward/Reverse Flye

This exercise works the pectorals, the anterior and posterior deltoids, the triceps, and the upper back.

1. Stand with your back straight, your shoulders back and your chest elevated, and your arms bent at shoulder height holding dumbbells. Imagine hugging a big tree and bring your arms forward in a semicircular motion. Contract your chest muscles when the dumbbells meet in front.
2. Now open your arms wide and push back, in line with your shoulders; contract the rear deltoid and back muscles. Repeat for desired reps.

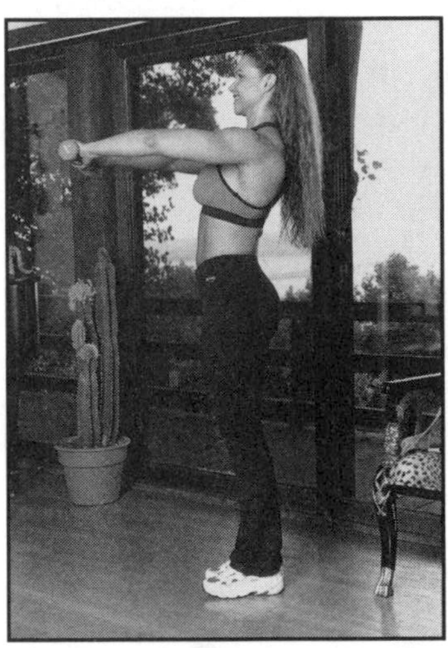

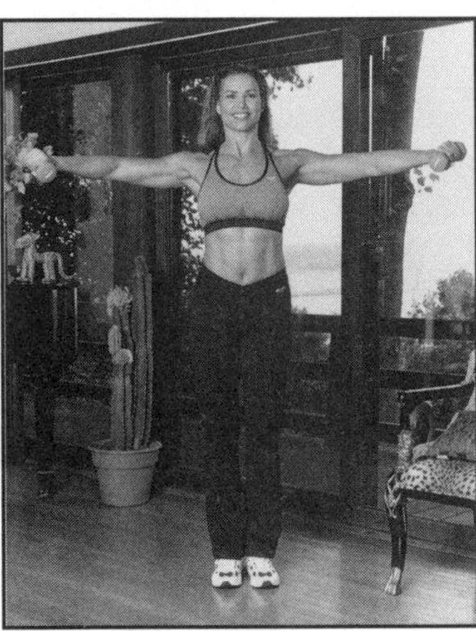

Bent-Over Row Super Set

This exercise works the upper back.

1. Start by standing with your feet hip-width apart and your back flat, and bend at the waist until you're almost parallel with the floor, with your arms hanging in front of you holding dumbbells.
2. Exhale and bring your arms back, leading with the elbows, and contract your back at top position. Lower slowly for a count of three seconds, and repeat for desired reps.

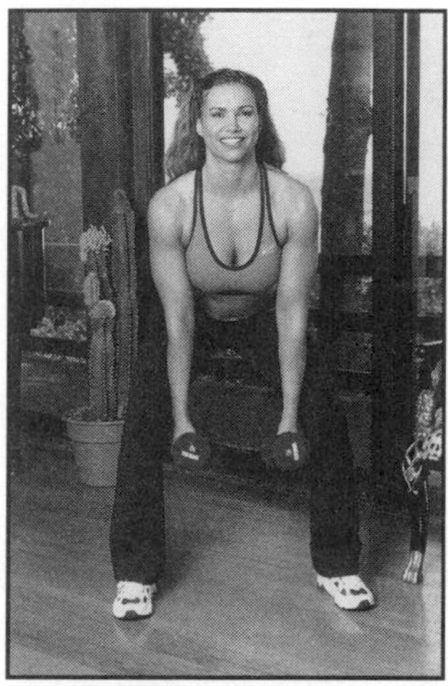
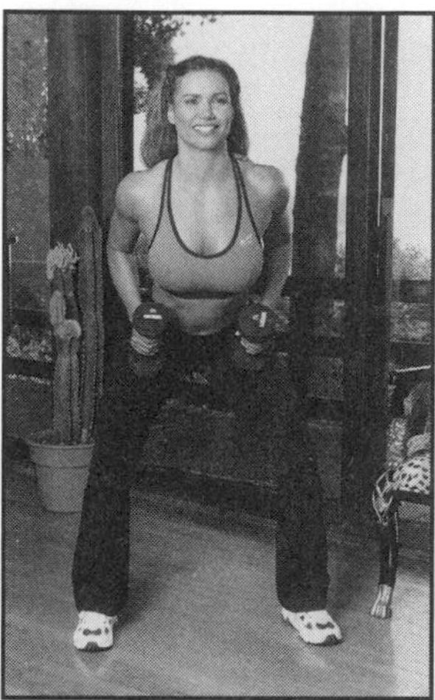

3. Now bring your feet together and turn the dumbbells so that your palms are facing up.
4. Bring the dumbbells back to waist level, and lower slowly. Repeat for desired reps. (Dumbbells should be an inch off your thighs all the way up and down during movement.)

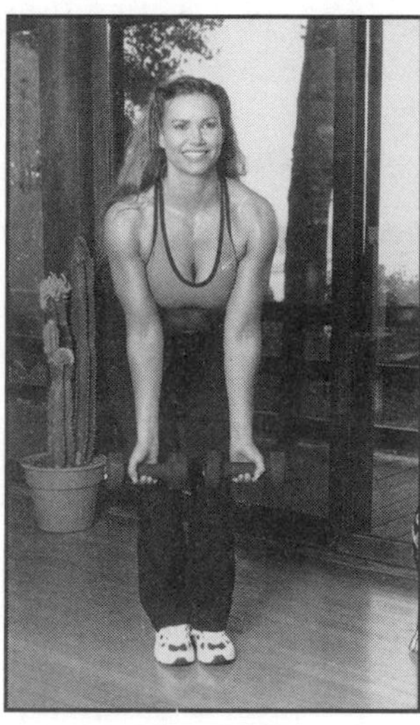
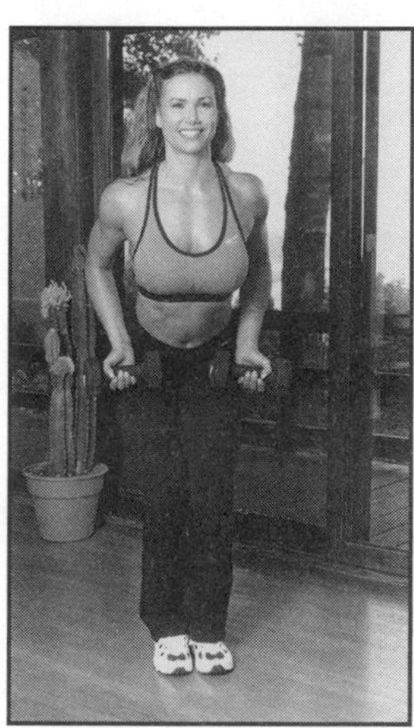

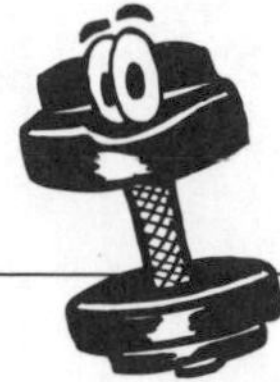

Hard-Body Headliners

Because you can't see your back while you're training, it's very easy to think that your back is doing the work when your arms actually are taking over. To prevent this, make sure that you feel your back contract on each rep. The rule of thumb is that if you feel it more in your arms, the weight is too heavy for your back to do alone.

Pull-Down Super Set

This exercise works the upper back and the biceps.

1. Start by sitting directly under the pull-down bar with your arms in a wide grip. The pull-down bar attachment is available for some weight benches and is a standard component of multi-station home gym systems.
2. Arch your upper back slightly, contract your back, and pull the bar to your upper chest. Try to touch your shoulder blades behind you while you lift your chest to meet the bar. This contracts the back muscles. Release slowly for a count of three seconds, and then repeat for desired reps.
3. Now grip the bar from underneath with your hands shoulder-width apart. Arch back, and pull the bar to your chest, as in step 2. Release slowly, and repeat for desired reps.
4. This combination can also be done using a pull-up bar (not shown). The difference is that now you're pulling yourself up to the bar. If you cannot lift your body weight, use a chair and lift yourself up to the bar. Hold this position as long as you can, and then lower as slowly as possible. Another way to build your strength level is to have a friend hold your feet so that you can press into his or her hands to assist your lift.

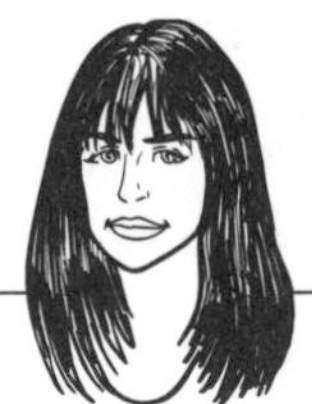

Jourdan's Gems

If your primary fitness goal is to build muscle size, do the exercises that are part of a superset separately with heavier weight for fewer reps.

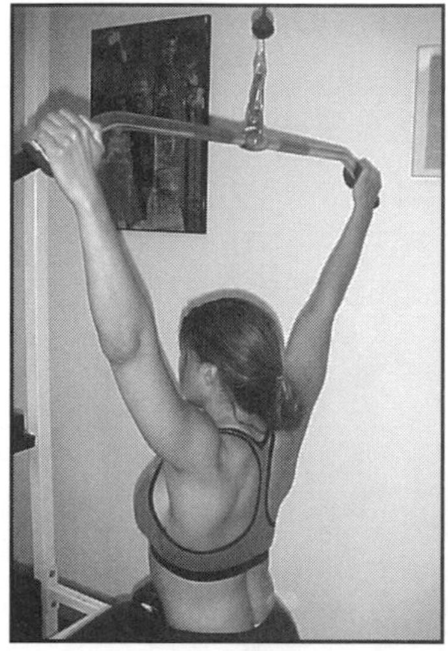

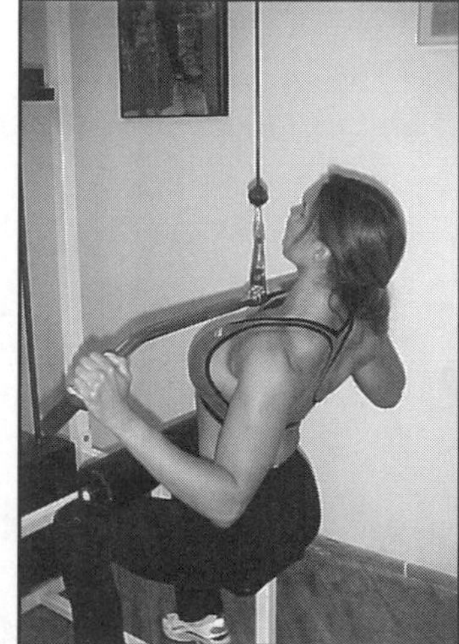

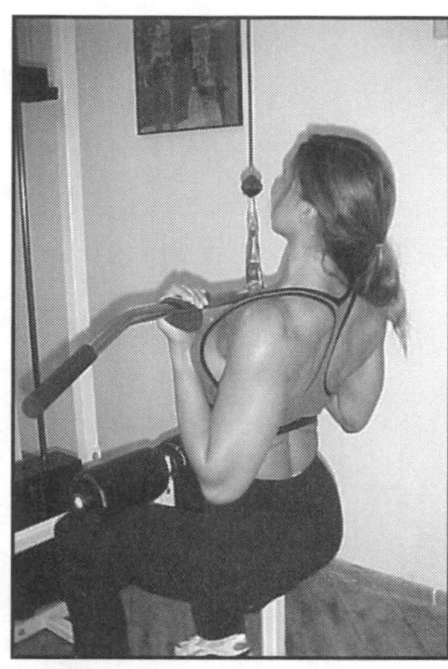

Delt Press Super Set

This exercise works the anterior and medial deltoids, as well as the triceps.

1. Start with your upper arms straight out to the side and your forearms making a 90° angle at the elbow (field goal position).
2. Exhale and raise the dumbbells until your arms are straight, outside your ears, and the dumbbells are almost touching in the center. Lift your shoulders to contract the muscles. Lower slowly for a count of three, and repeat for desired reps.

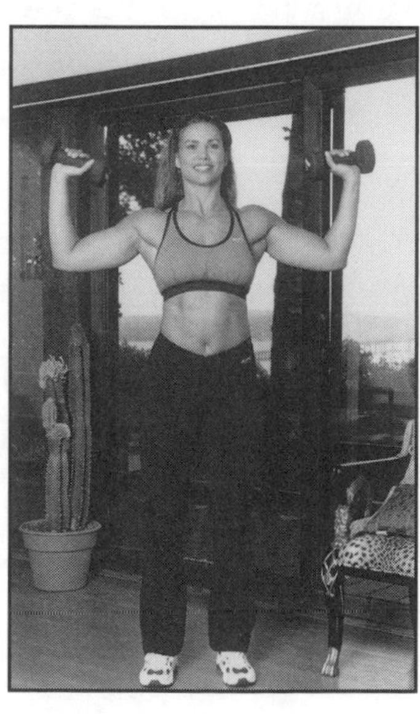

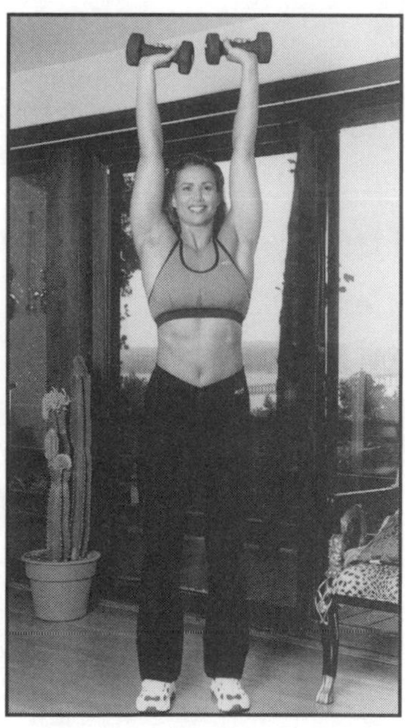

3. Now bring your arms in front of you.
4. Exhale and press the dumbbells up while turning your palms to face the front until your arms are straight yet unlocked. Lower slowly, and repeat for desired reps.

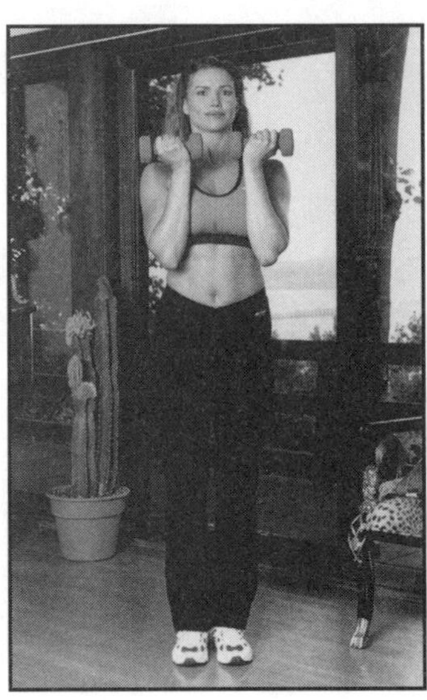

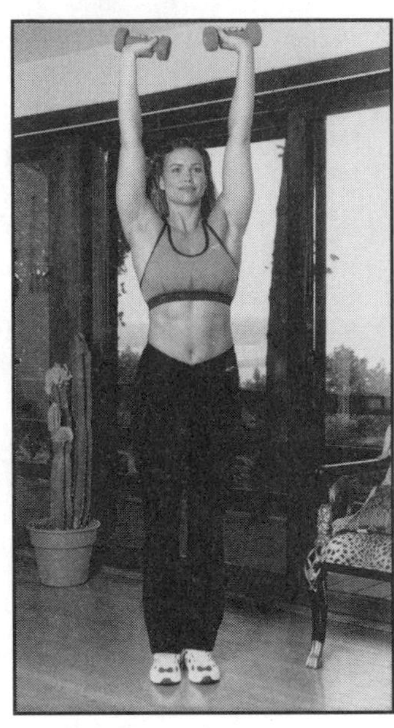

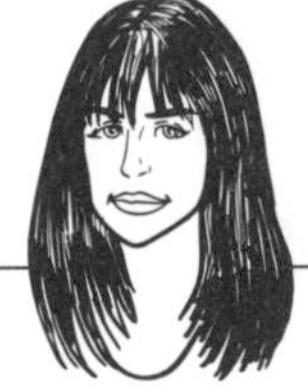

Jourdan's Gems

Drop setting lateral raises is my secret to building amazing medial deltoids. Having width and definition in your medial delts will be the crowning finish to your new lat shape.

Drop Set Lateral Raise

This exercise works the medial deltoids and the triceps.

1. Stand with your feet hip-width apart and your knees slightly bent to lower your center of gravity. Your back should be straight, your shoulders should be back, and your hands should be in front, holding dumbbells.
2. Raise the dumbbells out to the side to shoulder height on a count of one second. The shoulder, elbow, and wrist should all be in line.
3. At the top position, slightly tip the dumbbells down, as if you're pouring two pitchers of water. Lower slowly for a count of three seconds, and repeat for as many reps as possible (AMRAP) while maintaining perfect form.

4. When you can't lift it for another rep, immediately drop to a lighter weight and do AMRAP with that weight. Depending on your strength level, you can drop up to three times. Leave a few pounds difference between each drop (for example, 10 pounds, 5 pounds, 3 pounds).

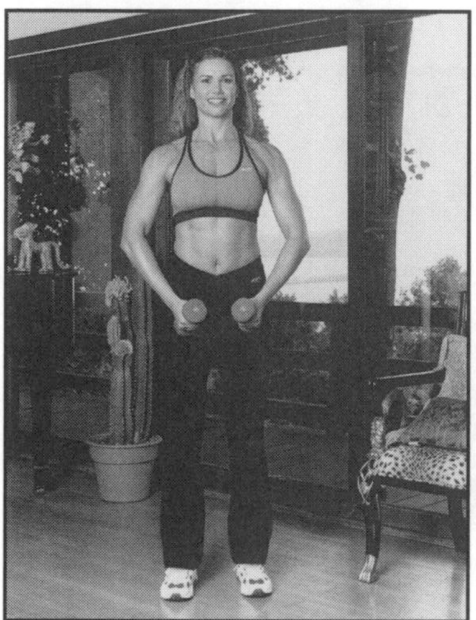

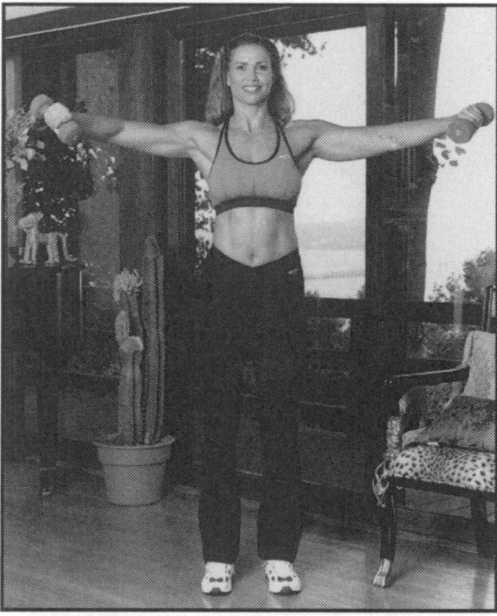

J Curl

This exercise works the biceps and the forearms.

1. Start by standing with your back straight, your shoulders back, and your arms by your sides, palms up.
2. Curl the dumbbells up to shoulder level.

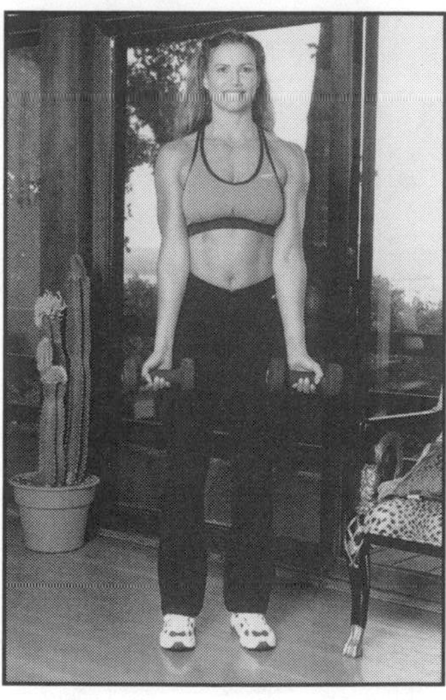

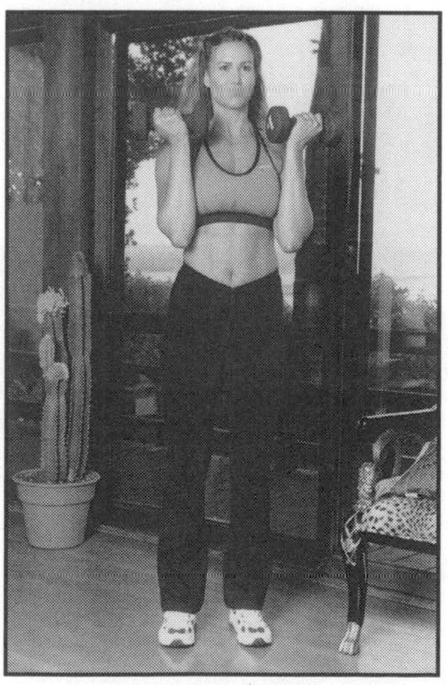

3. Turn the dumbbells so that your palms are facing down, and lower slowly for a count of three.
4. Now turn the dumbbells so that your palms are facing each other, and curl the dumbbells up to shoulder level and back down for a count of one second. Repeat for desired reps.

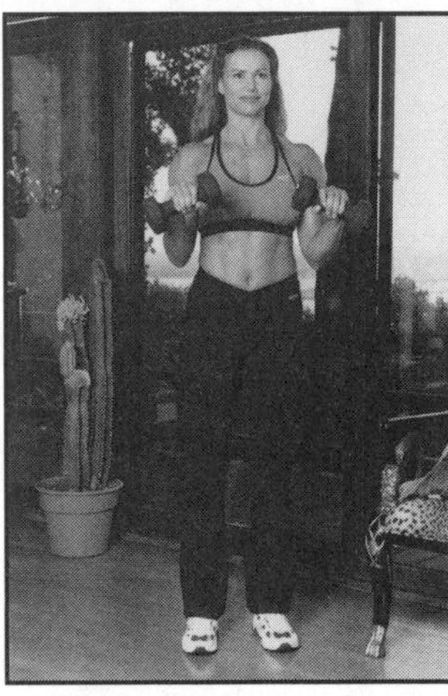
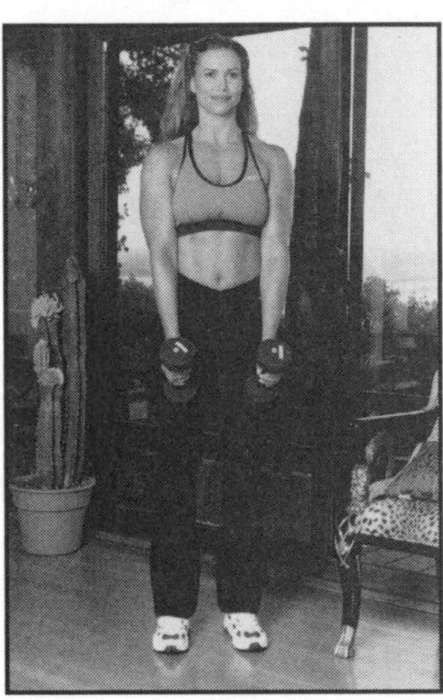

Side Curls

These work the biceps.

1. Stand with your back straight, your shoulders back, and your arms angled out to the side, with your elbows glued to your sides.
2. Curl the weight up to shoulder level, and contract your biceps. Lower slowly, and repeat for desired reps.

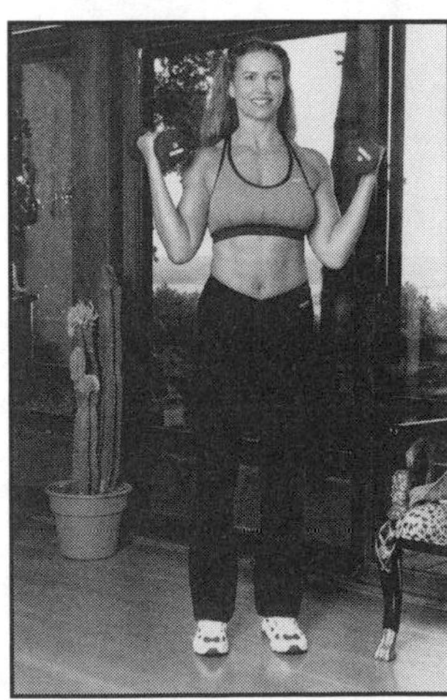
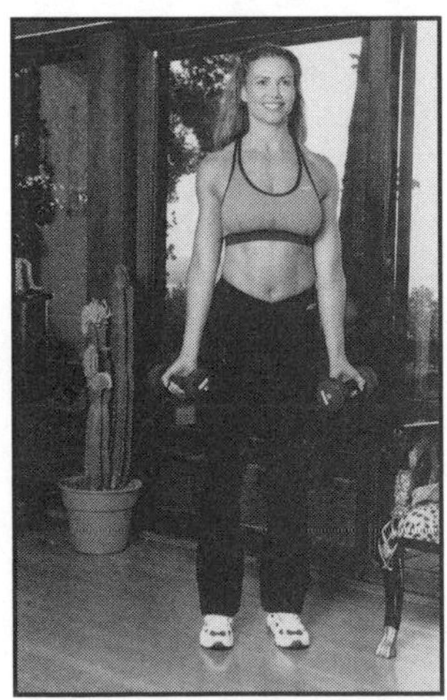

Forward Curls

This exercise works the biceps.

1. Start with your back straight, your shoulders back, and your chest forward, while holding dumbbells or a straight bar with your palms facing forward.
2. Exhale and curl the weight up to shoulder level, and contract your biceps. Lower slowly, and repeat for desired reps.

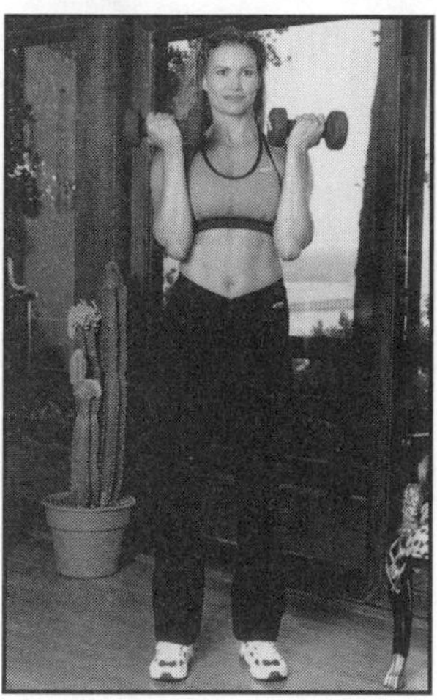

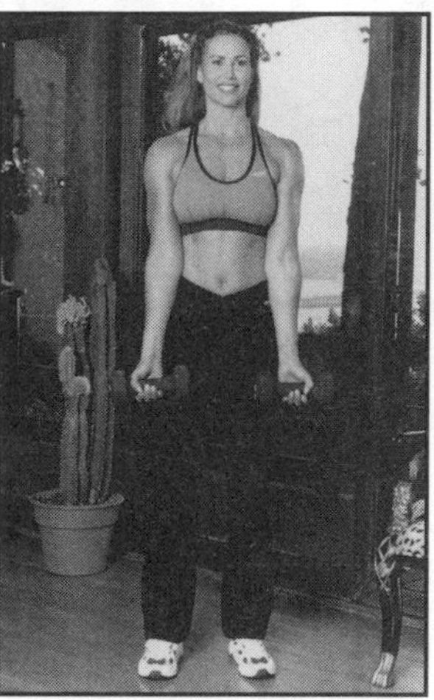

21's

This works the biceps.

1. Stand with your back straight, your shoulders back, your chest forward, and your hands holding a straight bar outside your hips.
2. Curl the bar halfway up to chest level, contract the biceps, and lower down. Repeat seven times.
3. Now curl the bar all the way up to shoulder level seven times. Finally, curl the bar halfway down from shoulder level to chest level seven times, completing a total of 21 reps.

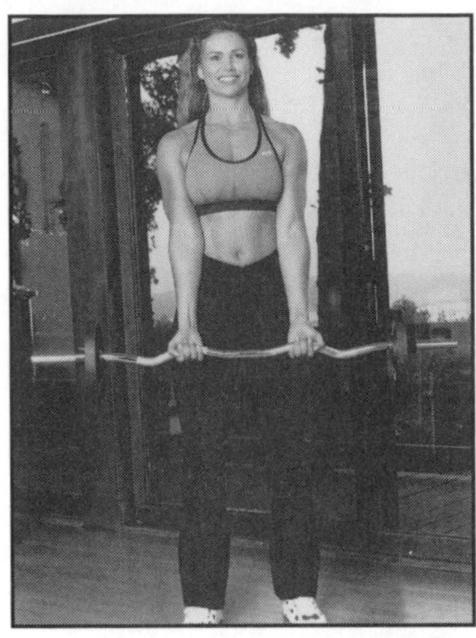

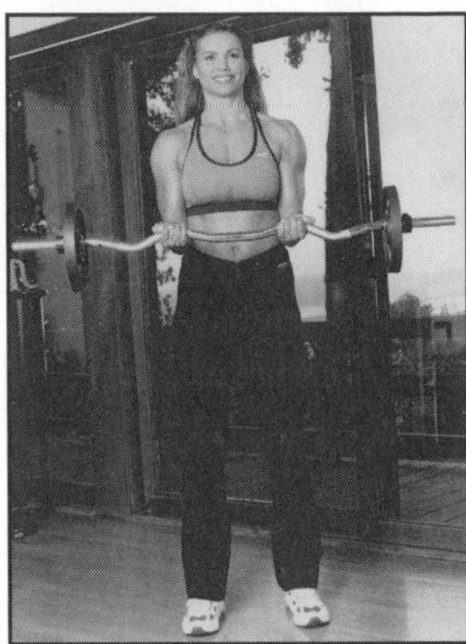

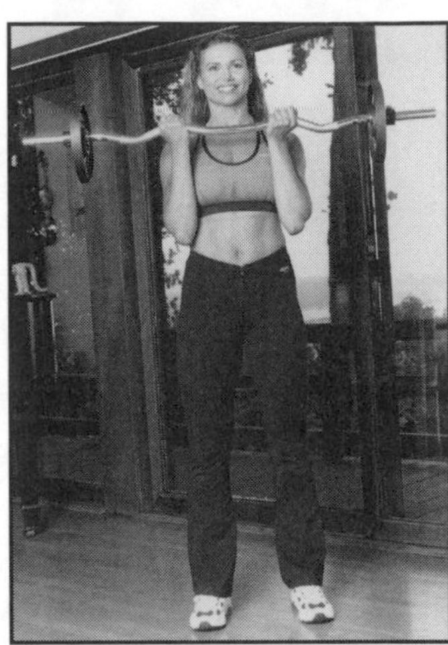

Dips

These work all three heads of the triceps.

1. Place your hands on either side of your hips, fingers forward, gripping the edge of the bench. Your feet should be straight with your heels on the floor or balanced one on top of the other.
2. While keeping your rear close to the bench the entire time, bend your elbows and lower until your upper arms are parallel to the floor.
3. Exhale and press up until your arms are straight. Contract your triceps. Repeat for desired reps.

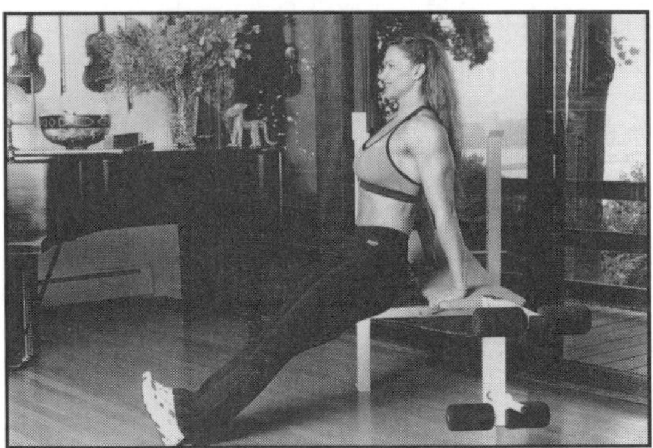

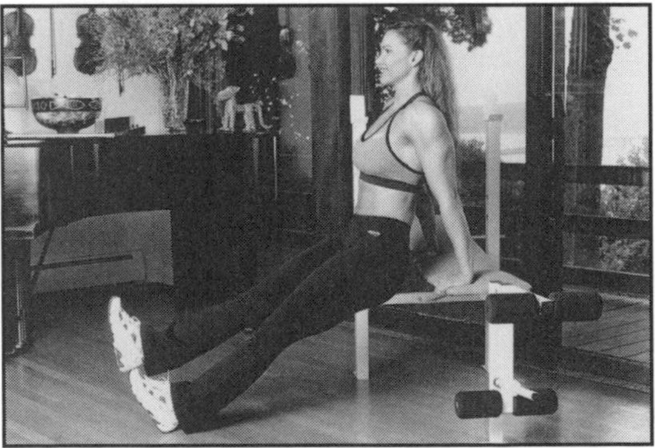

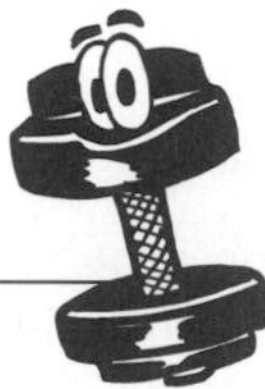

Hard-Body Headliners

Developed triceps make a big difference in total arm shape because they make up three quarters of your upper arm. Doing exercises for the long head of your triceps will help you avoid having an arm that swings in the wind when you wave.

Overhead Press

This exercise works the long head of the triceps.

1. Standing with your back straight and your feet hip-width apart, lift two dumbbells overhead. Lower the dumbbells behind your head, keeping the elbows close to your head.
2. Now lift the dumbbells overhead until your arms are straight yet unlocked. Contract your triceps, and then lower slowly. Repeat for desired reps.

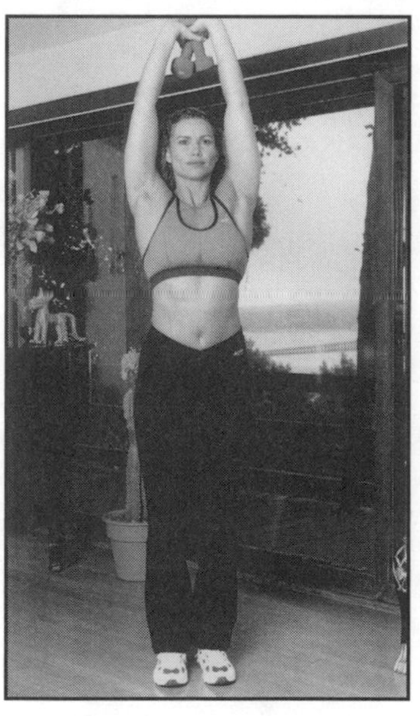

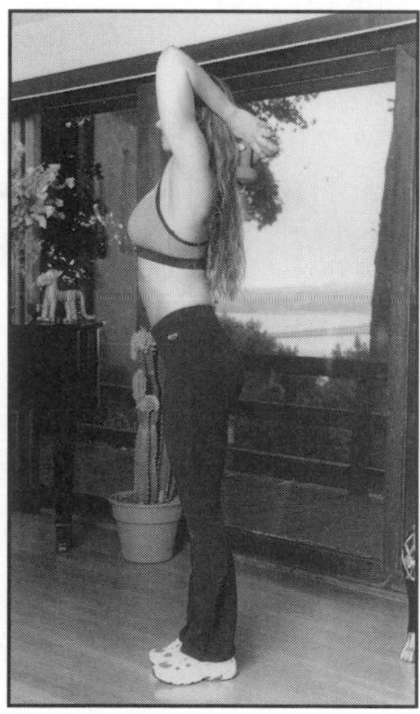

Kickback Variation

This exercise works the triceps, with a focus on the lateral head.

1. With a slight bend in the knees, bend forward from the waist with a flat back. Hold the dumbbells close to your sides.
2. Extend your arms to the rear, turning them midlift so that your palms face up at the top. Contract your triceps, and then lower slowly. Repeat for desired reps.

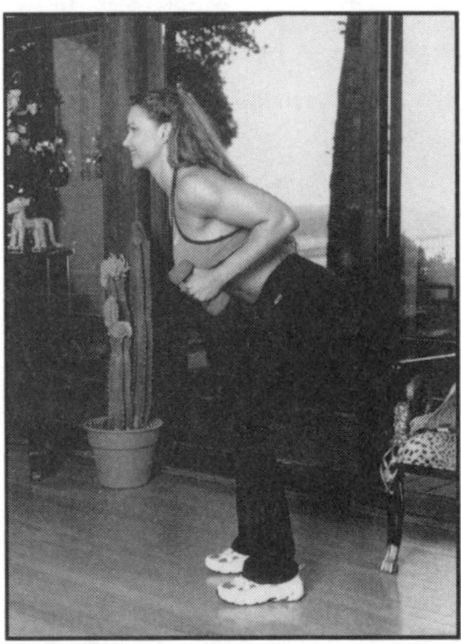

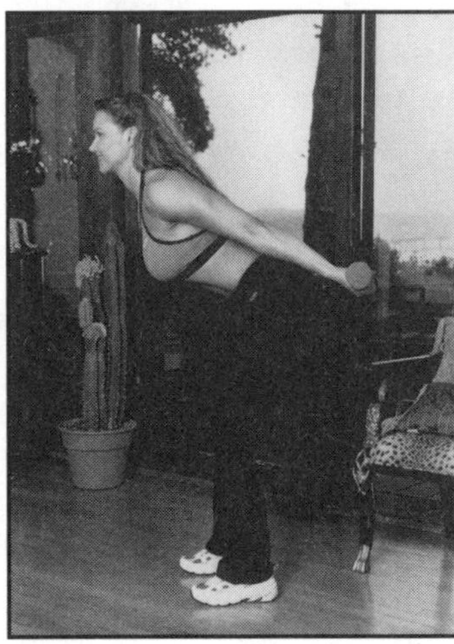

Pullover Press

This exercise works the triceps, the serratus anterior, and the lower lats.

1. Using a straight or E-Z bar (a bar that is bent in two places) with weight plates, lie on a flat bench with the bar just below chest level and your arms close to your sides.
2. Inhale and bring the bar over your head until you feel a good stretch. Exhale and return to the starting position.
3. Then extend your arms fully and contract the triceps. Lower to the starting position, and repeat for desired reps. (To really isolate your triceps, keep your elbows close to your sides at all times.)

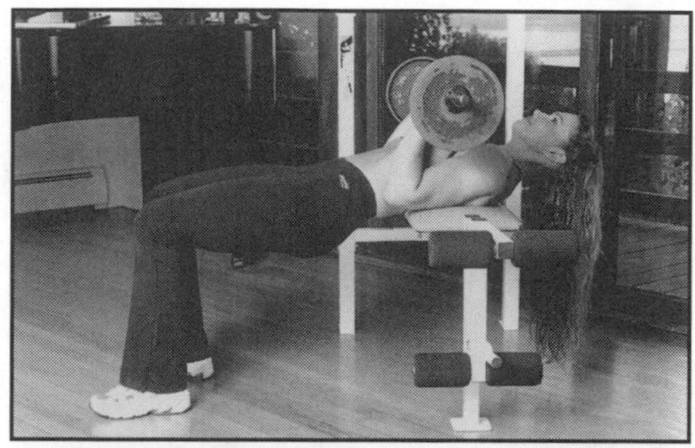

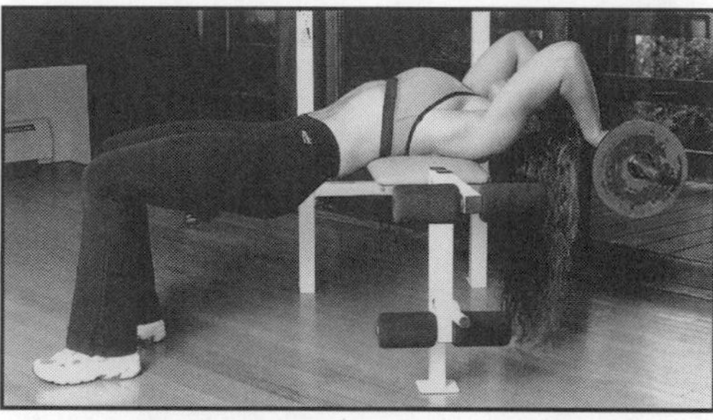

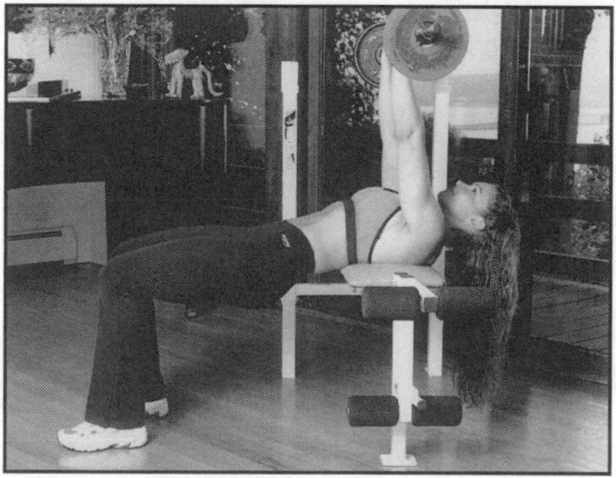

Dumbbell Pullover

This works the pectorals, anterior delts, triceps, serratus anterior, and lower lats.

1. Start by lying on a bench, with the back of your shoulders touching the bench and your chest elevated, holding a dumbbell hand over hand at chest level.
2. Inhale and lower the dumbbell overhead until you feel a stretch.
3. Exhale and bring the dumbbell back to the starting position. Elevate your chest and contract your lats when the dumbbell is over your chest. Repeat for desired reps.

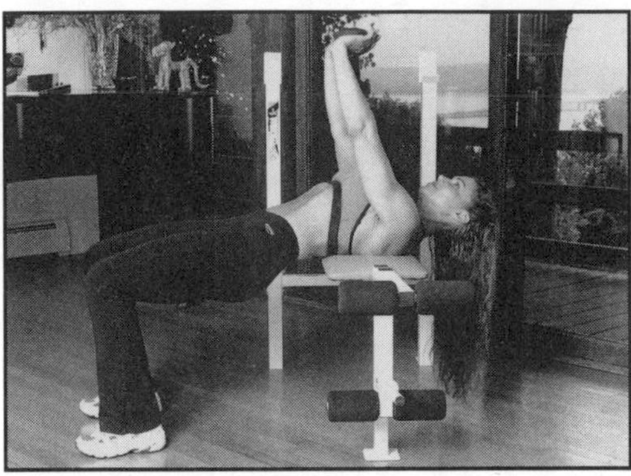

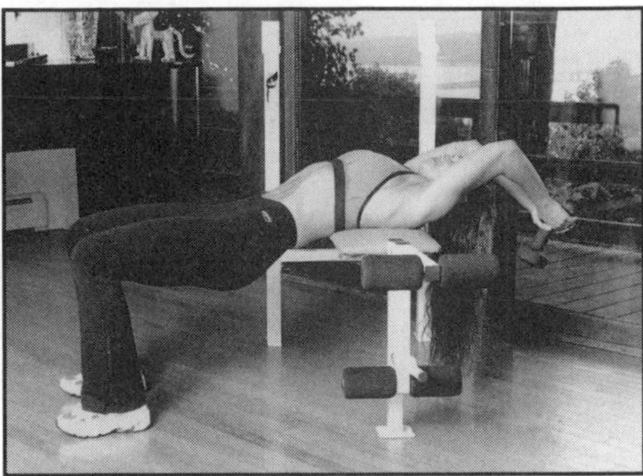

External Rotator Lift

This exercise works the external rotators.

1. Stand with your back straight and your feet hip-width apart, holding the dumbbells at shoulder height. Your elbows should be bent at a 90° angle, in line with your shoulders.
2. Slowly turn your arms upward until your hands are pointed straight up.
3. Lower to the starting position, and repeat for desired reps.

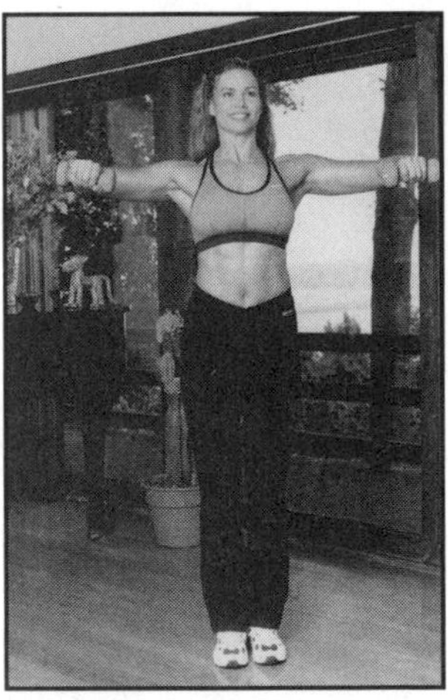

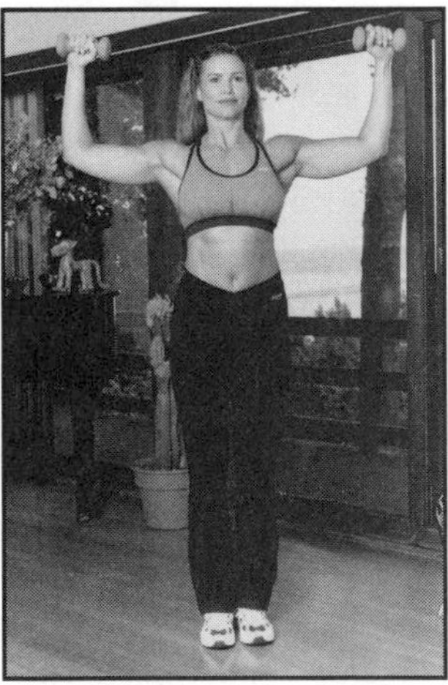

Rotator Press

This exercise works the external rotators.

1. Start by standing, holding a bar with a grip that is wider than shoulder width.
2. Lift the bar straight up, with arms straight, until it reaches chest height. Pause for one second.

3. Finally, raise the bar overhead. Reverse the steps back to the starting position, and repeat for desired reps.

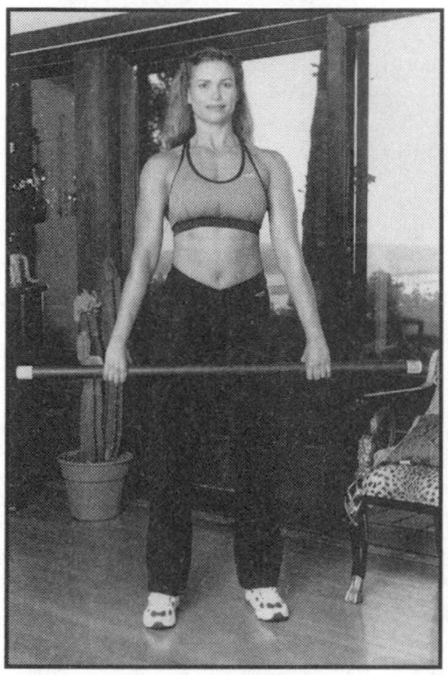
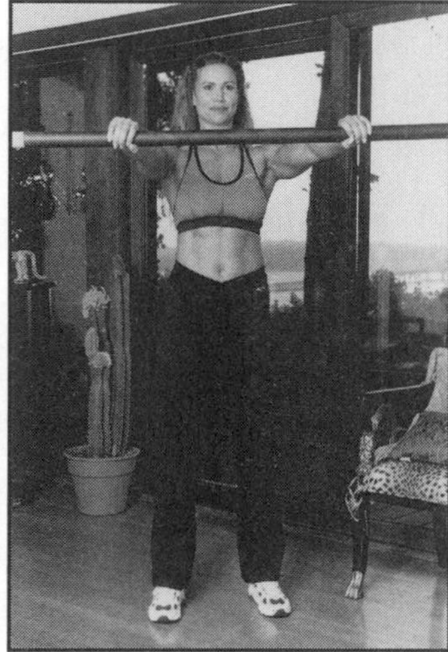
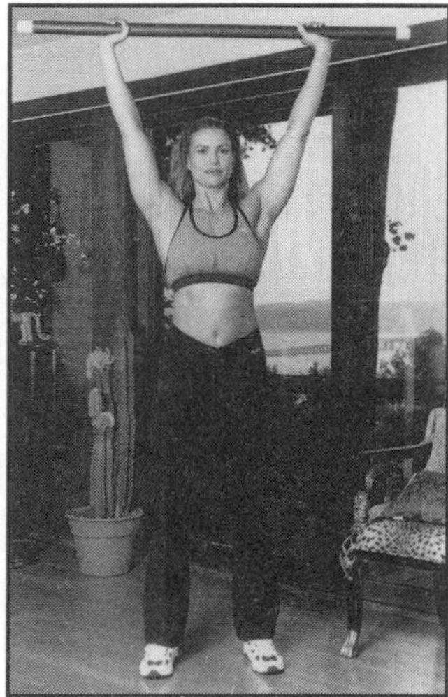

Rotator Abduction

This exercise works the external rotators.

1. Start by standing with your back straight, with an arm close to your body holding a dumbbell in front.
2. Rotate the working arm outward by pivoting only at the shoulder joint.
3. Return to the starting position, and repeat for desired reps. Switch sides, and repeat with your other arm.

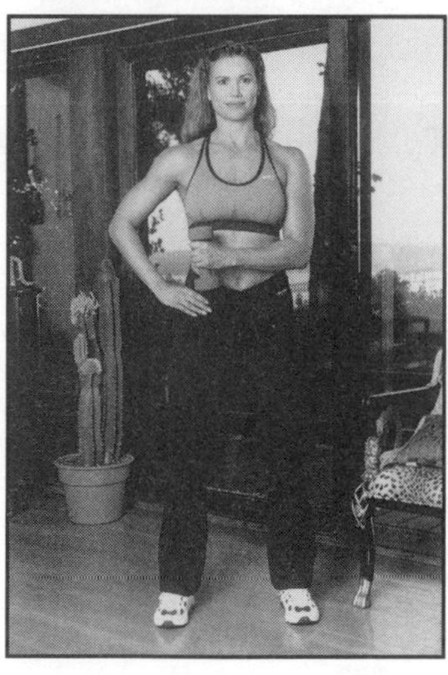
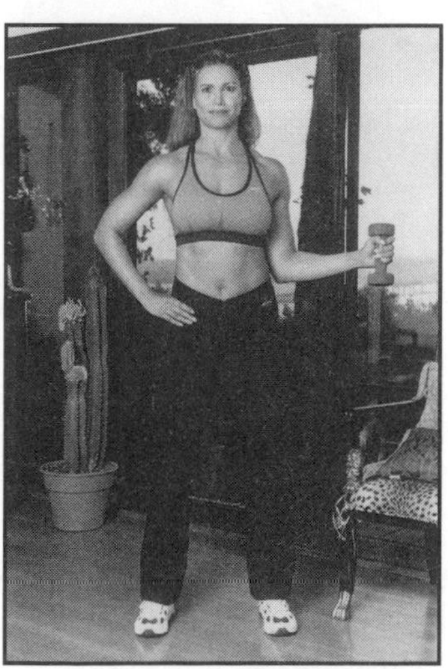

By following the transformation training keys, adding rotator training to your program, and utilizing your upper-body exercise encyclopedia, you can create the major changes in your upper body that'll give you hard-body, show-stopping symmetry.

The Least You Need to Know

- Separating primary and secondary muscle training increases results because muscles can be trained more often.
- Increasing the width of your lats makes your waist look smaller because the increase gives your upper body a V shape.
- Training your external rotators will positively affect your posture and back development.
- Because you can't see it, you must consciously feel your back contract during exercises. If you feel it more in your arms, lower the weight.

Chapter 9

Custom Home Hard Bodies

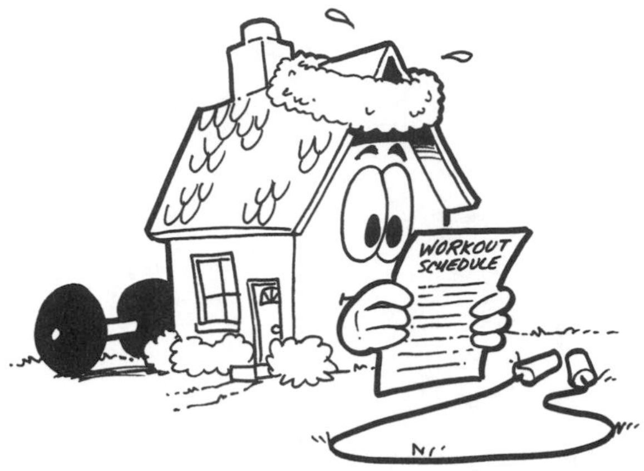

In This Chapter

- Beginning with the full body
- Hitting both highs and lows
- Making splits easy
- Laying out a daily half-hour plan

Even the best tools can't turn your shed into a mansion if all you know is shed building. You'll build a nice shed, but it is still a shed nonetheless. I know that you didn't come this far to wind up with a hard-body shed, nice or not, so I've brought out the hard-body heavy-hitters. These programs have successfully turned many a shed into a hard-body homestead.

To prevent any slowing down or strikes on your hard-body construction site, you need to vary your exercises and their order. Keeping your exercise encyclopedia handy will make it simple to have an endless supply of hard-body workouts at your fingertips.

Beginner Hard-Body Program

If you're just starting out, you first need to master the hard-body exercise form. Doing a full-body workout three times a week with one *compound movement* for each body part gives your body the opportunity to maximize its potential without overtraining. Start each day with a five-minute warm-up (see Chapter 5, "Warming Up!") and work up to three sets for each exercise. This program should be done a minimum of two to four weeks. After that, you should be able to advance to a three-day upper/lower training split.

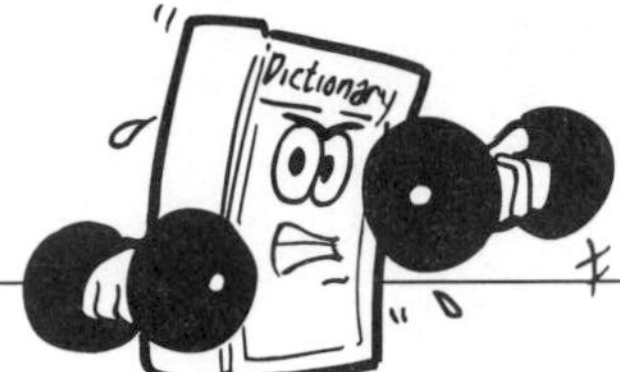

Workout Wisdom

A **compound movement** is an exercise that involves the movement of more than one joint at a time. Benefits of compound movements include working more than one muscle group at a time and burning more calories.

Beginner Hard-Body Program

Exercise	Sets	Reps
Day 1		
Free bar squats	2–3	10
Stiff-legged dead lifts	2–3	10
Chest press	2–3	10
Bent-over row	2–3	10
Calf raises	2–3	15
6-minute six-pack routine	2–3	15
Fit Ball Hypers	2– 3	10
Day 2		
Walking lunges	2–3 laps	
Step-ups	2–3	12–15
Push-ups	2–3	AMRAP
Flat dumbbell chest flye	2–3	15
Pull-downs	2–3	10–12
Calf raises	2–3	15
Lower back lifts	2	10
Weighted oblique reach sequence	2	10 each
Day 3		
Side squats	2–3	10
Flat dumbbell press	2–3	10

Exercise	Sets	Reps
Bent-over row super set	2–3	10
Dumbbell pullover	2–3	10
Calf raises	2–3	15
Fit ball crunches	2–3	10–15
Fit ball extension	2–3	10–15

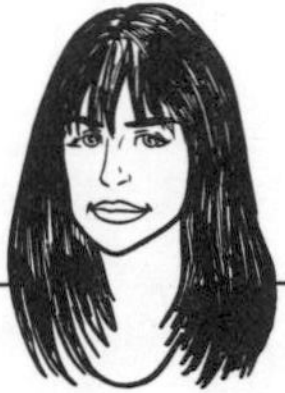

Jourdan's Gems

Training your abs and lower back (core muscles) together is an easy way to maintain even muscle balance and prevent posture and lower back problems. When you strengthen your core muscles you strengthen all the muscles in your body.

Four-Week Intermediate Hard-Body Program

The upper/lower training split divides your workouts into alternating upper- and lower-body workouts that are done three times a week (Week 1: upper/lower/upper; Week 2: lower/upper/lower). This is done so that you can expand your training to include *isolation exercises*. Trying to include all these exercises would make a full-body workout too long, and you wouldn't be able to maintain the same intensity for the smaller muscles.

This program can be done for four to eight weeks. Don't forget your five-minute warm-up each day. Switch to a four-day training split the last two weeks of your training cycle to get your body ready for the next level (Monday: upper; Tuesday: lower; Wednesday: off; Thursday: upper; Friday: lower).

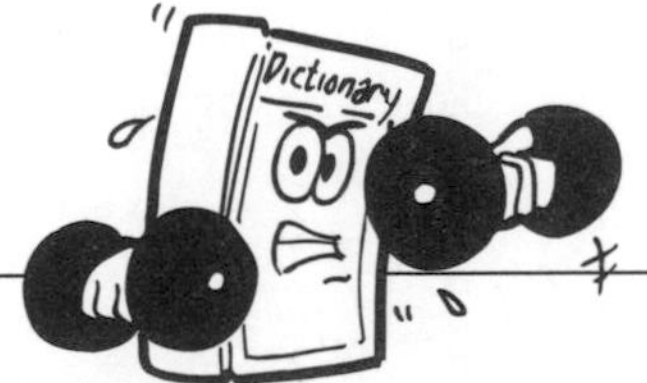

Workout Wisdom

Isolation exercises use only one joint; therefore, they focus on one muscle. These exercises are used to strengthen and add defined shape to individual muscles (for example, biceps curls). To create your best overall body symmetry, you need to add isolation exercises to your program.

Four-Week Intermediate Hard-Body Program

Exercise	Sets	Reps
Weeks 1 and 3: Day 1—Lower Body		
Single leg squats	3	10
Free bar squats	3	10
Walking lunges	3 laps	
Stiff-legged dead lifts	4	10
Hamstring lean	3	10
Calf raises	3	15
6-minute six-pack routine	3	15
Fit Ball Extensions	3	15
Day 2—Upper Body		
Incline dumbbell chest press	3	10–12
Flat dumbbell chest flye	3	15
Pull-downs	3	10–12
Bent-over row	3	10–12
Drop set lateral raise	3	AMRAP
Forward/reverse flyes	3	10
Curls (straight bar or dumbbell)	3	10
Overhead press	3	10
Kick backs	3	10
Fit ball hypers	3	10
Weighted oblique reach sequence	3	10 each
Day 3—Lower Body		
Leg curls	4	10
Stiff-legged dead lifts/step-ups	4/4	10/10
Side squats	3	15
Leg extensions	3	10
Calf raises	3	15
6-minute six-pack routine	3	15
Lower back lifts	3	10
Weeks 2 and 4: Day 1—Upper Body		
Incline dumbbell chest press	3	10–12
Flat dumbbell chest flye	3	15
Pull-downs	3	10–12
Bent-over row	3	10–12
Drop set lateral raise	3	AMRAP
J-curl	3	10
Pullover press	3	10

Exercise	Sets	Reps
Fit ball crunches	3	10
Fit ball hypers	3	10
Day 2—Lower Body		
Free bar squats (wide stance)	3	10
Walking lunges	3 laps	
Stiff-legged dead lifts/step-ups	4/4	10/10
Hamstring lean	3	10
Calf raises	3	15
6-minute six-pack routine	3	15
Lower-back lifts	3	15
External rotator lift	3	15
Day 3—Upper Body		
Flat dumbbell chest flye/press super set	3/3	10/10
Dumbbell pullover	3	10
Pull-down super set	3/3	10/10
Side curls	3	10
Tricep dips	3	10
Fit ball extensions	3	10
Weighted oblique reach sequence	3	10 each

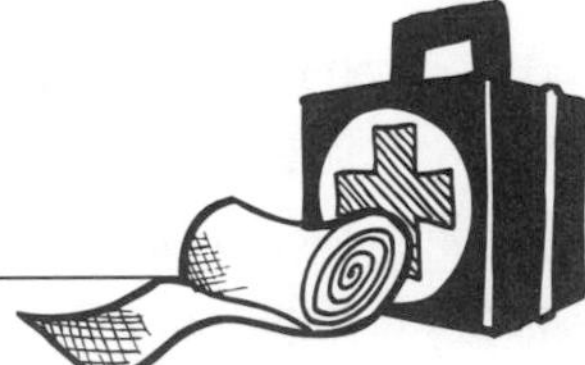

Safety Scoop

After the five-minute warm-up, do at least two light sets of the first exercise to further warm up your muscles before attempting your working weight. Doing this will warm up the specific muscles that are being worked so they will perform better. This will also help prevent injury from lifting too much too fast.

Four-Day Advanced Hard-Body Split Program

The four-day split divides your workouts by muscle group. The following is my favorite training split. Don't forget your five-minute warm-up each day.

Four-Day Advanced Hard-Body Split Program

Muscle Group	Exercise	Sets	Reps
Monday			
(Session 1) Legs	Free bar squats	4	10
	Walking lunges	3	laps
	Stiff-legged dead lifts	4	10
	leg extensions	3	10
	Calf raises	3	15
Abs/lower back	Weighted oblique reach	3	15
	Lower-backlifts	3	15
(Session 2—optional)	60 minutes kickboxing training		
Tuesday			
Chest/biceps	Incline press	4	10
	Flat flyes/press	3/3	15/10
	Pull-over	3	10
	Forward/reverse flye	3	10
	Straight bar curls	4	10
	Jourdan curls	3	10
Wednesday			
Abs/lower back	Lift and twist	3	10
	Fit ball crunches	3	10
	Fit ball hypers	3	10
	(Do 45–60 minutes cardio)		
Thursday			
Back/light legs	(Dead lift every two weeks)		
	Pull-down (pull-up) Super set	4	10
	Bent-over rows	3	10
	Side squats	3	15
	"Around the world" leg routine	3	20
	Calf raises	3	15
Friday			
Shoulders/triceps	Delt press super set	3/3	10/10
	Drop set lateral raise	3	AMRAP
	Dips	3	10
	Pullover press	3	10
	Overhead press	3	10
Abs/lower back	6-minute six pack routine	3	15
	Lower-back lifts	3	15

Hard-Body Split Options

To prevent plateaus in your training, your body needs variety. Variety can be achieved by changing exercises, order of exercises, or training splits. I keep the same split but change exercises and order every week. Training splits can be changed every four to six weeks. The thing to remember is not to train similar muscle groups too close together so that they have plenty of rest time. That means that chest day shouldn't be next to shoulder day, and back day shouldn't be next to biceps day, unless you're doing a push/pull split. Simply put, no rest means no results. Here are a few split options to get you started:

- Day 1: chest/back/abs. Day 2: off. Day 3: legs/abs. Day 4: off. Day 5: shoulders/arms/abs. Day 6: off.
- Day 1: chest/hamstrings. Day 2: back/biceps/abs. Day 3: off. Day 4: quads/calves/abs. Day 5: shoulders/triceps. Day 6: off.
- Day 1: chest/shoulders/triceps. Day 2: abs. Day 3: legs. Day 4: abs. Day 5: back/biceps.
- Day 1: quads/calves/abs. Day 2: chest/biceps/forearms. Day 3: abs. Day 4: hamstrings/back. Day 5: shoulders/triceps/abs. Day 6: off.
- Day 1: chest/hamstrings. Day 2: back/shoulders. Day 3: off. Day 4: quads/calves/abs. Day 5: arms/forearms. Day 6: off.

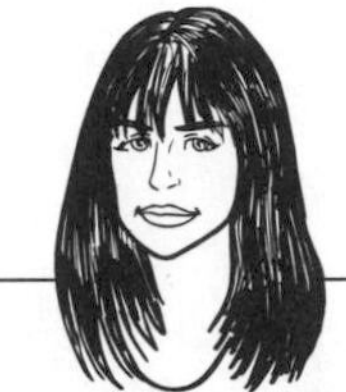

Jourdan's Gems

I like to train the chest with biceps exercises and delts with triceps exercises. Even though they are trained last, my biceps still get a good workout because they are an opposite muscle group. This way, my delts get two training sessions, one as a secondary muscle and one as a primary muscle.

Hard-Body Half-Hour Plan

The following week's split-shift schedule is great if you have only 30 minutes to tone. Also, if you're just starting out, you might want to start with 30 minutes so that you will be able to maintain the intensity. (See Chapters 13, "Ten-Minute Ticket to Tone," for all 10-Minute Ticket to Tone routines, and 16, "Return of the Couch Potato," for ideas on rest and relaxation.)

Jourdan's Ultimate Hard Body Half-Hour Plan

Monday	Tuesday	Wednesday	Thursday	Friday	Saturday	Sunday
10 minutes	10 minutes	60 minutes	10 minutes	10 minutes	Sleep in	Sleep in
Weight training legs routine #1	Weight training chest/back/abs	Cardio easy pace***	Weight training legs routine #2	Weight training delts/triceps/ biceps/abs	Breakfast	Rest and pamper yourself
20 minutes Cardio speed interval training*	20 minutes Cardio hill interval training**	Juice day	20 minutes Cardio speed interval training*	20 minutes Cardio hill interval training**	At least 60 minutes of any sport you love with friends	Breakfast
Breakfast	Breakfast	Breakfast	Breakfast	Breakfast		
Snack	Snack	Snack	Snack	Snack		Snack
Lunch	Lunch	Lunch	Lunch	Lunch	Lunch	Lunch
Snack	Snack	Snack	Snack	Snack	Snack	Snack
Dinner	Dinner	Dinner	Dinner	Dinner	Dinner	Dinner
(Eliminate starches)	(Eliminate starches)		(Eliminate starches)	(Eliminate starches)		
10 minutes Weight training legs routine #1	10 minutes Weight training abs/chest/back	Yoga practice with friend	10 minutes Weight training legs routine #2	10 minutes Weight training abs/delts/triceps	60–75 minutes Cardio moderate pace**** (Take a walk in the afternoon or evening with a friend.)	(Have one cheat meal today.)
20 minutes Cardio speed interval training*	20 minutes Cardio hill interval training**		20 minutes Cardio speed interval training*	20 minutes Cardio hill interval training**		

**After your warm-up, do 2 minutes of sprinting and a 2-minute slow jog or medium speed walk for four intervals.*

***After your warm-up, do 2 minutes of elevation at level 10 and 2 minutes of elevation at level 5 for four intervals.*

****65 percent of your maximum heart rate (maximum heart rate = 220 – your age).*

*****75 percent of your maximum heart rate.*

******Ultimate pamper suggestion: Try shopping and then get a massage. (Shopping burns calories, and the massage helps remove toxins and speeds up the recovery time.)*

Intensity levels are based on your own individual 1–10 point scale of exertion, with 10 being maximum effort.

The Least You Need to Know

- If you're new to training, start with a full-body program for at least two weeks to perfect your exercise form and get your body used to training.
- Doing an intermediate phase of upper/lower training will condition your body so that you'll be ready to split-train at an intense level.
- To change body shape and focus on specific areas, you need to split-train.
- Regularly changing exercises, exercise order, and training splits will help prevent hard-body plateaus.
- When split training, make sure that similar muscle groups have adequate rest time between training sessions.

Chapter 10

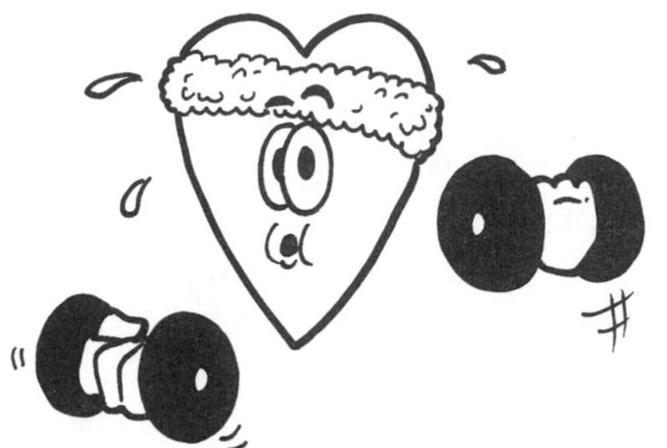

Home Is Where the Heart Gets Fit

In This Chapter

- Fuel for the hard-body engine
- Guidelines for cardio FITness
- Maximizing your cardio time
- The cardio smorgasbord

Aerobic training is the final component of your home hard-body program. Cardio is going to make it possible to see all that great muscle you've built by sweating off the unnecessary adipose tissue (nice word for *fat*) that's on top.

If you don't do cardio and weight training at the same time, you could start looking bigger. Remember, you're building muscle, and that will add some size and weight. Not to worry—muscle is heavier and more compact than fat, so if you get rid of the fat, you will look leaner and more defined even if you weigh more. My best advice is to use a scale to weigh your produce, not your home hard body. Measure your progress with body fat testing, clothes, and your mirror.

The biggest mistake people make in cardio training is working too hard to lose fat. (I don't know about you, but I'd be really mad if I knew that all the cardio work I was doing wasn't doing *exactly* what I wanted it to do.) The FIT guidelines are designed to make sure that you know which target heart rate is right for strengthening your heart muscle and which is right for kicking your fat to the curb.

Cardio Fuel Facts

Your car runs on fuel, and so do you. The difference is that, instead of gasoline, your body uses adenosine triphosphate (ATP) for fuel. The energy that's released from ATP is what runs your body's functions. Because the quantity of ATP in your body is limited to only about three ounces at one time, it has to be constantly remade to provide you with a continuous supply of energy.

ATP is produced in the muscle cells in two ways—with oxygen (aerobic), and without oxygen (anaerobic). When ATP is produced anaerobically, your body uses its supply of *glucose*. When ATP is produced aerobically, a combination of glucose and fat is used.

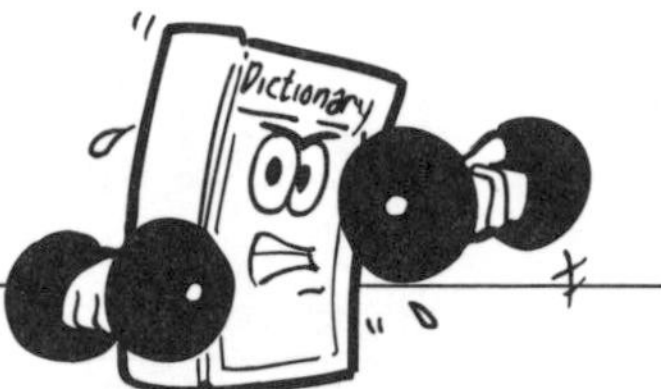

Workout Wisdom

Glucose is a simple sugar that is a vital energy source in the human body. Glucose is stored in the muscles and liver as a substance called glycogen. Glucose is produced from the breakdown of carbohydrates.

Factors that determine the type of fuel that your body uses during exercise include these:

- Intensity of exercise
- Duration of exercise
- Fitness level
- Diet composition

The breakdown of fat to ATP is a slow process and doesn't supply ATP fast enough to provide sufficient energy for high-intensity exercise. To make sure that fat is being used as fuel, you should decrease the intensity of the exercise (between 60 and 70 percent of your maximum heart rate) and increase the length of time that you exercise (a minimum of 20 minutes, not including warm-up and cool-down).

When you exercise longer, you are reducing your supply of glucose, so your body has to use more fat for fuel. The increased endurance level also increases the body's ability to use more fat as a fuel source.

The percentage of carbohydrates in your diet determines how much glucose will be available for fuel. Because any leftover glucose is stored as body fat, and because having no glucose at all won't even get you on the treadmill, a diet too high or too low in carbohydrates in not advisable.

Cardio FIT Guidelines

Your cardio FIT (frequency/intensity/time) guidelines are based on your cardio fitness goal and current fitness level. Your cardio goal could be to strengthen your heart muscle and to increase your endurance level, or to lose body fat. Figure out your FIT guidelines, and log that information in your Home Hard-Body Journal. A sample cardio log page appears in Chapter 17, "Dear Diary."

Frequency

Your cardio frequency is the number of exercise sessions have you do each week. The American College of Sports Medicine recommends 20 to 60 minutes of continuous aerobic exercise every day, at 60 to 90 percent of your maximum heart rate.

For conditioning, you will need to do a minimum of three cardio sessions a week.

For weight loss, you will need to do five to six sessions a week. If you're a beginner, then start with two to three sessions a week and work up gradually. Intermediates can start with three to four sessions. Advanced levels can start with four to five sessions. When your body feels ready, you can add another session until you reach the desired frequency for your goal. When you reach your desired weight, you can reduce your cardio to three sessions for maintenance. If you start to gain weight, then add one cardio session.

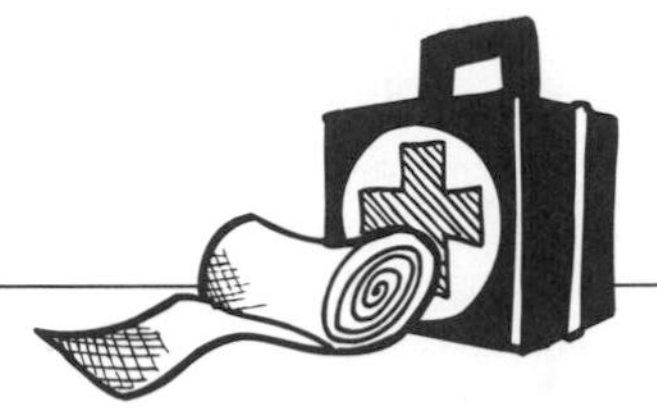

Safety Scoop

If you're just starting and haven't done much physical activity, it's important not to overdo it. If you experience loss of appetite, chronic fatigue, loss of sleep, mood swings, or extreme muscle soreness, you could be overtraining. Reduce the amount of training until your energy level starts to return to normal, and proceed from there.

Intensity

Intensity is how hard you're going to work during your cardio session. This is where most people fall off the fitness path by thinking that if they work harder, they'll lose more weight. What can wind up happening is that they might actually gain weight because the increased amount of exercise will cause them to eat more. Knowing your different heart rate ranges and monitoring your heart rate during cardio work will ensure that you stay on the right hard-body track.

The first thing you need to do is figure out your *maximum heart rate*. This is done with the following formula (I have used mine as an example):

220 – your age = your max heart rate

220 – 37 = 183 (my max heart rate)

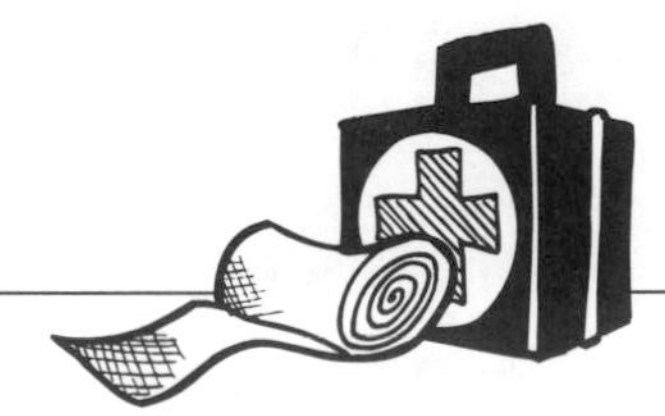

Safety Scoop

A quick test to see if you're working too hard is to try talking. If you can speak without sounding out of breath, then most likely you're not working too hard. Slow down the intensity if you're out of breath, and stop exercising if you feel dizzy or lightheaded.

Now you need to figure out your different *heart rate ranges*. Your fitness goal will determine what range you need to maintain during your cardio session. Log your heart rate ranges in your Home Hard-Body Journal. The following table outlines the various ranges that you will use during your hard-body training.

Heart Rate Ranges			
Healthy range	50% to 60% of max HR	92 bpm to 110 bpm	(10 for 6-second count)
Fat-burning range	60% to 70% of max HR	110 bpm to 129 bpm	(13 for 6-second count)
Aerobic range	70% to 80% of max HR	129 bpm to 147 bpm	(15 for 6-second count)
Anaerobic range	80% to 90% of max HR	147 bpm to 166 bpm	(17 for 6-second count)
Intense range	90% to 100% of max HR	166 bpm to 184 bpm	(18 for 6-second count)

Time

Your current fitness level will determine the length of your cardio sessions. It's an unrealistic expectation if you're a beginner to try to do 60-minute sessions. Not only would you not be able to keep it up, but you also could risk possible overuse injury. Remember, the goal is to train smart so that you can keep training for a long time. Beginners should start with 10- to 20-minute working sessions. (Warm-up and cool-down times are not included in the working session time.) Intermediates can start with 20- to 45-minute working sessions. Advanced exercisers can start with 30- to 60-minute working sessions.

Cardio Maximizer Tips

For maximum fat burning during your cardio sessions, the following are the best times to do your cardio:

- First thing in the morning on an empty stomach
- Right after your weight-training session
- In the evening, after your last meal

When you do cardio first thing in the morning, your body is low on glycogen because it has used most of its supply while you were sleeping. (You've got to love the fact that we burn fat while we sleep.) This is especially true if you didn't have any starches for dinner and did cardio afterward. Wait after your meal, and then do some light cardio, such as walking, for 30 minutes.

When you do your cardio after weight training, your body has used most of its glycogen by that time, so it

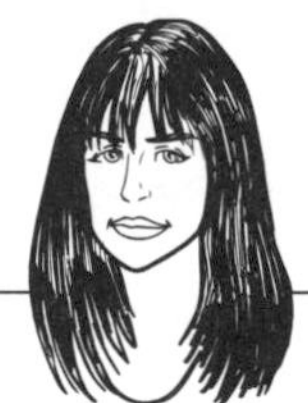

Jourdan's Gems

One of your best investments will be a heart rate monitor. This eliminates the guesswork and makes checking your heart rate much simpler than checking your wrist or neck with your fingers. See Chapter 4, "Home Grown," for sources to purchase monitors.

gets to the fat sooner. Also, your heart rate is already elevated, so you'll reach your fat-burning threshold quicker.

Doing your cardio after your last meal of the day will use up glycogen so that while you sleep, you'll burn a larger amount of body fat. An evening cardio session will also make it possible for more fat to be burned in your morning cardio session.

Cardio Calorie Counting

Energy is measured by calories. The following chart lists various home hard-body activities and how many *calories* are burned per minute of activity. Multiply the number appropriate for your weight by the number of minutes you exercised to figure out the amount of calories you've burned.

Energy Expenditure of Various Home Hard-Body Activities

Body weight in lbs.	*115*	*125*	*135*	*145*	*155*	*165*	*175*	*185*	*200*
Hard body activity	**Calories burned per minute of activity**								
Aerobics: low impact	5	6	6	6	7	7	8	8	9
Aerobics: high impact	6	7	8	8	9	9	10	10	11
Bicycling: moderate	6	7	8	8	9	9	10	10	11
Bicycling: vigorous	10	11	11	12	13	14	15	16	17
Calisthenics: moderate	4	5	5	5	6	6	6	7	7
Calisthenics: vigorous	7	8	9	9	10	11	11	12	13
Elliptical trainer	8	9	10	10	11	12	13	13	14
Jumping rope	9	10	11	12	12	13	14	15	16
Kickboxing	9	11	11	12	12	13	14	15	16
Rowing machine: moderate	6	7	8	8	9	9	10	10	11
Rowing machine: vigorous	8	9	9	10	11	11	12	13	14
Running: 5 mph (12 min/mi)	7	8	9	9	10	11	11	12	13
Running: 7.5 mph (8 min/mi)	12	13	14	15	16	17	18	19	20
Running: 10 mph (6 min/mi)	15	17	18	19	20	22	23	24	26
Step: low impact	6	7	8	8	9	9	10	10	11
Step: high impact	9	10	11	12	12	13	14	15	16
Stretching, Hatha Yoga	4	4	4	5	5	5	6	6	6
Tai Chi	4	4	4	5	5	6	6	6	6
Weight lifting: moderate	3	3	3	3	4	4	4	4	5
Weight lfting: intense	6	6	6	7	7	8	8	9	10

Home Hard-Body Cardio Options

In the workout quiz in Chapter 4, "Home Grown," you found out what types of exercises best suited your personality. If you still aren't sure, the following sections outline a cardio option list that includes benefits and training tips and can help you find the best cardio match for your fitness goals.

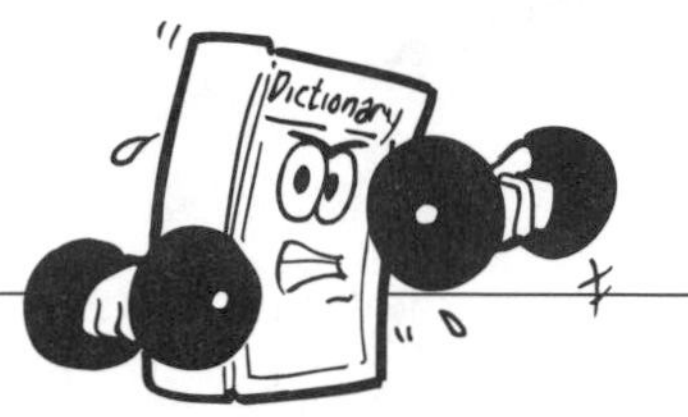

Workout Wisdom

Calorie is the amount of heat required to raise the temperature of one kilogram of water one degree Celsius; also called kilocalorie.

Treadmills

Advantages Strengthens lower body. (Walking) Is low-impact, so involves less joint stress. (Running) Lessens the impact of running with its belt.

Training tips Maintain good posture. Increase intensity by pumping your arms. Try to increase your pace so that it takes less time for the same distance. Elevating the machine will work hamstrings more. Vary elevation/intensity levels for interval training.

Elliptical Trainers

Advantages Simulates running with calorie-burning benefits. Low-impact, so puts less stress on joints (impact is lower than on treadmills). Increases coordination and balance. Good for stability work.

Training tips Increase tension so that you're able to work without holding on, to increase intensity and strengthen your core muscles. Vary elevation levels to work different leg muscles. Going backward works quadriceps muscles.

Stationary Bikes

Advantages Good for beginners and overweight people. Puts less stress on the back. Strengthens quadriceps.

Training tips Work on increasing your exercise duration. Vary rpm/intensity levels for interval training. Always keep some tension on the bike to support your knees.

Aerobic Dancing

Advantages Works the entire body. Has a large variety of workout options available through video tapes. Can be done in a low-impact format. (Call Collage Video at 1-800-433-6769 to get a catalog with over 300 exercise video options.)

Training tips Include a warm-up and cool-down. Aerobic session should be a minimum of 20 minutes. Start with a beginning workout. Slow down if you feel out of breath.

Rowing Machine

Advantages Strengthens the upper body.

Training tips Keep your back straight while rowing. Try to increase distance each workout.

Urban Rebounding

Advantages Puts less stress on joints. Increases balance and coordination. Provides ability to do plyometric drills without shock to joints. Strengthens upper- and lower-body muscles. Is good for stabilization work. Enables you to work harder and longer because no energy is used to absorb floor shock.

Training tips Do standard free-weight exercises with weights to strengthen the upper body. Simulate exercises with arm movements during aerobic moves for total-body conditioning. Use basic bounce between exercises to help eliminate lactic acid.

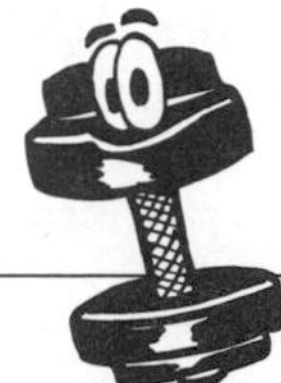

Hard-Body Headliners

Research has shown that wearing the "Burke Spencer Leg and Butt Buster" while exercising on a treadmill, men can burn 50 percent more calories, and women can burn 20 percent more calories. Just wearing it without exercising can also result in up to 50 percent more calorie burning.

Step Aerobics

Advantages Strengthens lower-body muscles. Improves coordination. Is low-impact.

Training tips Step on the bench with the whole foot to prevent slipping. Raise intensity by holding hand weights. Use light steps to avoid joint stress (if it sounds loud, you're stepping too hard). Master basic moves first. Videotapes make good visual aids to learn of combinations of steps.

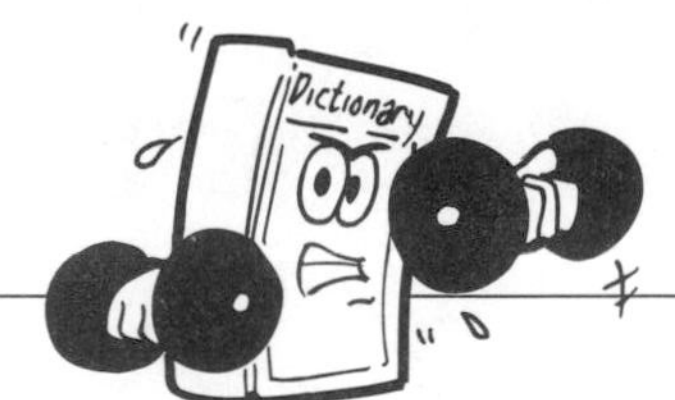

Workout Wisdom

Interval training is short, high-intensity exercise periods alternated with periods of rest (such as a 100-yard sprint and a 1-minute walk, repeated six times).

"Burke Spencer's Leg and Butt Buster"

Advantages It increases exercise intensity, strengthens upper-/lower-body muscles, and is great for people with joint problems or injuries.

Training tips Wear while walking, running, or even doing housework to increase leg strength and burn more calories.

Cool Cardio Routine

Interval training burns more calories in a shorter period of time. That's the first reason I like interval training. The second is that it gives me variety in my cardio workout so that I'm not bored to tears. Finally, my attention is focused on when to change intervals instead of thinking, "When will this be over?"

My whole treadmill routine, including warm-up and cool-down, takes only 25 minutes. Excluding the warm-up and cool-down, I maintain a brisk walking pace during the entire routine. It's also important to note that my routine intervals reflect an advanced fitness level.

The Least You Need to Know

- ➤ Aerobic exercise burns glucose and body fat as fuel, while anaerobic exercise burns only glucose.
- ➤ The type of fuel that your body uses is determined by the intensity of exercise, the duration of exercise, your current fitness level, and your diet composition.
- ➤ Monitoring your target heart rate will keep your cardio work on track.
- ➤ For maximum fat burning, cardio should be done first thing in the morning on an empty stomach, right after weight training, or in the evening after your last meal.

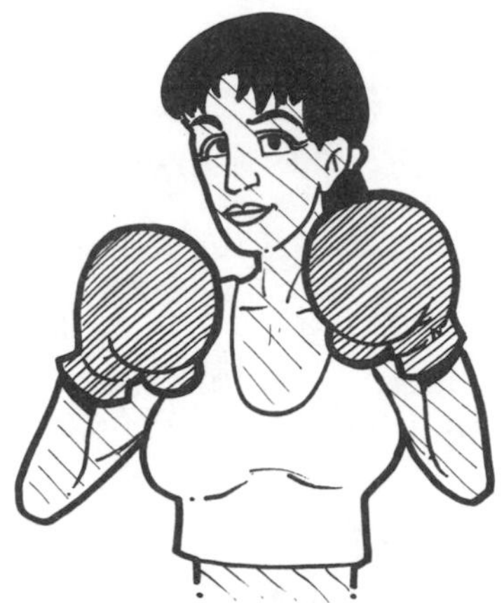

Chapter 11

Hard-Body Knockouts

In This Chapter

- Gearing up right
- Learn hard-body punching and kicking skills
- Putting it together: combination drills

To me, a great workout gets you fired up and leaves you feeling like you can do anything. (You've got to love those endorphins.) Kickboxing is the ticket to main event exercise that'll get your entire hard body into the action. A kickboxing workout builds muscle, burns fat, teaches you how to kick some butt, and releases major amounts of stress. (If you want proof, just picture the source of your stress in front of you, and see what happens.)

In addition to giving you a great workout, punching and kicking drills give you better balance and coordination. Pads and heavy bag work give you the feeling of hitting an opponent. The best thing is, no matter how hard you hit, it won't hit back. (Finally there's an outlet for the knockout king in all of us.)

To start you off, I've made sure to thoroughly break down the basics so that you'll have the best foundation for your hard-body knockout training and the best opportunity to become a hard-body kickboxing master. You can easily pick out the masters in a crowd—they're the ones who've mastered the basics.

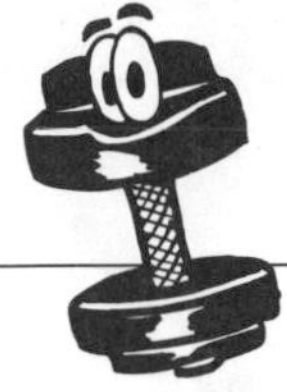

Hard-Body Headliners

Add baby powder to the inside of your gloves and let them air-dry after each use to keep them smelling fresh.

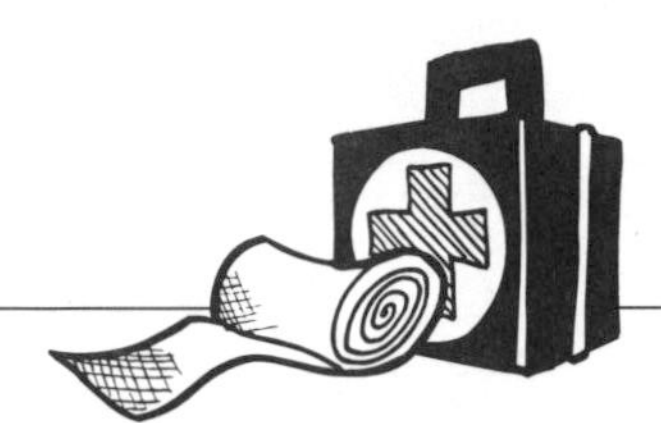

Safety Scoop

To protect your hand when hitting a bag (or your opponent), it's important to make a tight fist and to hit with the first two knuckles. Aiming the glove slightly downward makes this easier.

Gear Up Right

Whether your goal is to sweat some calories or turn your basement into Rocky's boxing gym, you need the right gear. Having the right gear will make your workouts more enjoyable, will make your performance better, and will protect you from injuries that could occur from oven mitt-type boxing gloves. Most people don't realize that getting the right gear isn't a serious blow below the money belt if you know what to look for.

Fits Likes a Glove

There are two types of training gloves: sparring gloves and bag gloves. Because my hard-body knockout program doesn't include getting into the ring, you will be using bag gloves. The difference is that bag gloves have extra padding around the knuckles to protect your hands. Of all the gloves I've tried (and I've tried many), I'd recommend the Contender bag glove by Ringside—it's a great fit at a great price.

Jump and Sweat

Jumping rope improves your agility, coordination, and timing while giving you one heck of a cardio workout. Ropes come in leather or plastic. I have a plastic rope, but either will get the job done right, so the choice is yours. Getting the right size is crucial if you don't want to keep getting slapped in the shins with the rope. (I speak from experience on this one.)

Rope Length	User's Height
7.5 feet	Up to 5 feet, 5 inches
8.5 feet	5 feet, 5 inches to 5 feet, 8 inches
9.5 feet	5 feet, 8 inches and up

Heavy Bag Heavy Hitters

Hitting the heavy bag gives you the feeling of hitting an opponent that doesn't hit back—the best kind. Bag work develops your strength and hitting power. There are two types of heavy bags: the kind that you hang from the ceiling on a big chain, and the kind that stands on its own. You also have the choice of a bag that's filled with sand or water. The thought of hitting something filled with water in my house makes me nervous, so I choose bags that can be filled with sand or water. Bags come covered in canvas, vinyl, or leather. For a bag that will last, pick vinyl or leather—both last about the same length of time. For the best bargain, however, vinyl is clearly the champ.

Kicking Shield

Practicing your kicks into a shield gives you powerful kicks. Unlike kicking a heavy bag, the shield remains stationary with the assistance of a training partner.

Wrap It Right

I cannot stress the importance of wrapping your hands right, especially when you start hitting hard. The numero uno reason to wrap is to protect the bones in your hand from breaking due to the impact from punching. If you just plan to shadow box, then chances are really high that you won't hurt yourself punching air, but if you're tempted by bag work, then it's time to wrap.

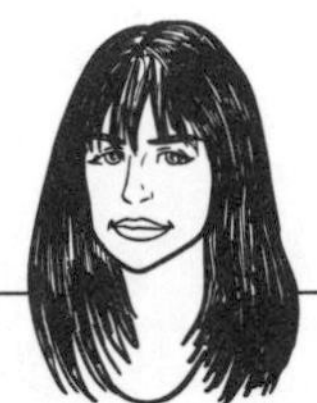

Jourdan's Gems

When holding shields, give some resistance but don't absorb the kick's full power. Your best bet when training with shields is to find a partner close to your strength level to prevent unnecessary stress to the body—and to the friendship.

When you wrap, you want to make sure that your wrist has good support. Wrap your thumb, in between each finger, and your knuckles firmly, but not too tight. If your fingers are starting to turn white or you can't open your hand inside the glove, it's time to rewrap. For a better fit, use a wrap that has elastic in the fabric. There is no one right way to wrap. The method that follows is the one that my sensei uses on me.

1. Put your thumb in the loop, and pull the wrap across the back of your hand away from your thumb.
2. Wrap around your wrist three times for support. Make sure that the wrap is snug, not tight.

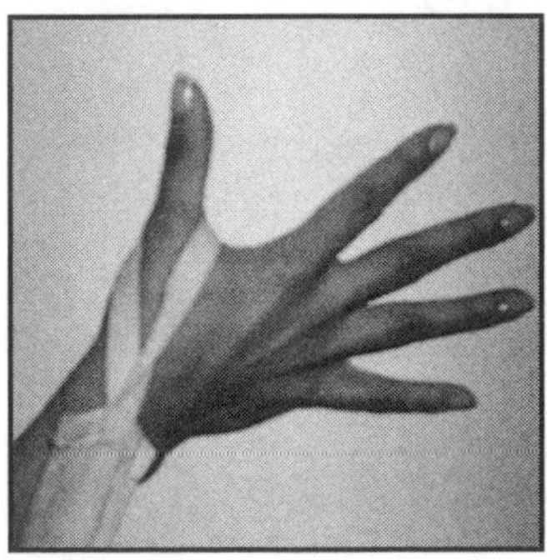

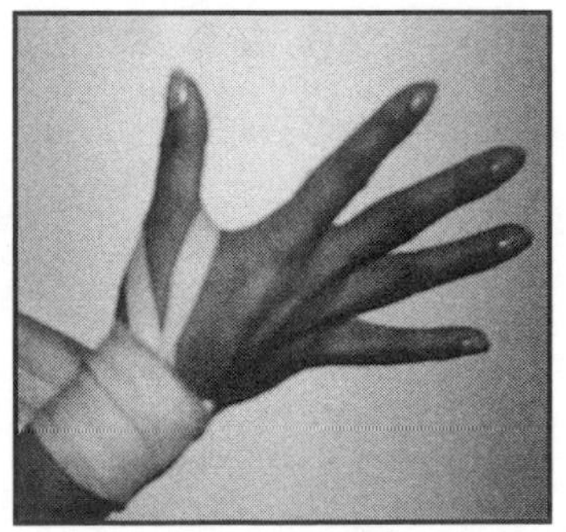

3. Bring the wrap toward your knuckles. From the backside, wrap your knuckles three times. Your knuckles should be completely covered.
4. Starting with your pinky, weave-wrap between each finger, running the wrap down your palm between each weave tightly.

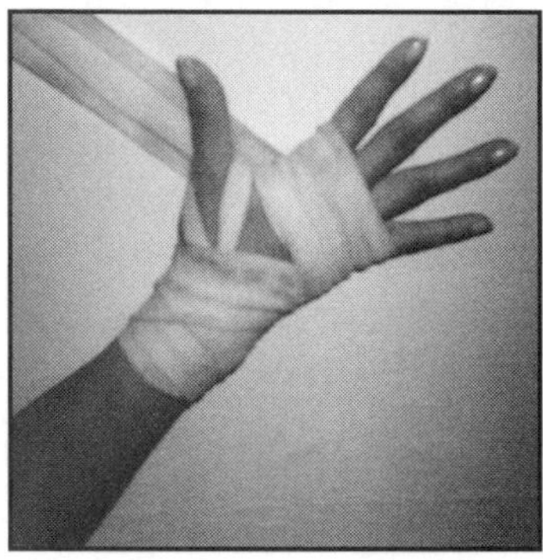

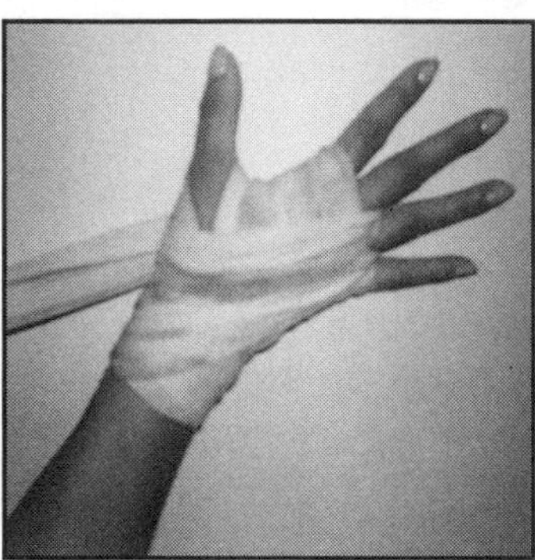

5. Bring the wrap up to your knuckles, and wrap your knuckles five times.
6. Wrap around your wrist once, and then circle-wrap around your thumb from behind once.
7. Circle your wrist with the remaining wrap, and then use Velcro to close the wrap.

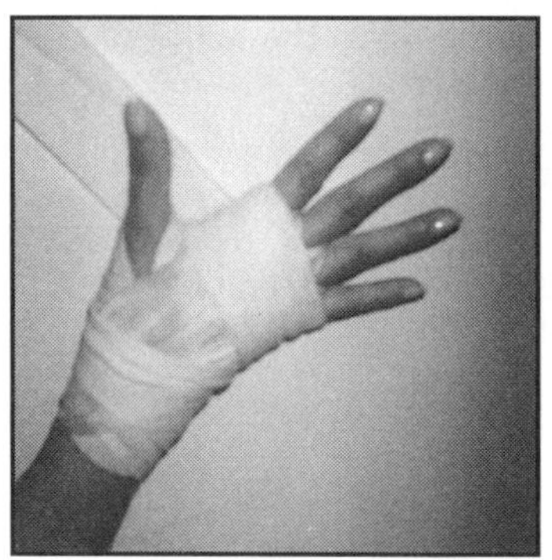

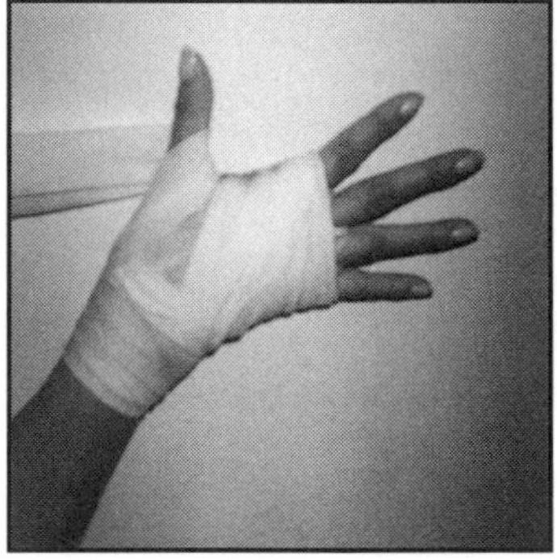

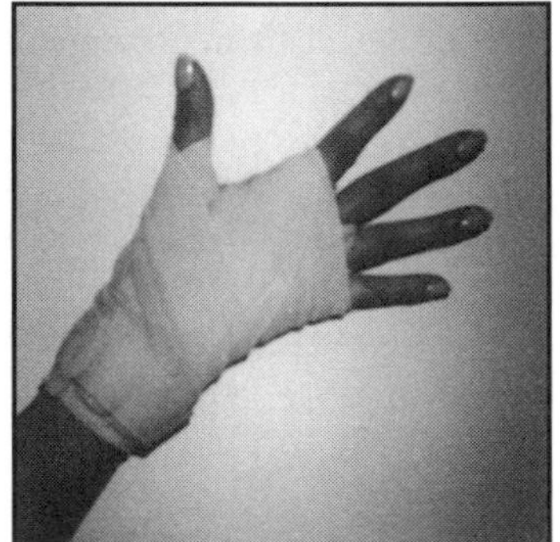

Hard-Body Punching

If done properly, punching can give you a buff upper body, help you sweat off fat, and stop an opponent cold in his tracks. Sloppy form will do you no good and could get you hurt.

The Fighting Stance

This is the position that you throw punches and kicks from and the position that you return to after each technique is executed. Your fighting stance should make you as small of a target as possible and should protect your body and head from oncoming blows. Whether you're a lefty or a righty determines whether you fight from a left or a right stance. For training purposes, you will be doing your techniques on both sides. I complained about being awkward on one side until I realized the advantage I would have being equally proficient on both sides. Now when asked what side I fight from, I can honestly answer, "Both."

Correct fighting stance Stand with one foot in front of the other hip-width apart, with your knees bent to lower your center of gravity, and your weight evenly distributed between both legs. Your body should face 2 o'clock, and your head should be facing 12 o'clock. Your hands are up, ready to protect the front and side of your head, and your arms are in tight to protect your body.

Incorrect fighting stance The gunslinger pose makes you an easy target.

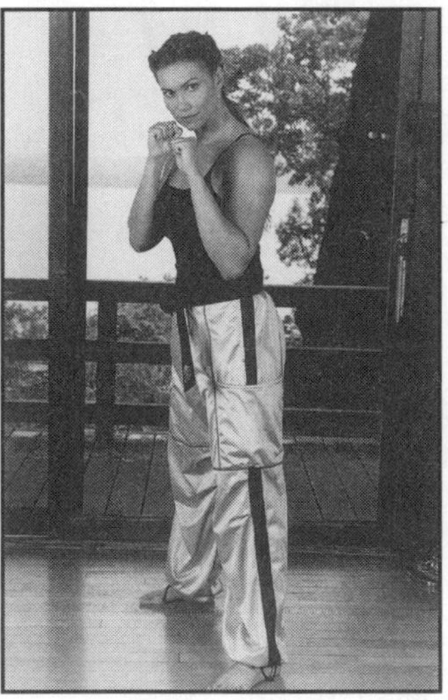

Correct fighting stance.

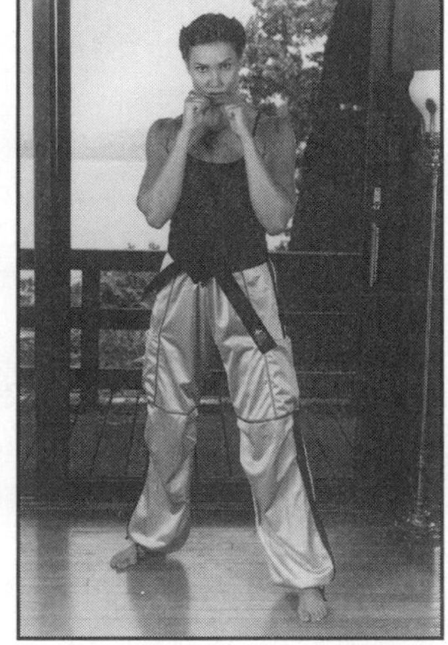

Incorrect fighting stance.

The Jab

The jab is usually used to set up most punching and kicking combinations. It is also used to keep distance between you and your opponent.

1. Assume a fighting stance.
2. Step forward with your left foot, and extend your left arm forward while turning your fist (like a cork screw) so that the palm is facing down. Your hand, elbow, and shoulder should be in line with a bend in the elbow. Strike target with your fist using a snapping motion.
3. Return to the fighting stance.

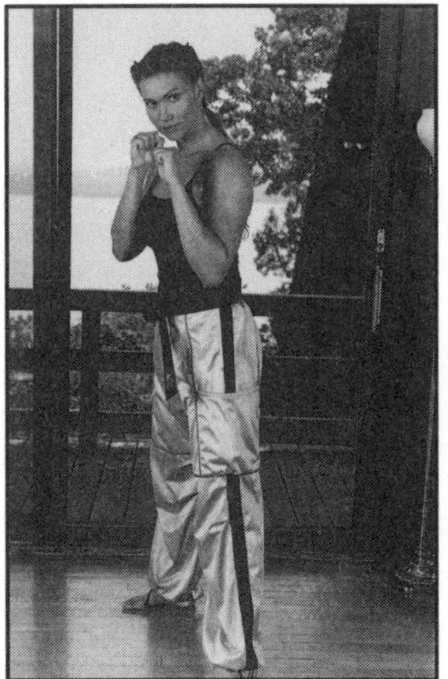
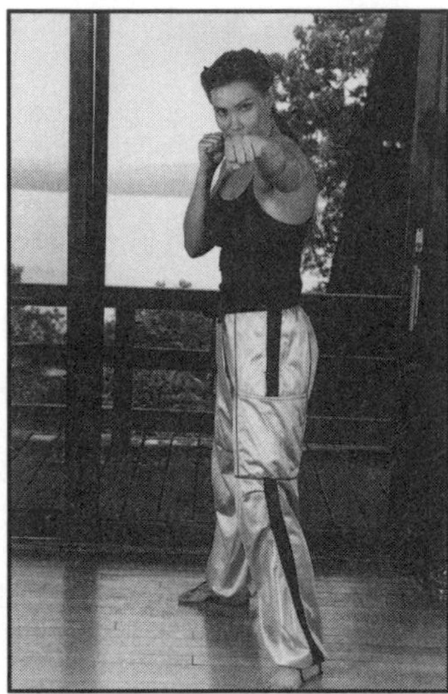
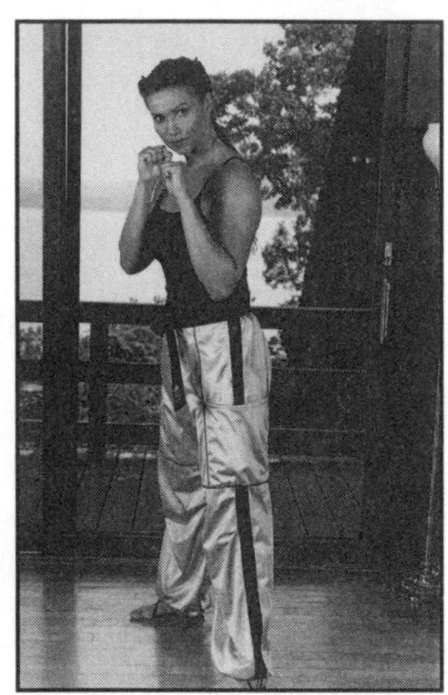

The Cross "Power Hand"

The cross after the jab is usually the second most-thrown punch. Unlike the jab, whose snapping power comes from the shoulder, the cross uses your entire body strength to deliver punches with knockout power. Turning your body in a whiplike motion as you punch is what turns your body into the driving force behind the cross.

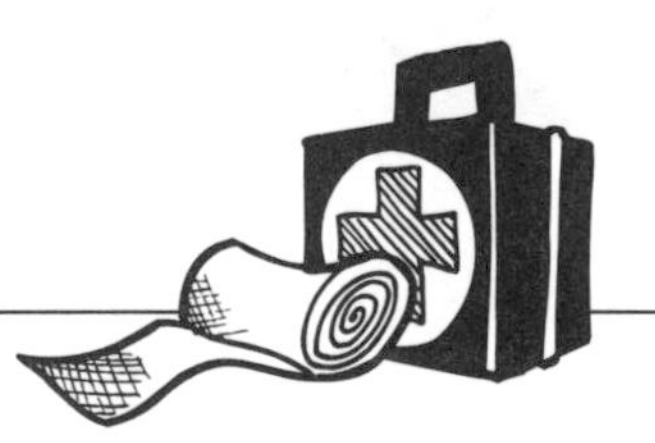

Safety Scoop

Joint injuries can occur when elbows are locked. It's important to always leave a slight bend in the elbow whenever you punch.

1. Assume a fighting stance.
2. Extend your right arm forward as you pivot on the ball of your back foot. Shift your weight to your front leg by driving your rear leg, hips, back, and shoulder forward. Your shoulder, bent elbow, and fist should be in line. Strike the target.
3. Return to the fighting stance.

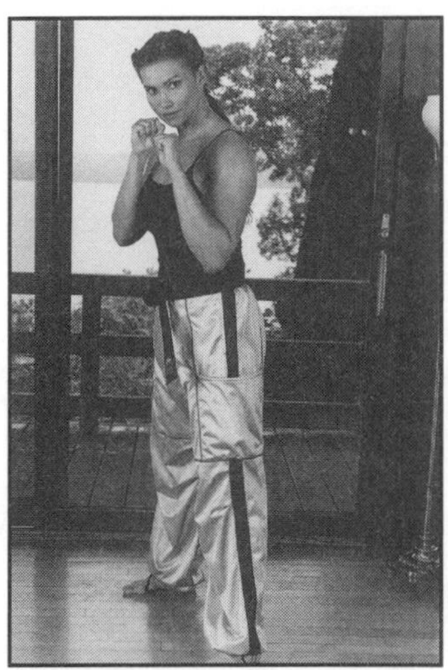
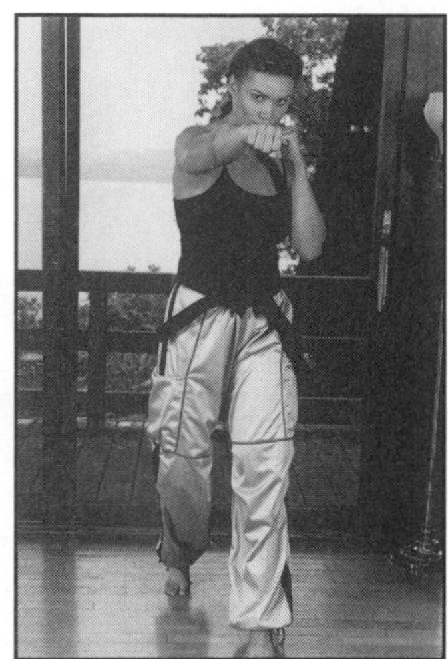
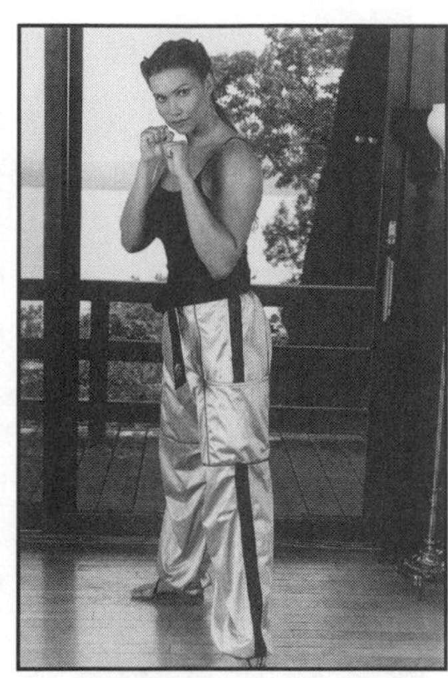

The Hook

Once mastered, the hook punch can also become a killer knockout punch. The hook can be thrown from the lead or rear hand. There are two acceptable ways to throw a hook punch—palm facing down or palm facing you. I like the second variation because it feels more natural and has more hitting power.

1. Assume the fighting stance.
2. Extend your left arm forward, and turn so that your forearm is horizontal and parallel to floor. Your palm should be facing you, with your fist not extended past your nose, and your elbow pointed away. Pivot on the ball of your left foot, and use body torque as the driving power force behind your punch. Strike the target.
3. Return to the fighting stance.

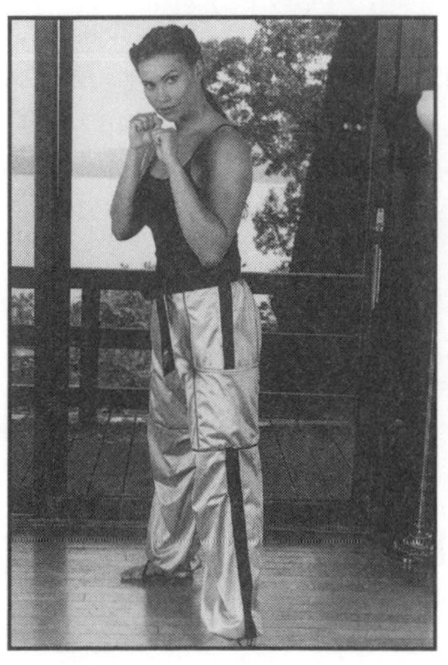
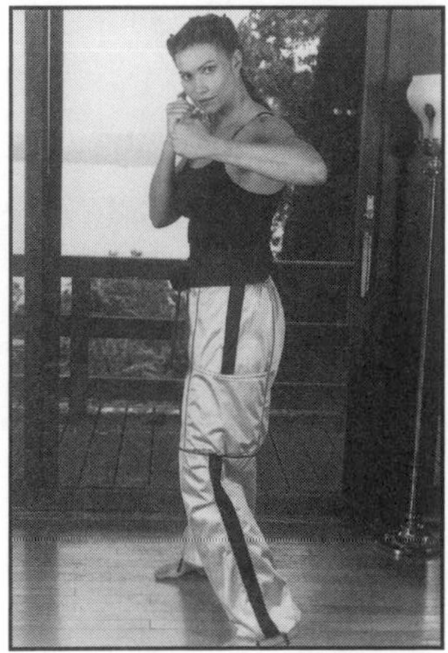
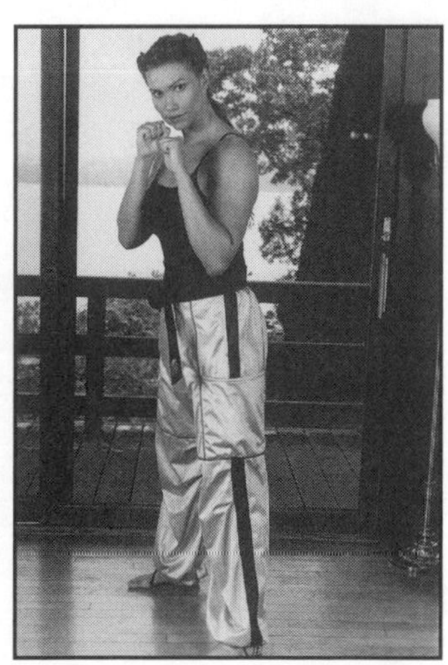

The Upper Cut

The upper cut is your best friend when you're in close range. Upper cuts aim for the chin and the body. A good upper cut to the body can make your opponent drop his hands so that you can then deliver a knockout cross.

1. Assume a fighting stance.
2. Bend your knees and fire right straight up (palm should be facing you) as you pivot on the ball of your right foot, using your body to drive power up into the punch. Strike the target.
3. Return to the fighting stance.

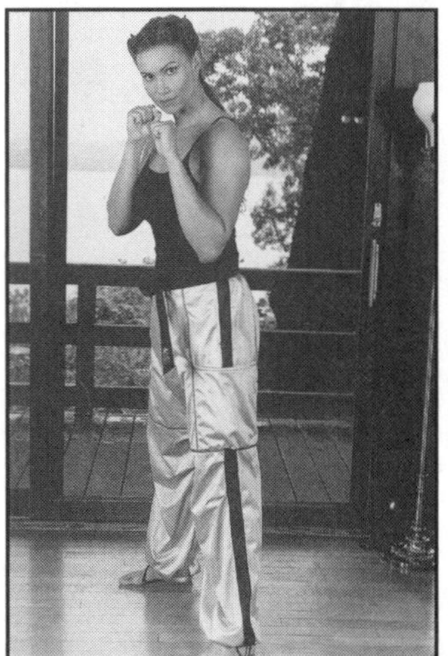

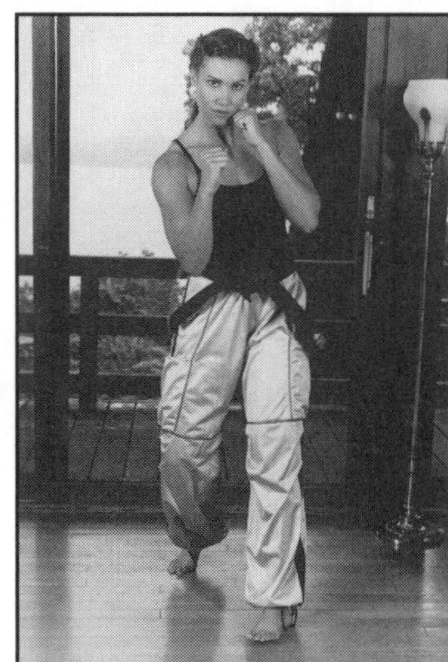

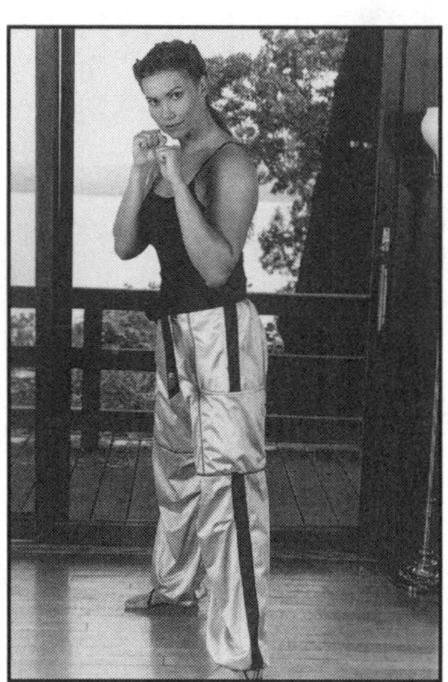

Power Punching Drills

Practice punches very slowly first in front of a mirror to work on perfect form. Make sure that your body is working together as one unit and that you're not just arm-punching. Next, increase the tempo so that each punch is one count, and work on punching a rhythm. Finally, work on snapping punches. Practice your punches separately and in combinations using the following drill. Do 10 reps of each on both sides:

- Jab
- Cross
- Hook
- Upper cut
- Jab/hook (lead hand)
- Jab/cross

- Jab/cross/hook
- Jab/cross/hook/upper cut
- Jab/cross/hook/cross

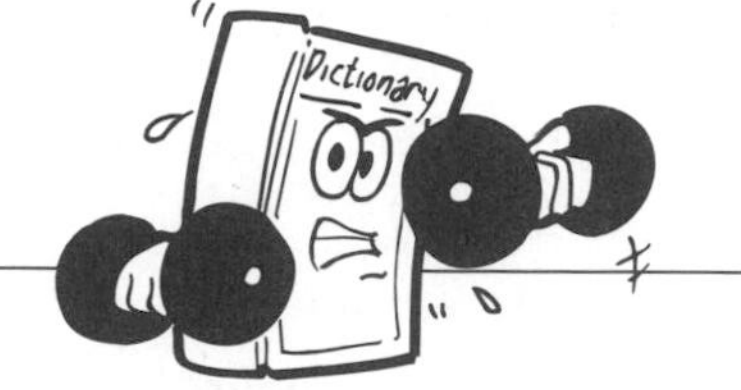

Workout Wisdom

The **chamber position** is the position that your leg goes to before you kick and the position that your leg goes to after completing the kick and before it lands on the ground. The height of the kick will be determined by the height of the chamber position.

Hard-Body Kicking

If it's done right, kicking will give your legs a lean and tone appearance and give you two more weapons in your fighting arsenal. I've given you three kicks to get your hard-body, knockout legs started.

Front Kick

The front kick is the easiest to learn and can be delivered by either the lead or the rear leg. The thrusting motion of the hip is what gives a front kick its power.

1. Assume a fighting stance.
2. Lean on your forward leg, shifting weight to this leg. Chamber your rear leg up above waist level with the suspended foot by a stationary knee.
3. Push your hip forward while snapping your foot forward, striking the target with the ball of your foot.
4. Bring your leg back to *chamber position.*
5. Return to the fighting stance.

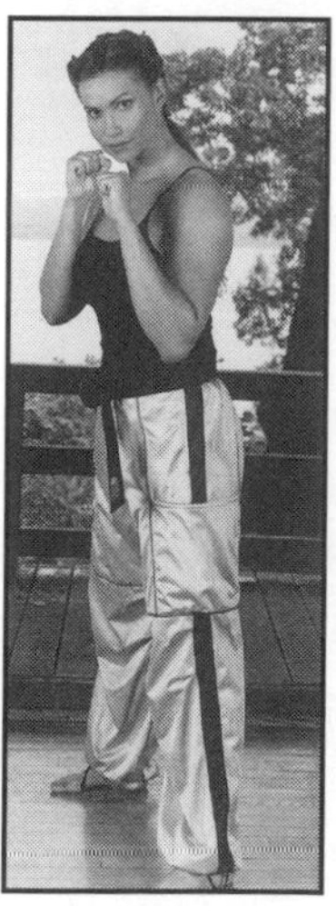
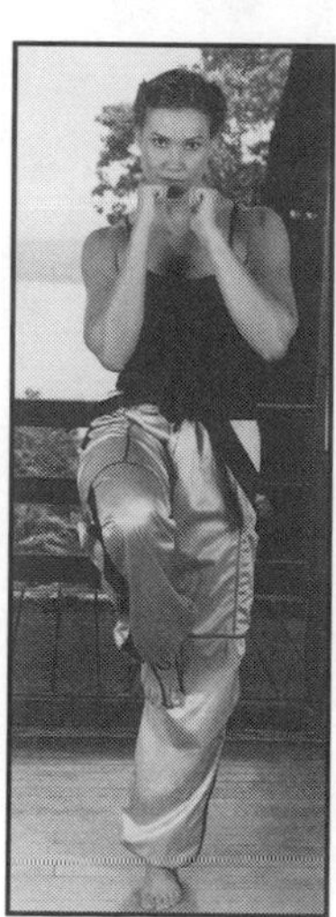
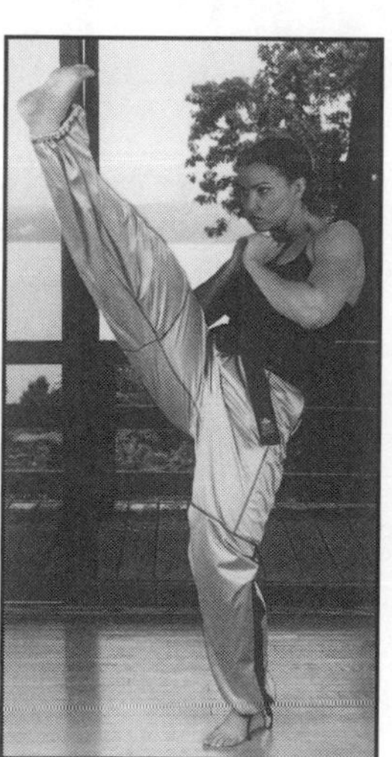
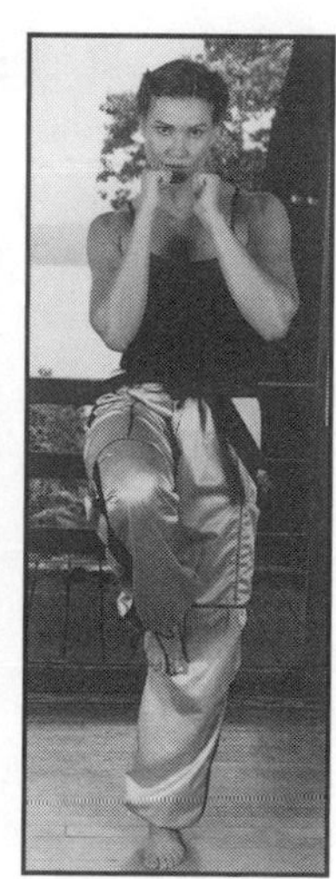
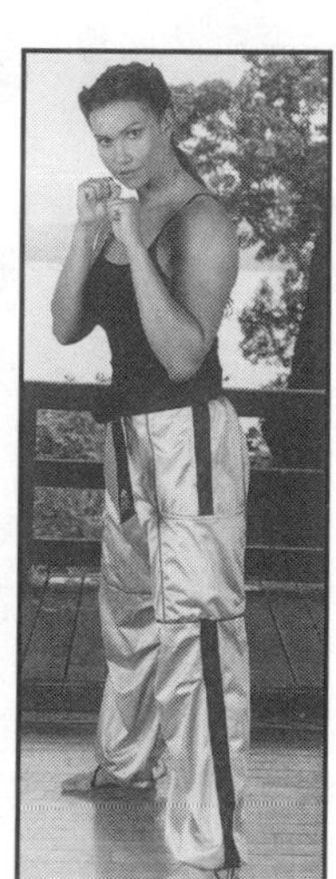

Side Kick

The side kick, utilizing the outer edge or blade of the foot, is one of the most frequently used kicks in all styles of karate because of its great range and force.

1. Assume a fighting stance.
2. Bring your leg up and across your body, with your foot flexed so that the bottom of the heel faces your target. Pivot the support foot out so that the heel is toward your target.
3. Snap your leg out and turn your hip into the kick. With the heel higher then the toe, strike your target with your heel.
4. Return to the fighting stance.
5. Bring your leg back to the chamber position.

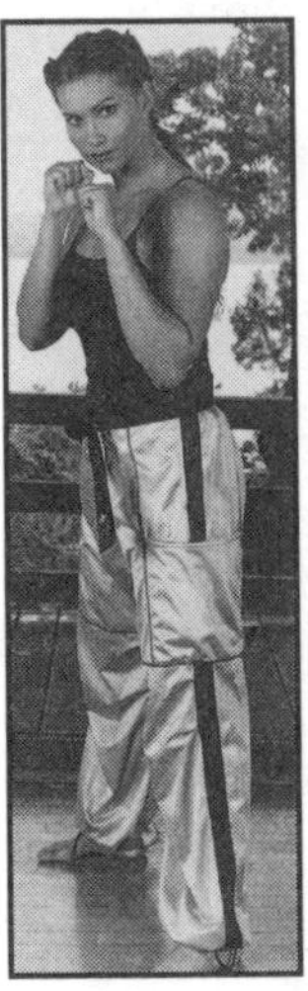
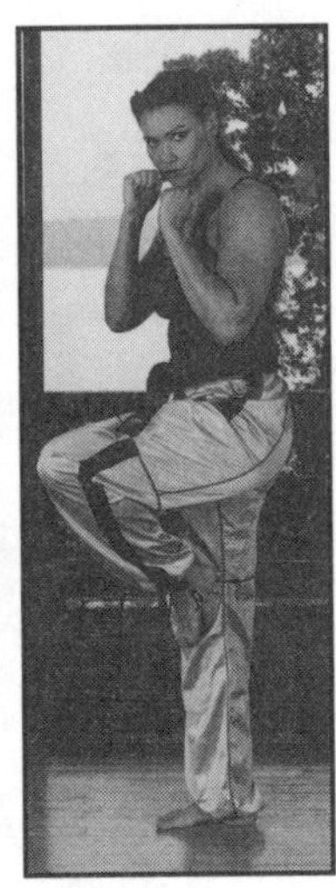
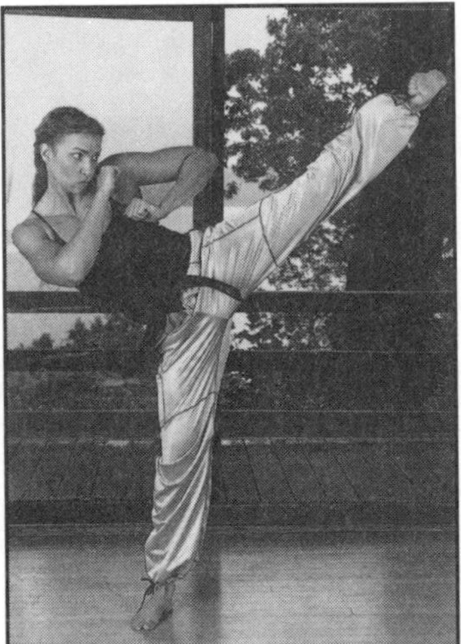
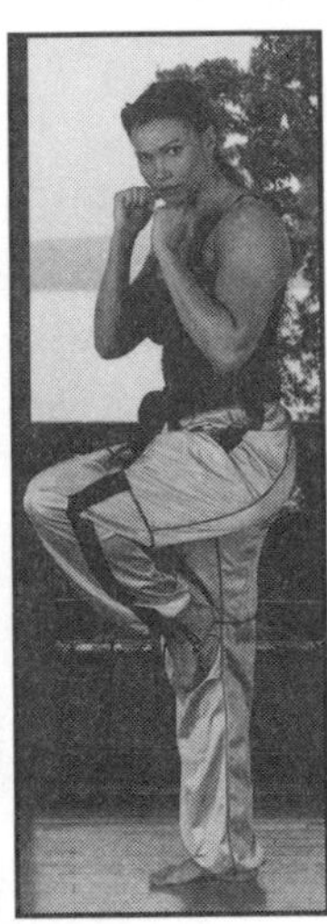
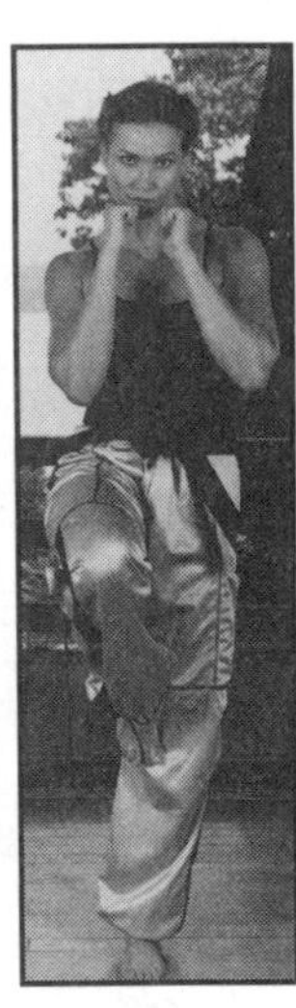

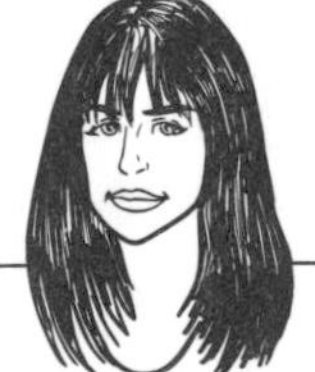

Jourdan's Gems

To maximize your axe kick and increase your leg development, use your hamstring and glute muscles to drive the kick downward.

Axe Kick

1. Assume a fighting stance.
2. With a straight leg and your foot flexed, bring your rear leg forward, up, and around. (Imagine going clockwise around the edge of a clock.) When your heel reaches 1 o'clock, push your hip forward and drive your heel downward to strike your target.
3. Return to fighting stance.

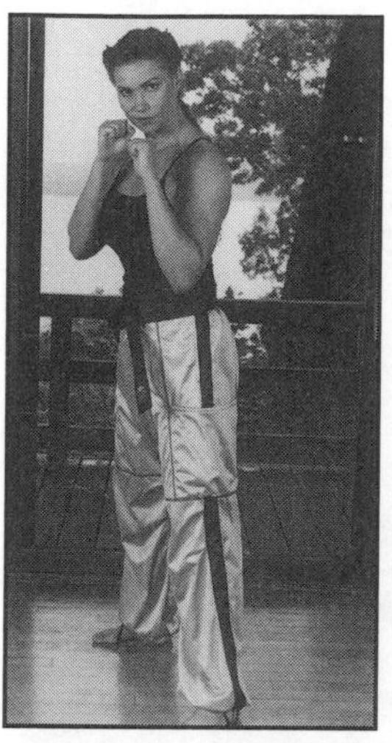
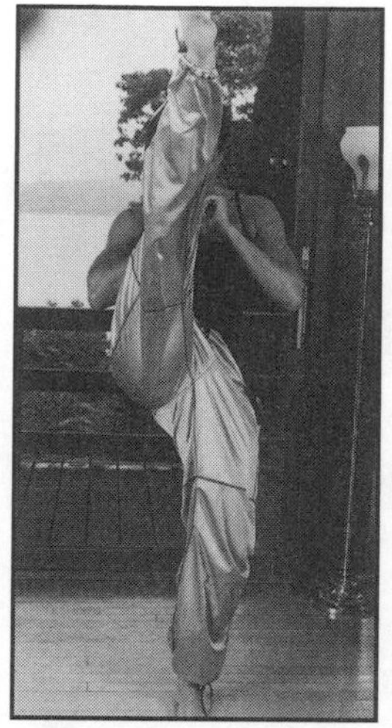
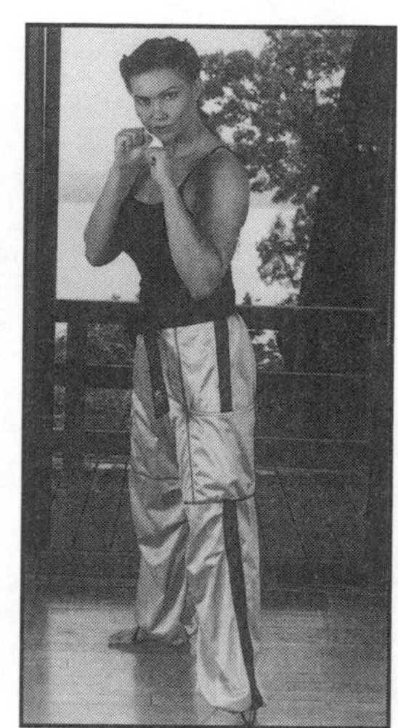

Power Kicking Drills

Always warm up and do light stretching before kicking drills. Start by doing kicks slowly to work on form, making sure that the leg is chambered before and after kicking. After you have mastered the kicking form, you can increase the kicking speed.

Do each drill 10 times slowly and 10 times with a quicker, controlled tempo, for a total of 20 reps on each side.

- Front kick
- Side kick
- Axe kick
- Front kick (lead leg)/front kick (rear leg)
- Front kick (rear leg)/axe kick
- Side kick (lead leg)/front kick (rear leg)
- Front kick (lead leg)/axe kick/side kick (lead leg)

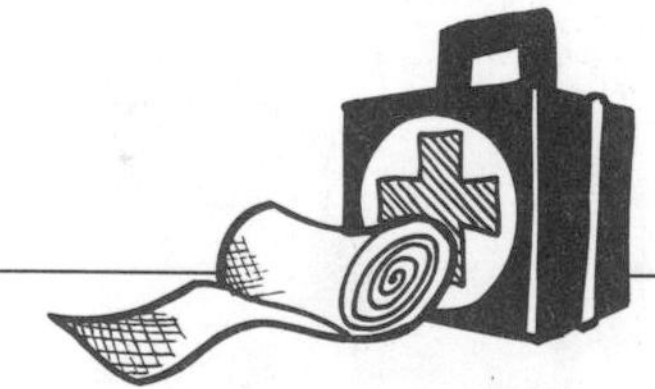

Safety Scoop

To protect knee joints, always keep your legs and knees strong during kicks. Flinging legs will cause knees to jerk and absorb a high level of stress.

Hard-Body Combinations

Now it's time for the hands and feet to join forces and work together. Do the following combinations 10 times slowly and then 10 times at a quicker, controlled tempo, for a total of 20 reps on each side. (Remember to return to a fighting stance between each combination.)

Jab/Cross/Front Kick (Rear Leg)

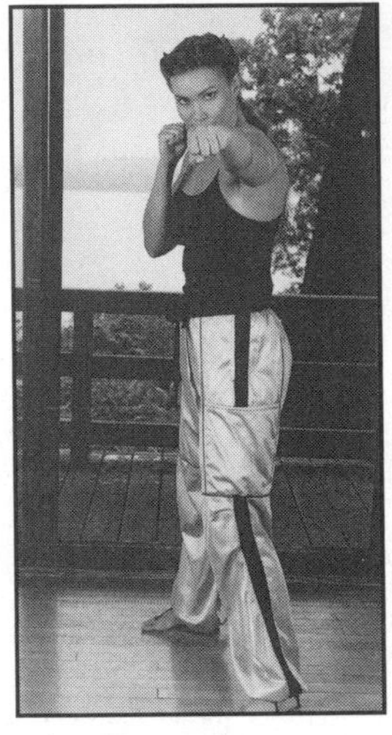

Jab.

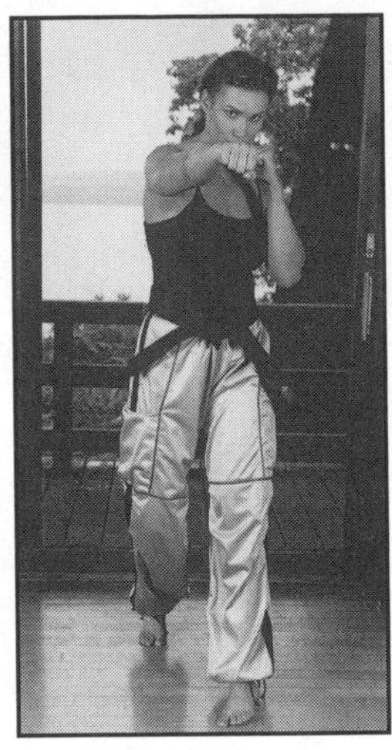

Cross.

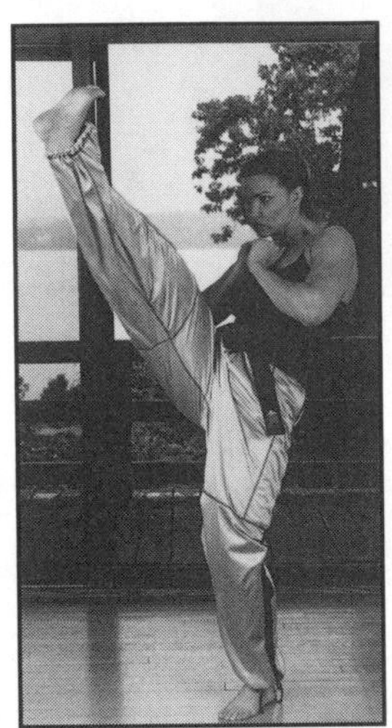

Front kick (rear leg).

Side Kick (Lead Leg)/Jab/Cross/Front Kick (Rear Leg)

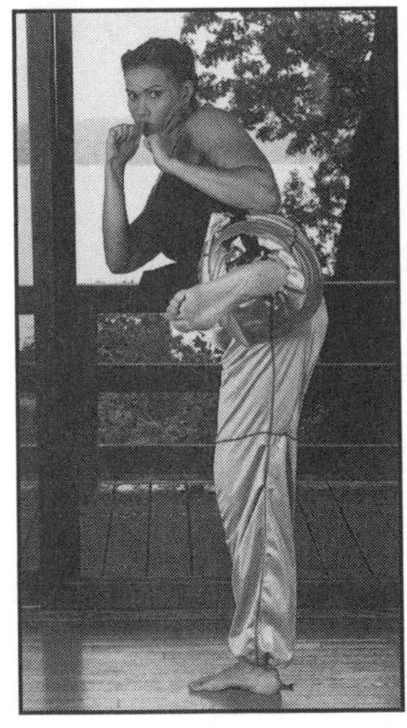

Side kick (lead leg).

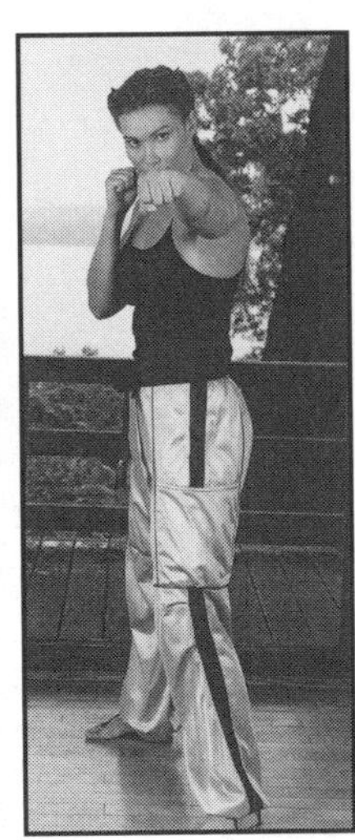

Jab.

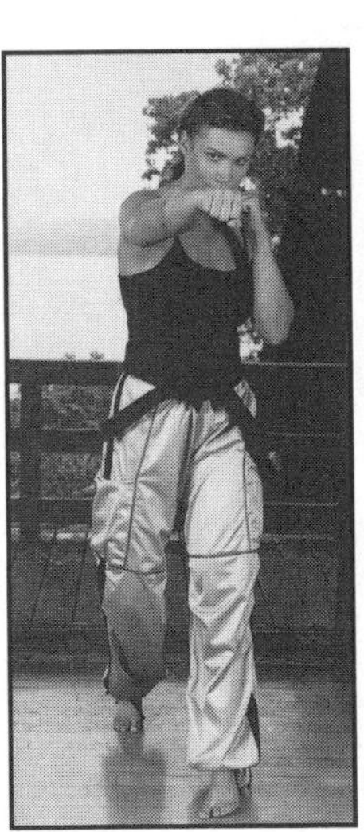

Cross.

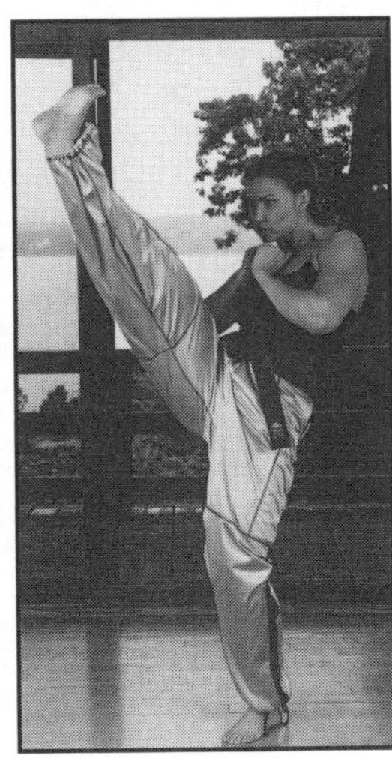

Front kick (rear leg).

Jab/Cross/Hook/Fronthouse Kick

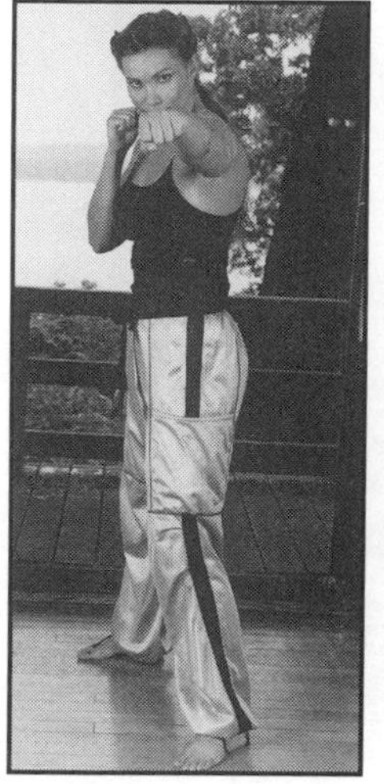

Jab.

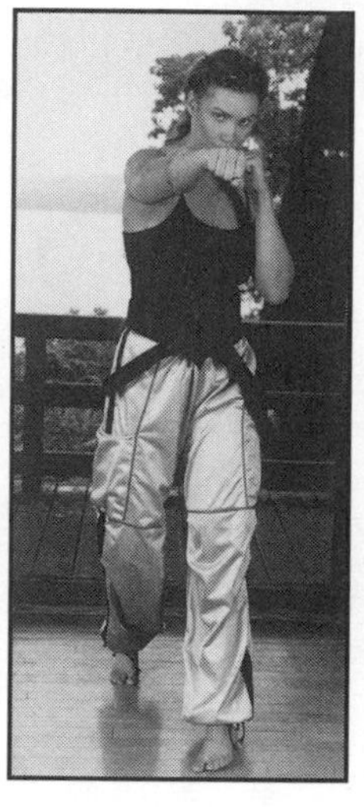

Cross.

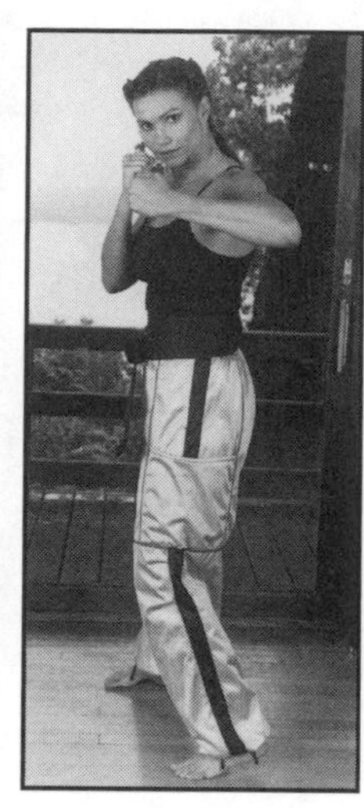

Hook.

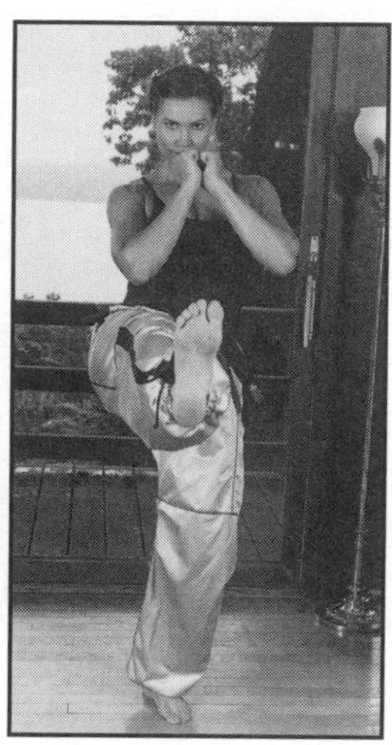

Front kick.

Side Kick (Lead Leg)/Jab/Cross/Hook/Upper Cut/ Axe Kick

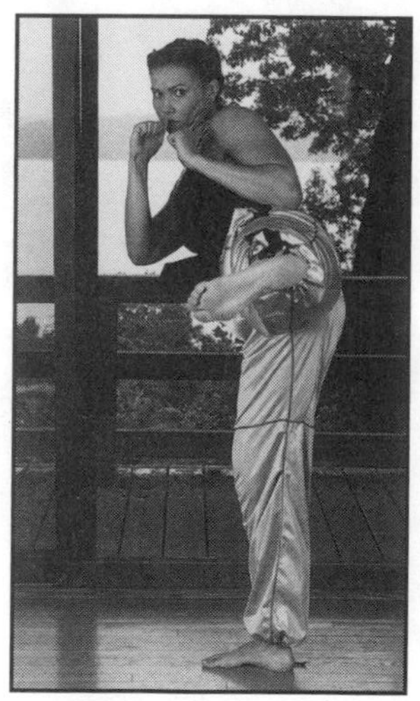

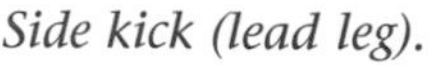

Side kick (lead leg).

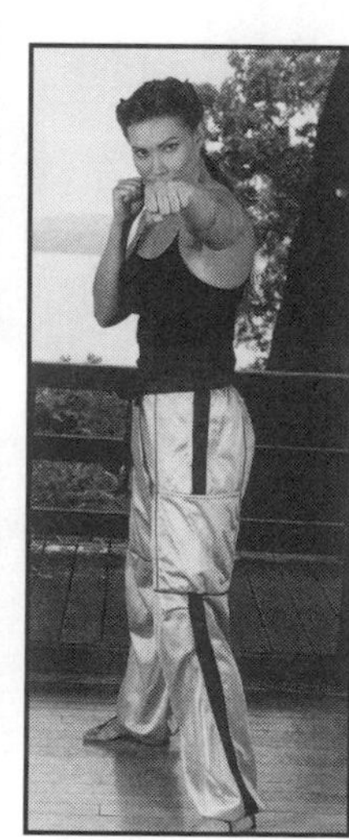

Jab.

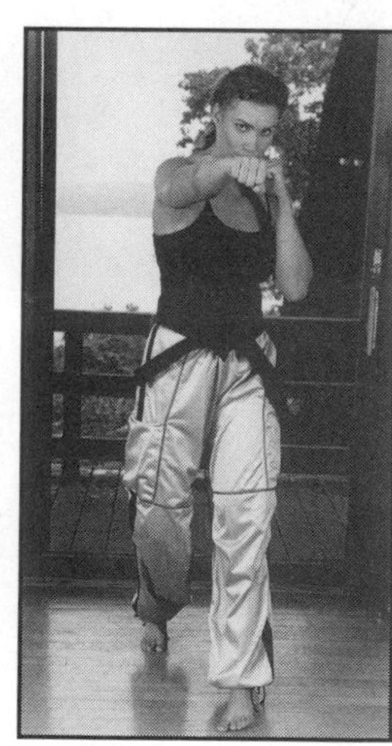

Cross.

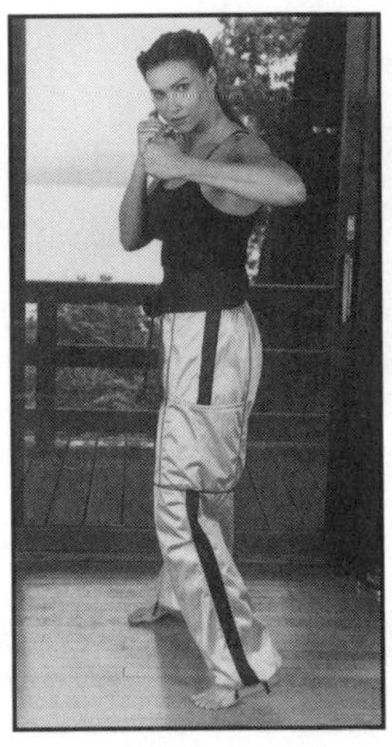

Hook.

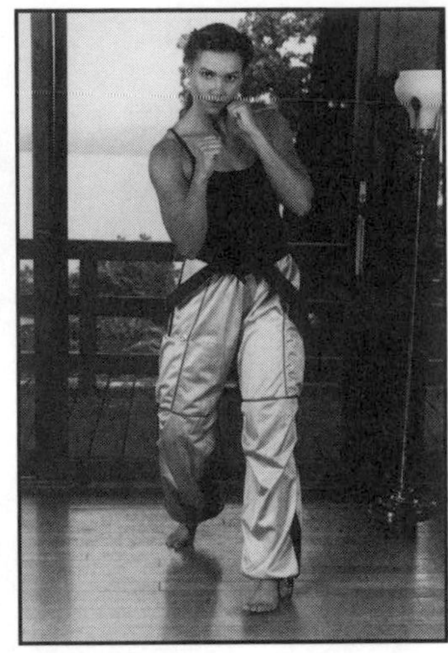

Upper cut.

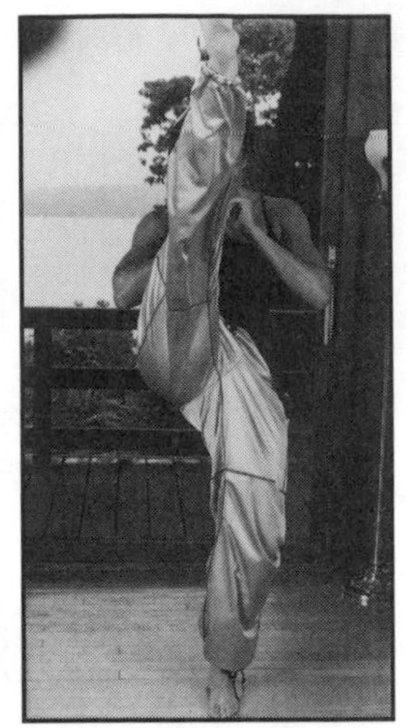

Axe kick.

Jab/Upper Cut/Hook/Front Kick (Rear Leg)

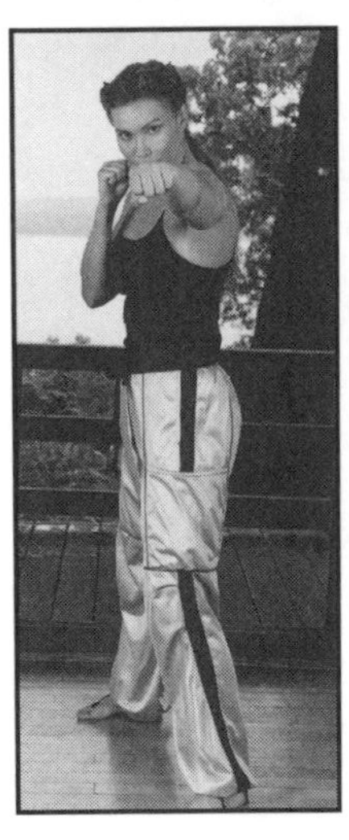

Jab.

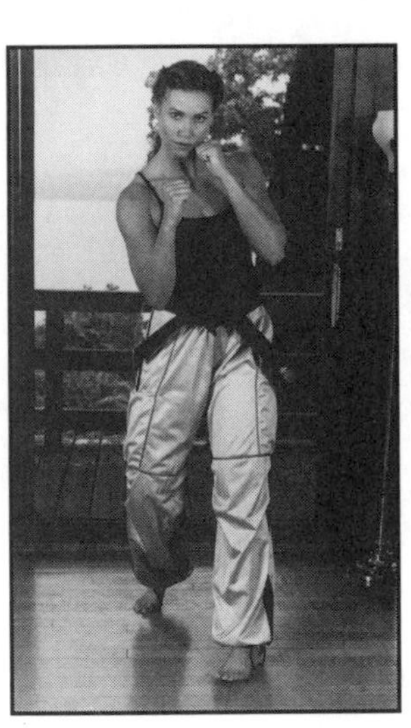

Upper cut.

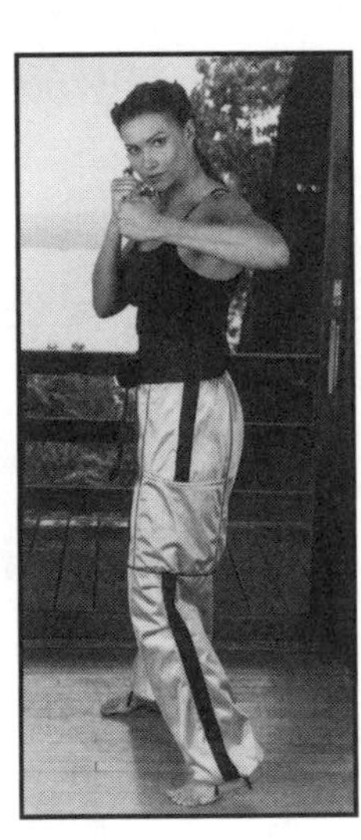

Hook.

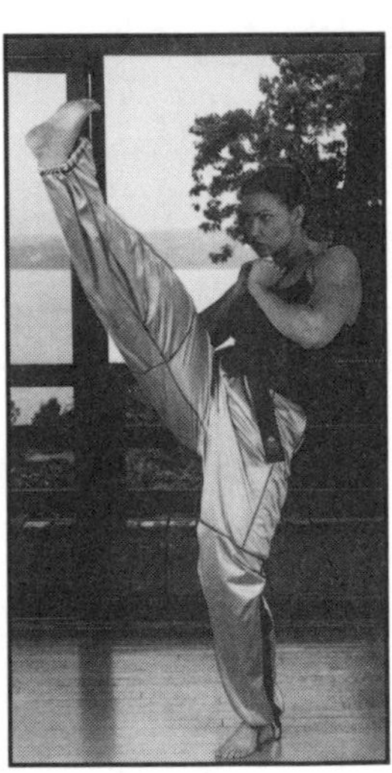

Front kick (rear leg).

The Least You Need to Know

- Kickboxing strengthens upper and lower muscles while delivering a great cardio workout.
- The right gear greatly increases the quality of your workout and greatly decreases the likelihood of injury.
- When punching, hit with your first two knuckles and leave a slight bend in your elbow so not to hyperextend it.
- Kicking height is determined by your flexibility level and the height of your chamber position.
- To increase your speed, start slow and practice, practice, practice.

Chapter 12

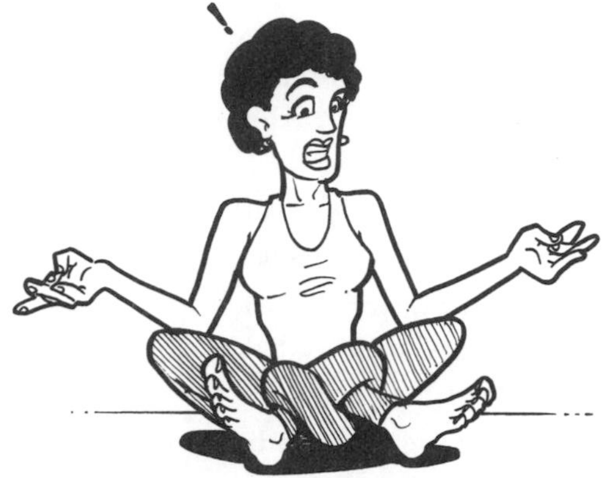

Have Floor, Will Lotus

In This Chapter

- Yoga elements
- Breathing exercises
- Hard-body asanas
- Hard-body yoga cool-down

When it comes to strength, flexibility, or cardio training, yoga has it all. Trust me, you'll sweat more body fat in a vigorous yoga practice then on any treadmill. In addition to its great workout benefits, yoga can soothe even the most savage stress beast. No matter how stressed out you may feel, a good practice will quickly put out the fuse to your time bomb. It doesn't surprise me because the purpose of yoga is to unite the mind, body, and spirit so that you can go with the flow of life's energy instead of fighting it upstream all the way. (I think that's better left to salmon.)

The goal in yoga is to achieve balance between strength, flexibility, and peace of mind. Enlightenment is yours when you become the master of balance on a daily basis. So, break out the mats—the only way to become a master is to practice.

Yoga Elements

A yoga practice session consists of five elements:

- **Proper breathing.** Focuses on nasal breathing techniques to release energy. The exercises concentrate on the exhalation to cleanse the lungs of stale air and toxins.
- **Proper relaxation.** Releases tension and keeps the body healthy. Each session should start and end with relaxation. Relax between poses to release energy.
- **Proper exercises.** Done in the form of *asanas*. The purpose is to create a balance in the body between strength and flexibility.
- **Positive thinking and meditation.** Puts you in touch with the real you that others might not see. Positive thinking clears your mind so that you have conscious control over your instincts.
- **Proper diet.** Made up of natural foods that keep the body strong and the mind calm. An ideal yoga diet is a vegetarian one.

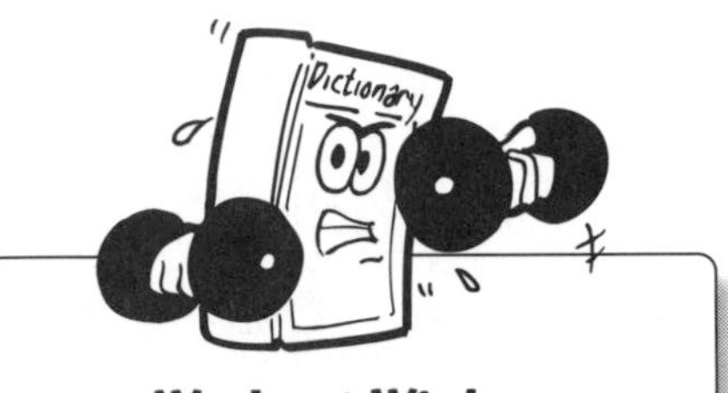

Workout Wisdom

Asanas are the exercises or poses in yoga that are designed to help you get control over your body.

Breathing Exercises

Most people use only about one third of their breathing capacity. By learning to use full breaths, you connect with your power source and automatically increase your energy level. Yoga breathing exercises, or pranayama, will help you gain control of your breath. They are done through the nose with the accent on exhalation to cleanse the lungs.

- **Full breathing.** Practice full breathing by sitting with your back straight, your shoulders back, and your legs crossed. Place one hand on your abdomen and one on your lower rib cage. As you take a breath, you should feel your abdomen and chest expand. (Imagine filling your abdomen, then your chest, and finally your upper back with air.) Do not let your body collapse as you exhale.
- **Single-nostril breathing.** Sit with your back straight, your shoulders back, and your legs crossed. Lower the second and third fingers of your right hand, keeping the others extended. This is called the Vishnu Mudra position.

1. Close your left nostril with your thumb, and inhale through your right nostril for a count of four. Exhale for a count of eight. Repeat four times.
2. Now close your right nostril with the two end fingers. Inhale through your left nostril for a count of four. Exhale for a count of eight. Repeat four times.

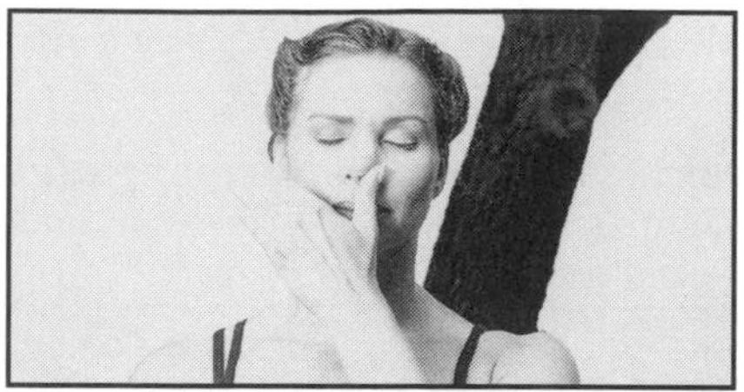

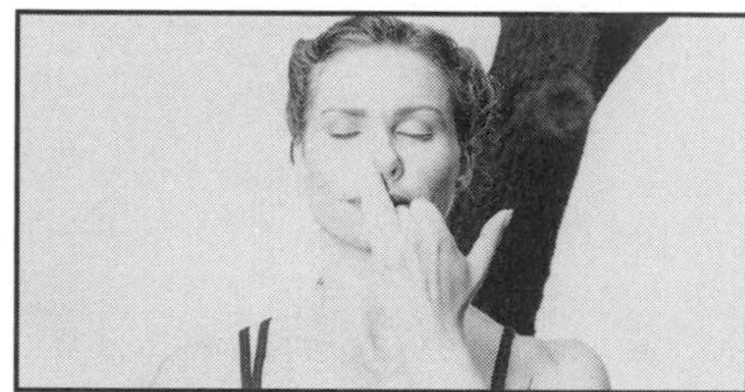

- **Alternate-nostril breathing** is done after single-nostril breathing exercises. Close your right nostril with your thumb, and inhale through your left nostril for a count of four. Close both nostrils and hold your breath for eight counts. Exhale through your right nostril for a count of eight. Close your left nostril with your two end fingers, and inhale through your right nostril for a count of four. Close both nostrils and hold your breath for eight counts. Exhale through your left nostril for a count of eight. Repeat the entire sequence a total of four times.
- **Kapalabhati** uses rapid breathing as a power cleanser. Force air out of your lungs by rapidly contracting your abdomen muscles. Do 4 rounds of 20 rapid pumps.

Hard-Body Sun Salutation

The Sun Salutation is the warm-up for your yoga session. Like any good warm-up, the Sun Salutation gets your body ready for yoga by raising your core temperature and lightly stretching your muscles. Do five to six Sun Salutations at the start of every session.

1. Inhale and extend your arms straight overhead.
2. Exhale, bend forward from the waist, and bring your palms to the floor.
3. Inhale look up, lift your chest, and flatten your back.

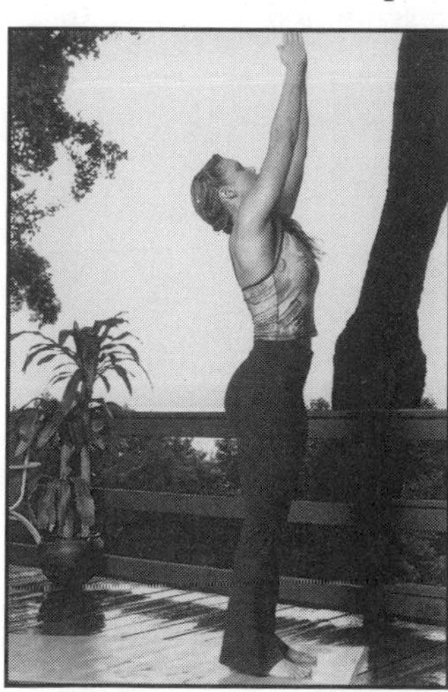

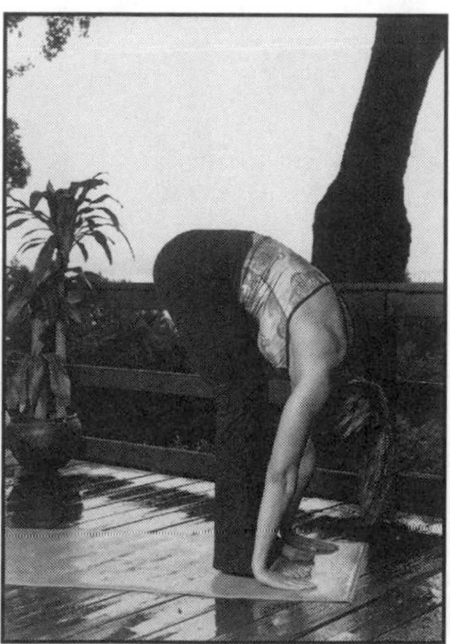

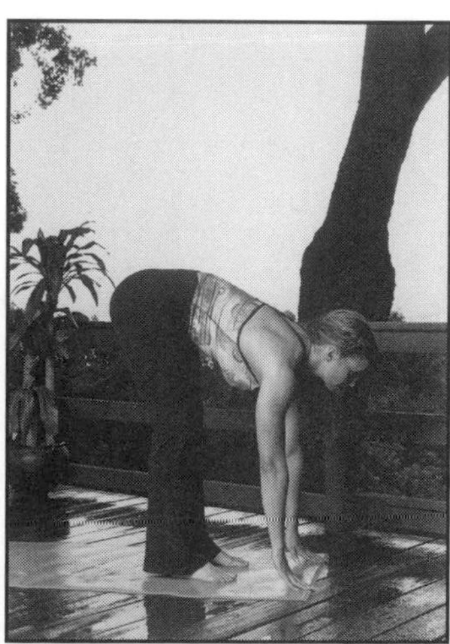

4. Exhale, shift your weight to your hands, and jump back extending your legs. You should be in a push-up position.
5. Inhale, lower your upper body by bending your elbows, and then push your upper body straight up (upward dog pose).

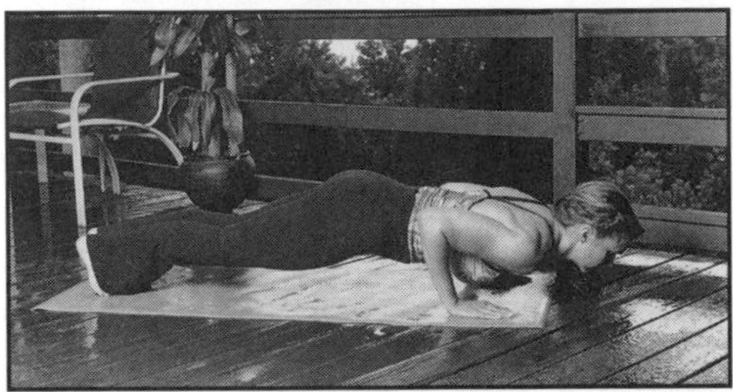

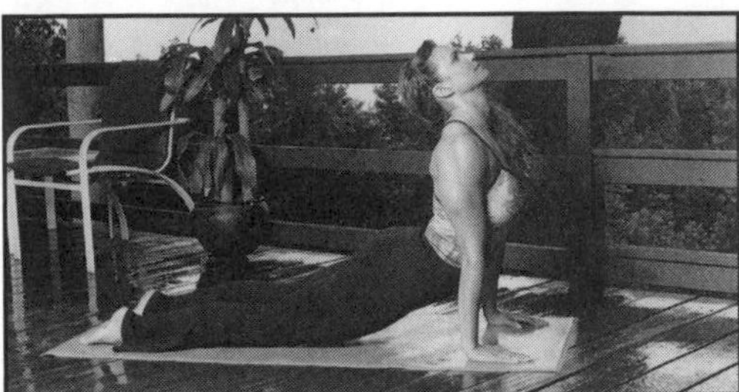

6. Exhale, turn your toes back under, and push up and back into an upside-down V (downward dog pose). Take five breaths in this position.
7. Inhale, look up, jump back up between your hands, and look up. (Land softly.)

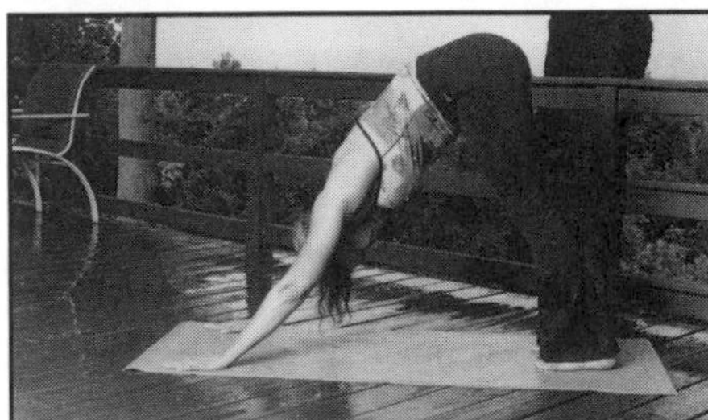

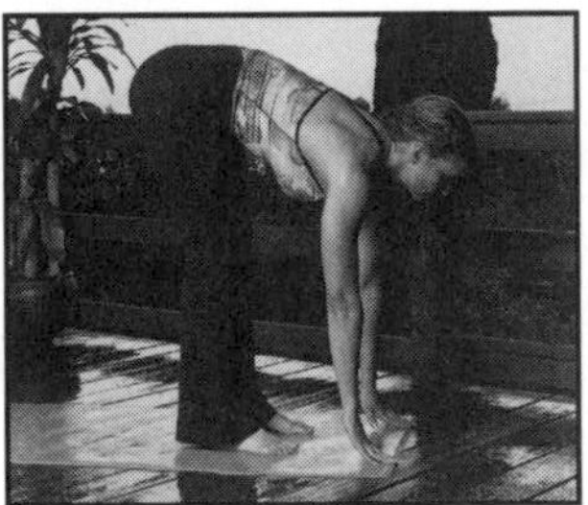

8. Exhale and bring your chest as close to your thighs as possible.
9. Inhale and power your arms straight up. Repeat entire sequence five more times.

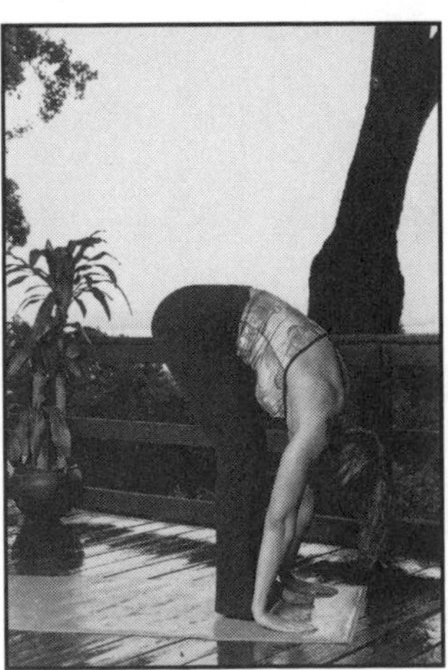

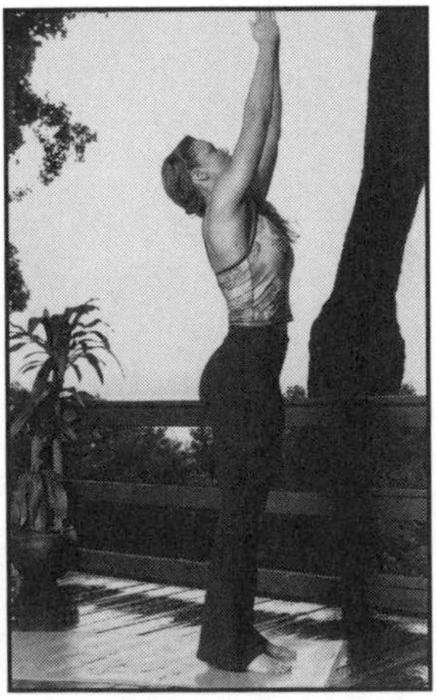

Standing Asanas

The standing poses develop strength and flexibility in your legs, hips, and spine, and improve overall balance. Do the three standing poses in the following order as a sequence.

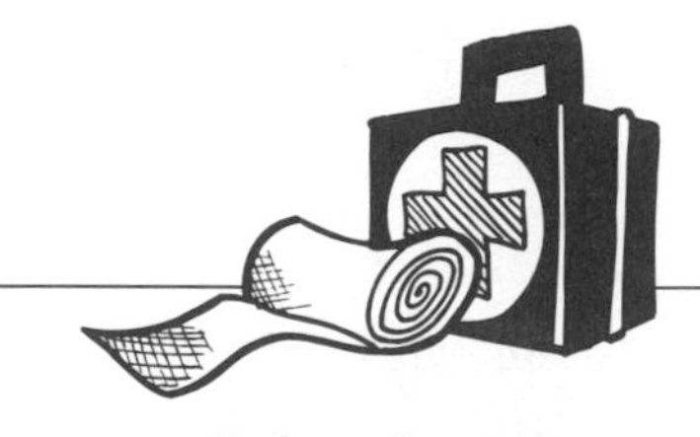

Safety Scoop

Make sure that your knee is pointed in the same direction as your foot in each pose.

Extended Triangle Pose

1. Inhale as you jump or step so that your feet are three feet apart. Turn your right foot out 90°. Turn your left foot in 30°. The heel of your right foot should line up with the arch of your left foot. Extend your arms out.
2. Exhale and bend to the right, with your arms, shoulders, and hips all in line. Grab your big toe with your first two fingers. Look up at your left thumb. Hold for five breaths. Inhale, come up with your arms out to the sides, and reverse your feet, with your left foot turned out 90° and your right foot turned in. Exhale and repeat the pose on the left side. Hold for five breaths.

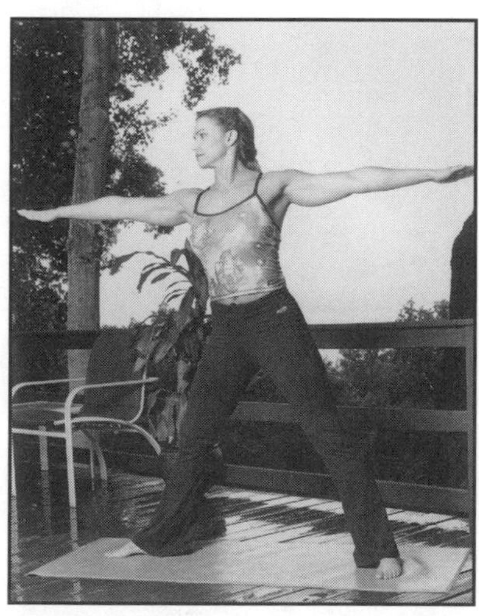

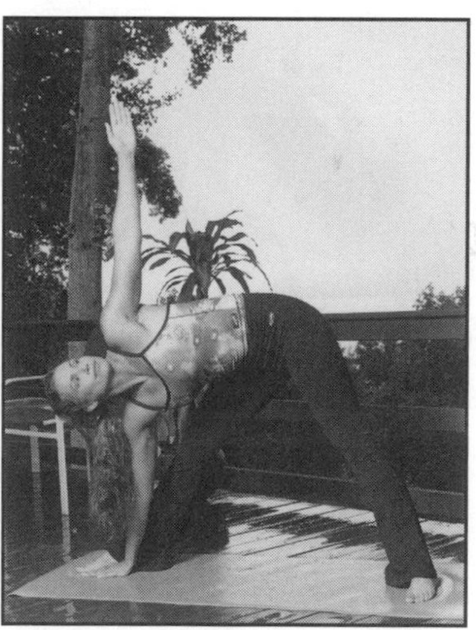

Side Angle Pose

1. Inhale, and jump or step into a wide stance with your feet parallel. Extend your arms out to the side. Your right foot is turned out 90°, and your left foot is turned in 30°. Your right foot and knee should point in the same direction as the extended hand. Exhale and lower into the pose by bending your right knee over your right ankle.

2. Place your right hand on the floor outside your right foot. Reach over your left ear with your left arm. Look up to your left hand. Hold for five breaths. Inhale and come up, with arms to your sides, and reverse feet. Exhale and repeat the pose on the left side. Hold for five breaths.

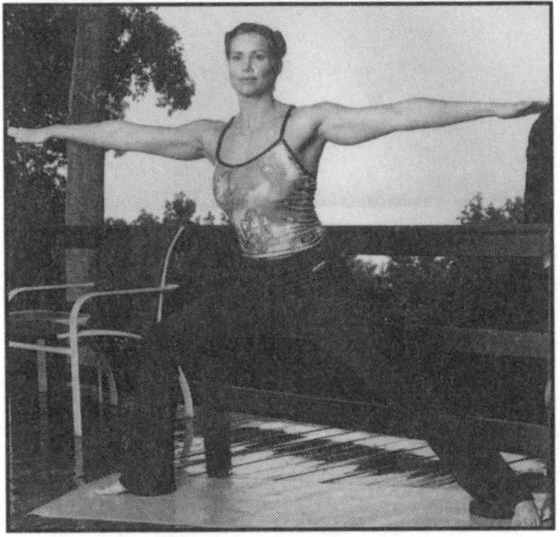

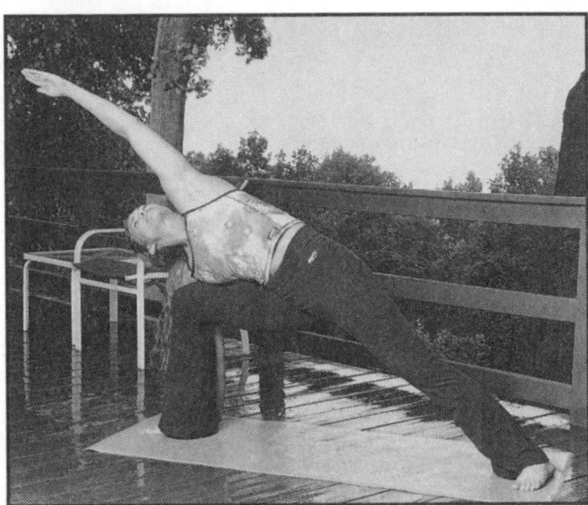

3. Inhale and come up, with arms straight to the sides. Turn your feet parallel, and face front.
4. Exhale and jump back to attention.

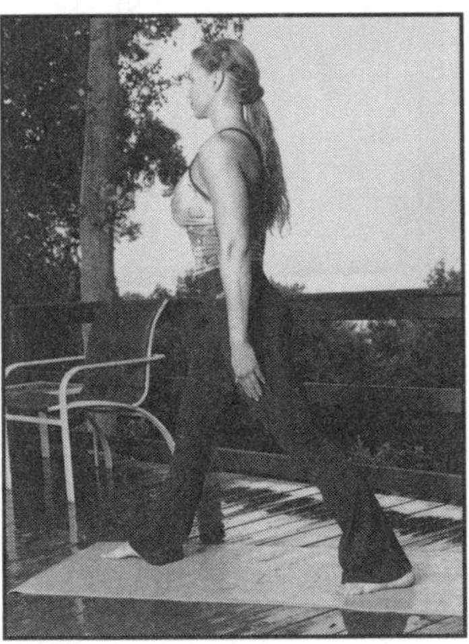

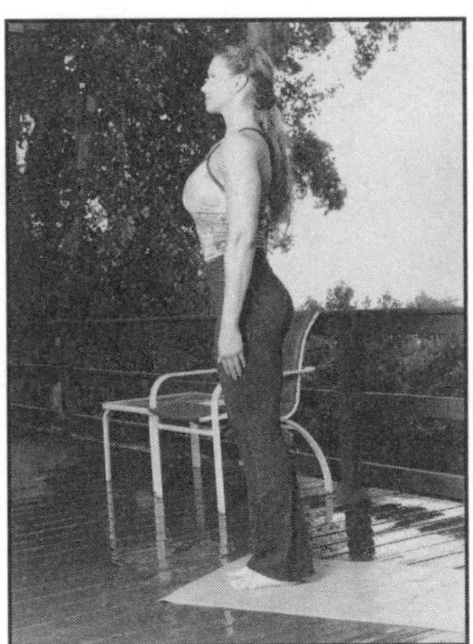

Backward-Bending Asanas

To be strong and flexible, your back has to be able to bend backward as well as forward. These poses will strengthen your back and spine muscles. Do wheel poses in the following order as a sequence:

1. Start lying flat on your back, with your knees bent, your feet flat on the floor near your glutes, and your hands grasping your ankles.
2. Exhale and push your hips up. Hold for five breaths. Inhale and lower to the starting position. Repeat two more times, and then go to step 3.

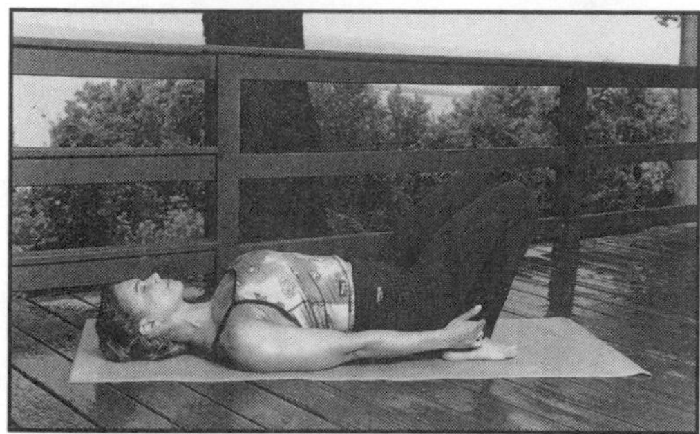
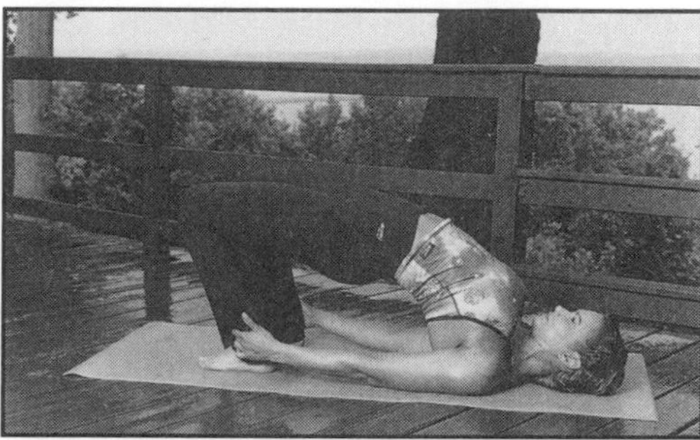

3. Lie flat on your back, with your knees bent and your feet close to glutes. Bend your arms, and turn your hands so that your fingers point toward your shoulder blades. Lay your hands flat on the floor behind your shoulders.
4. Exhale, lift your hips, arching your entire spine, and drop your head back. Hold for 10 breaths. Bend your arms and legs, and lower down slowly, shoulders first. Repeat two more times.

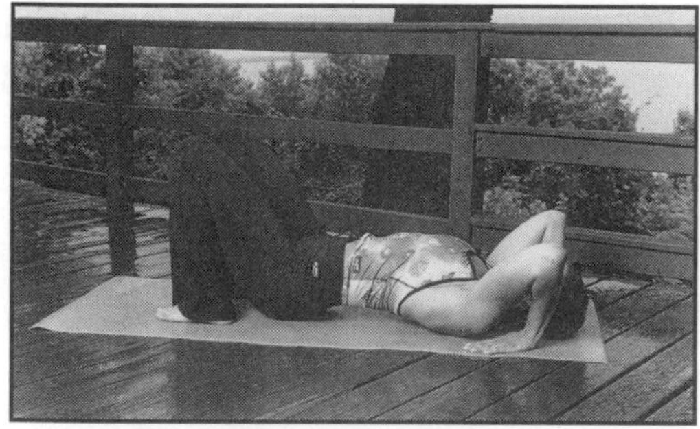
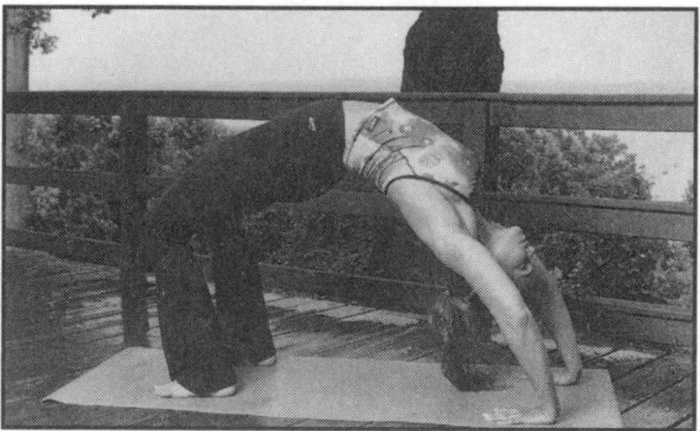

The Shoulder Cycle

The following poses will strengthen your entire body and improve the flexibility of the spine. Do the three poses in the following order as a sequence.

1. Start by lying flat on your back, with your arms by your sides. Inhale and bring your legs straight up.
2. Bring your hands under your glutes, with your fingers pointing toward your spine. Exhale and raise your body by letting your hands walk up your back and push you into position.

3. Continue to move your hands up your back until you are resting on your shoulders. Breathe normally, and keep your legs straight. Hold for 30 seconds.

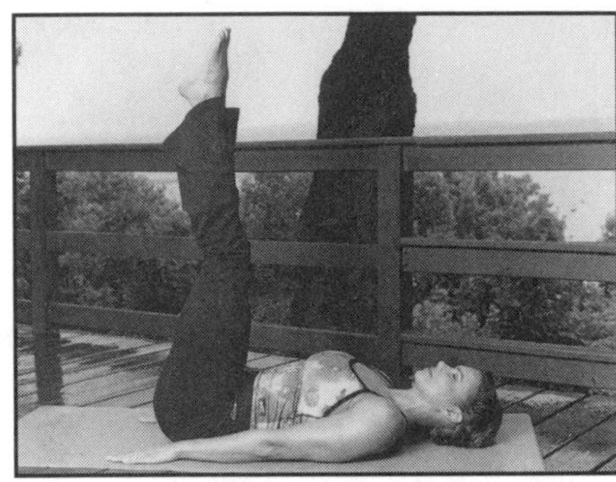

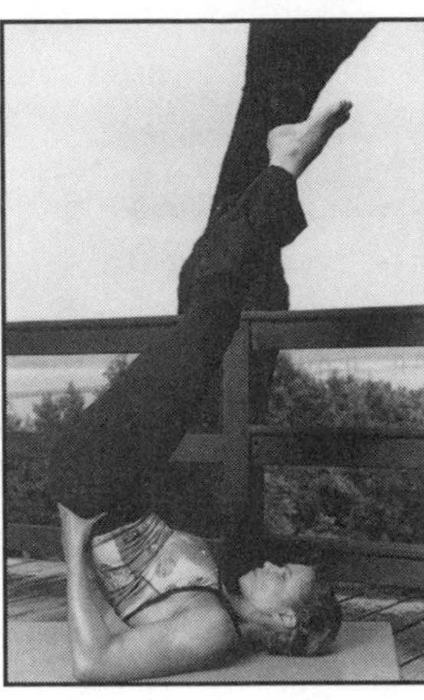

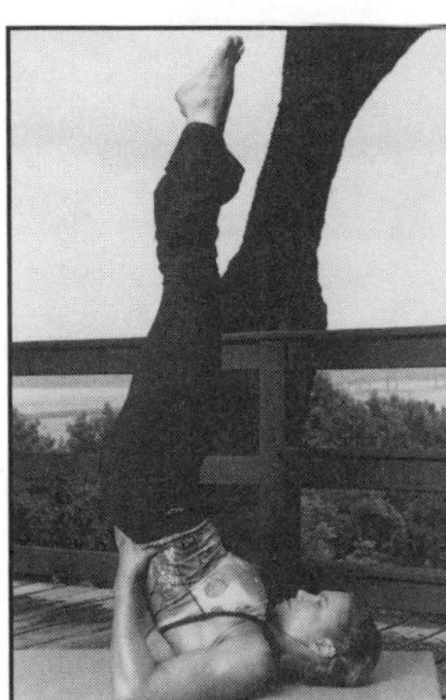

1. From a shoulder-stand pose, exhale and lower your feet to the floor behind your head.
2. Rest your toes on the floor, and then lay your arms down flat. Hold for 30 seconds. (If you can't lower to the floor, keep your hands on your back for support.)
3. Lower your knees to the floor by your ears. Hook your arms over your legs. Hold for 10–30 seconds. Straighten your legs and do a reverse plough order. When in a shoulder stand, roll out slowly one vertebra at a time until you're lying laying flat on the floor.

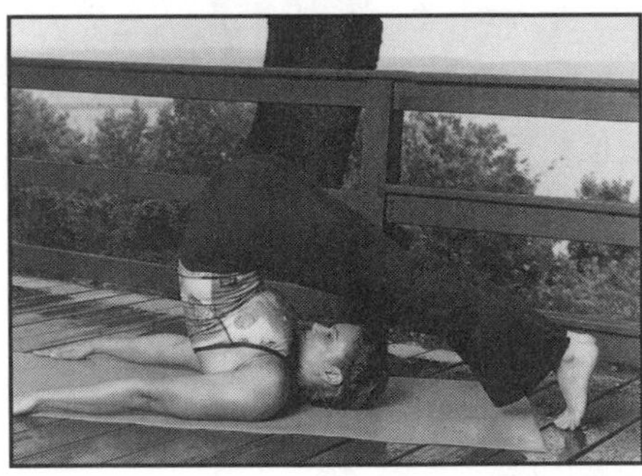

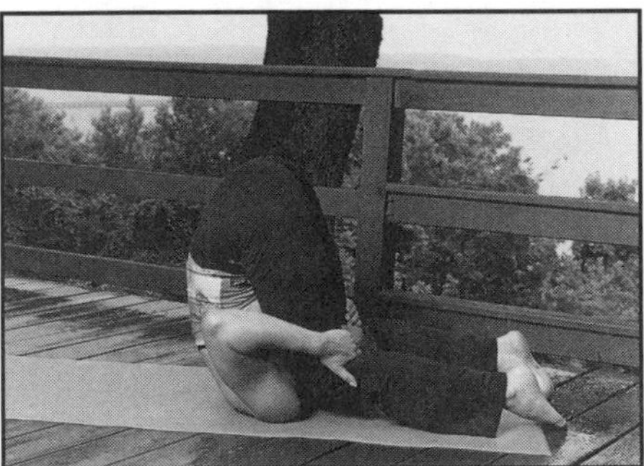

Hard-Body Yoga Cool-Down

My cool-down routine will relax your body, calm your mind, and energize your spirit. I love this routine so much that I used it in my *Body Enlightenment* video series and currently use it to end all my classes.

Start by centering yourself. Focus on your breath as you move in and out of each pose. Imagine moving through water so that each movement is slow and fluid. This cool-down routine can be done at the end of any workout session.

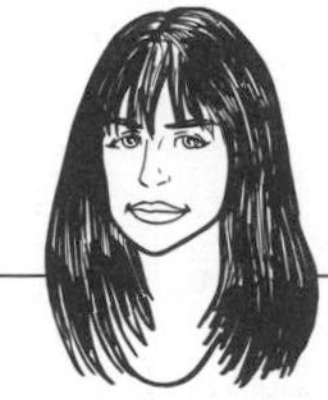

Jourdan's Gems

Doing a yoga routine as a cool-down after weight training will increase your muscles' range of motion and also speed up their recovery time.

1. Start by taking three deep breaths to center yourself.
2. Exhale and let your arms float out and up to the sides until they meet in the center overhead. With your palms touching, lower your hands in front to chest level, and hold them in a prayer pose.
3. Inhale. Exhale and raise your hands up. Reach up to lengthen the spine, and then arch back. Hold for five breaths.

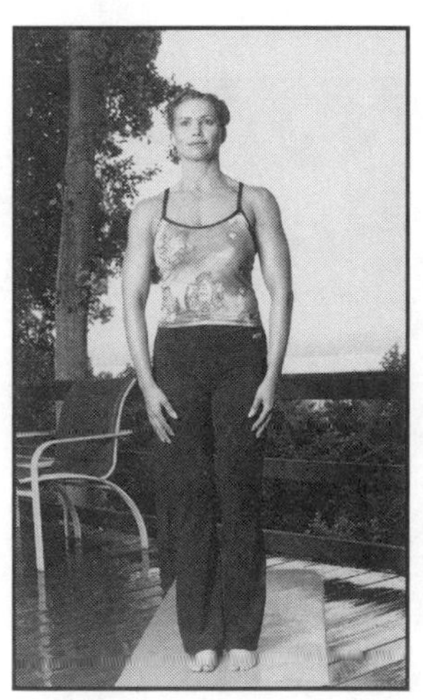

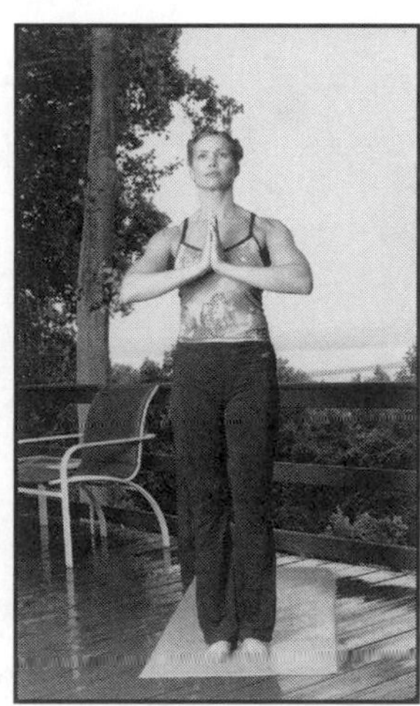

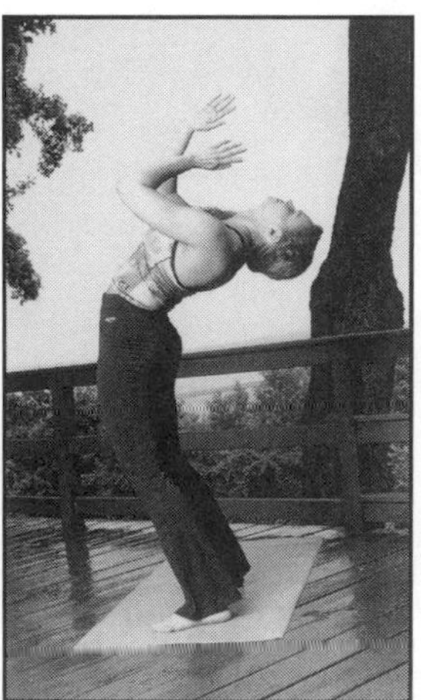

4. Exhale and reach up, reach forward, and reach down, placing your hands flat on the floor on either side of your feet.

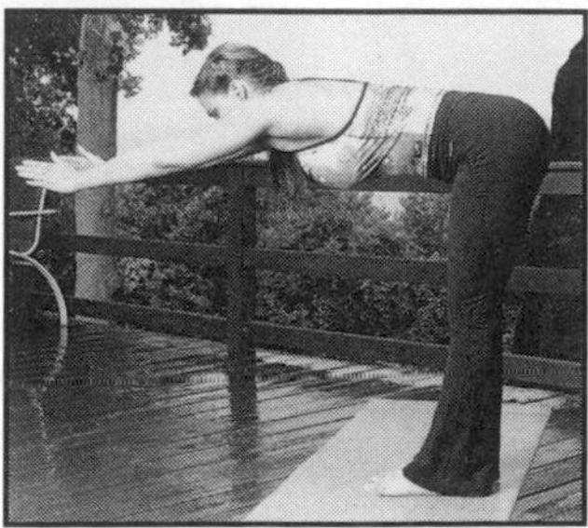

5. Inhale. Exhale and extend your right leg back into a deep lunge. Hands are outside the left knee, and head is up.
6. Inhale. Exhale and extend your left leg back and place it next to your right leg. Hold for five breaths.

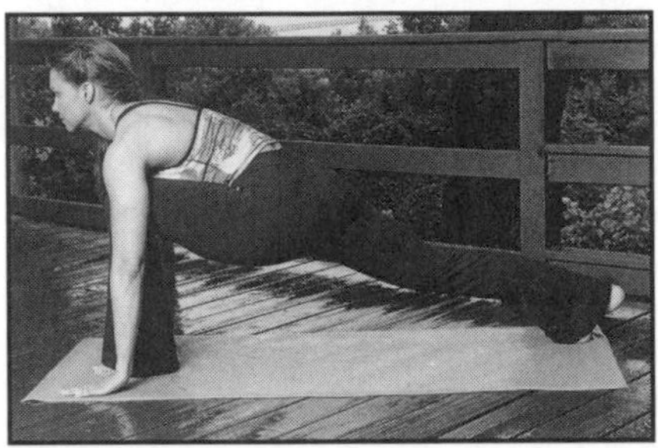
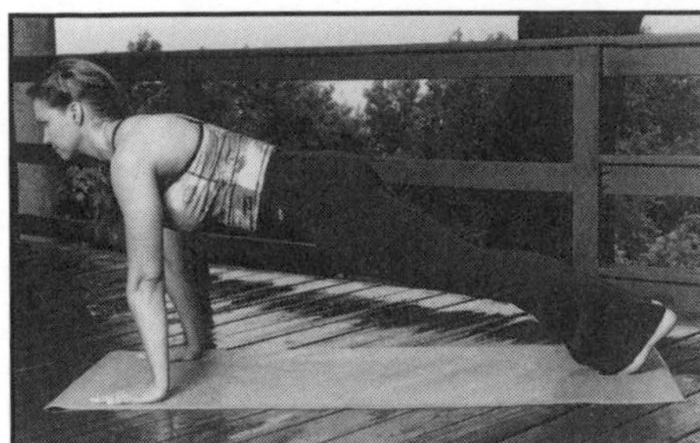

7. Inhale and lower your upper body down.
8. Exhale and press up. Repeat strength moves two more times.

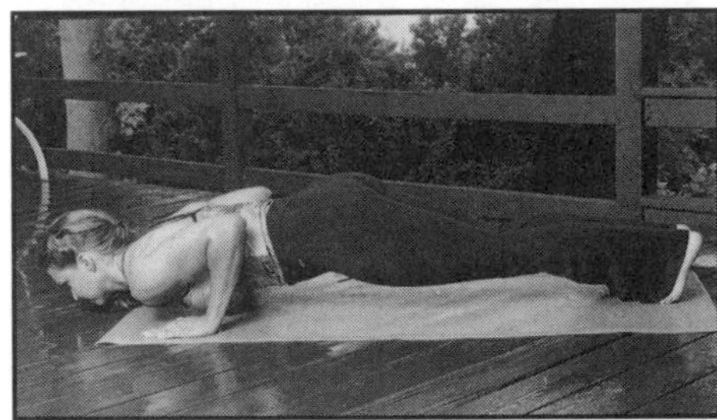
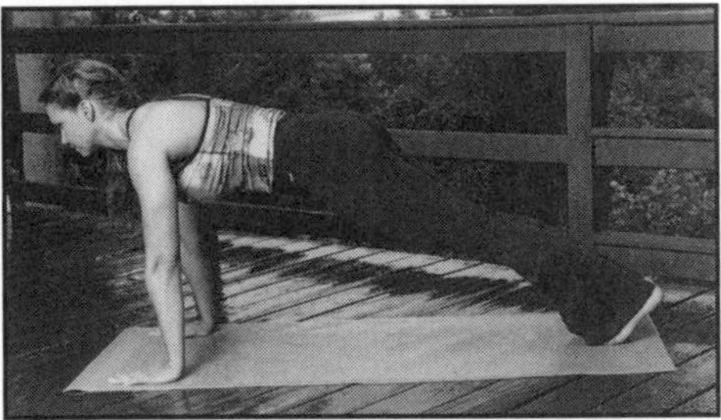

9. Inhale and lower your body down and up into an upward dog pose.
10. Exhale and press back into a downward dog pose. Hold for five breaths.

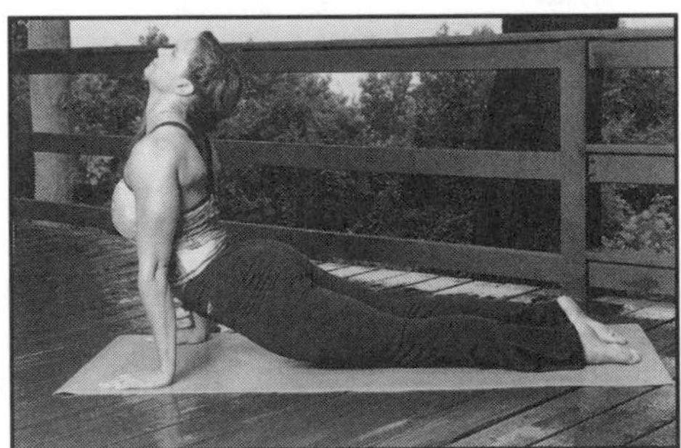
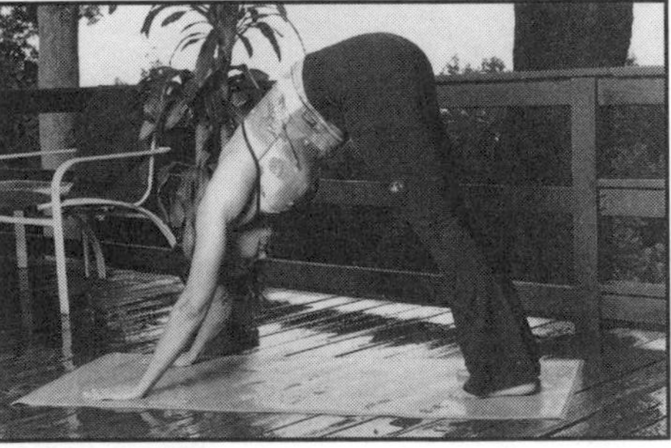

11. Exhale and step forward with your right leg. You should be in a lunge position, with your hands on either side of your right knee.
12. Inhale. Exhale, and bring your left leg up and place it next to your right leg.

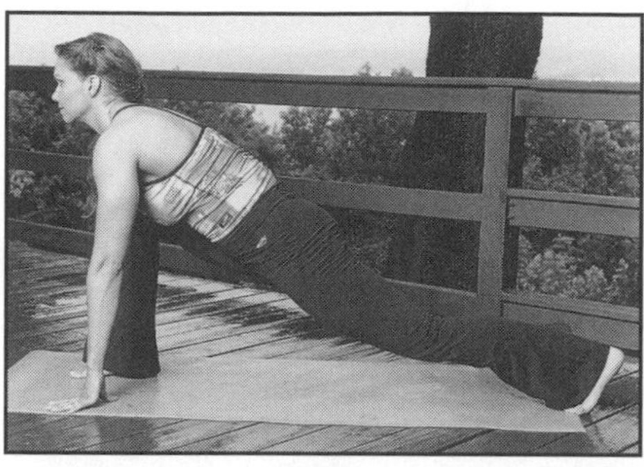

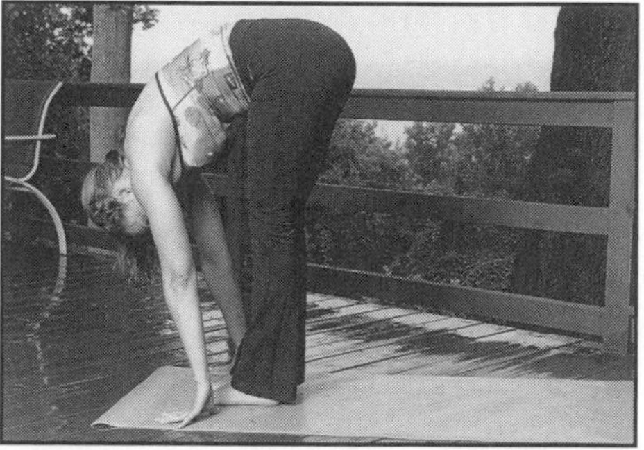

13. Inhale. Exhale, bend your knees, and lower down. Sit down on the floor and extend your legs forward. Your back, legs, and arms should all be straight.
14. Inhale. Exhale and raise your arms out and up. Bend forward from waist, and grasp the outer edge of your feet; bring your chest as close to your thighs as possible. Hold for five breaths.

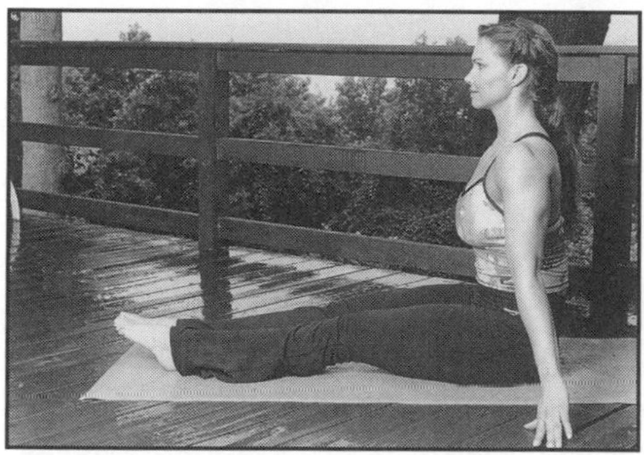

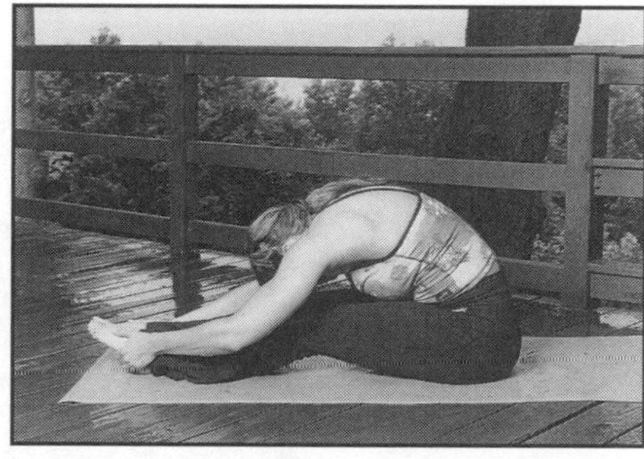

15. Exhale and rise up. Bring your hands behind you, with fingers pointing away from you.
16. Inhale. Exhale and raise your hips as high as possible, with weight evenly distributed between your hands and heels. Hold for five breaths.

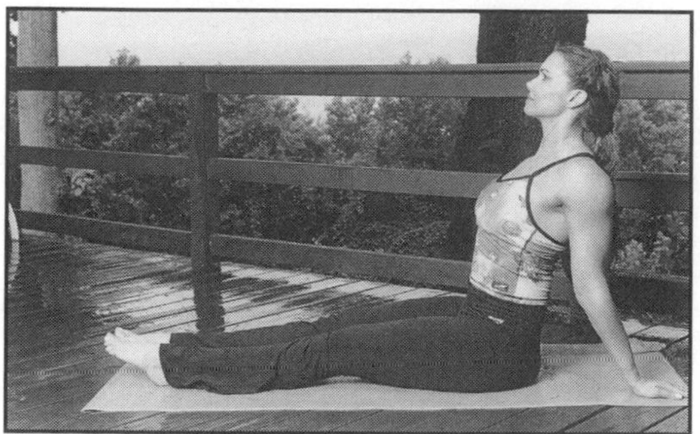

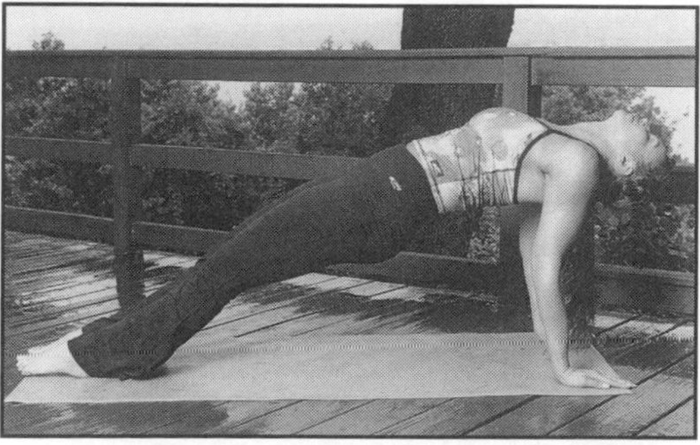

17. Exhale and lower down. Bring your legs into a straddle position, with your back straight and your hands inside your legs.
18. Inhale. Exhale and walk your hands to the side as far as your range of motion allows. Hold for five breaths.

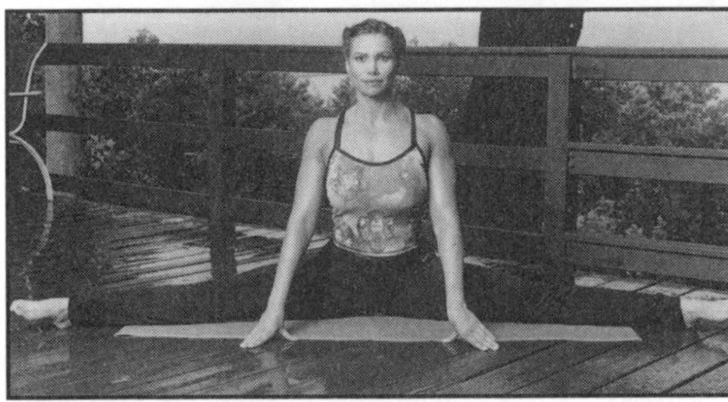

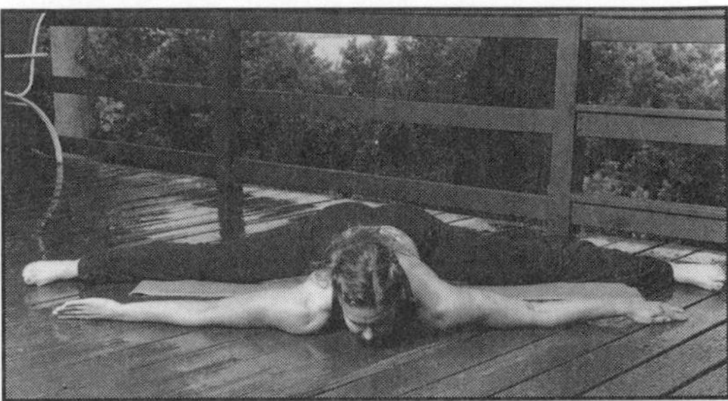

19. Exhale and walk your hands back. Bring your feet in and place them sole to sole, with your knees out to the side. Inhale. Exhale, pull your feet in, and push your shoulders back. Hold for five breaths.
20. Exhale and extend your legs forward. Cross your left leg over your right, and place your right arm inside your left knee. Inhale. Exhale and twist your upper body to the left as far as you can. Hold for five breaths.
21. Exhale and counter-twist your upper body to opposite side. Release and uncross legs. Do a spinal twist to the left side, hold for five breaths, and then counter-twist to the right.

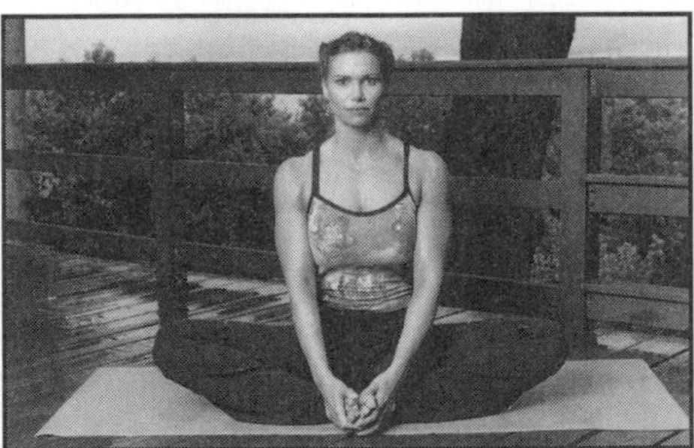

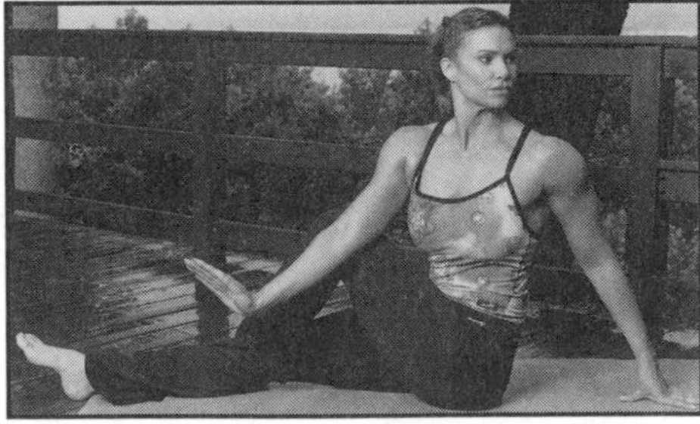

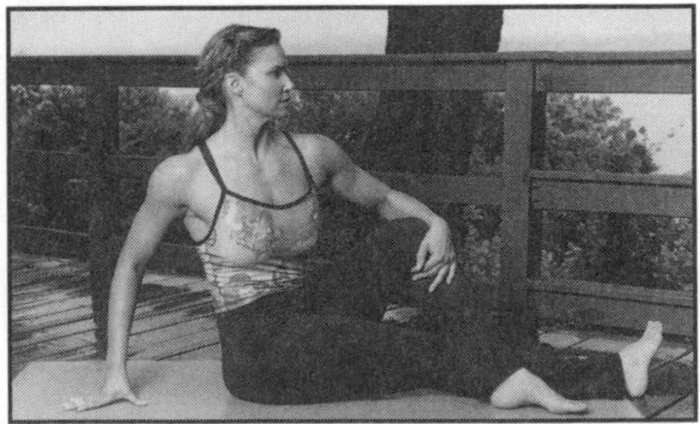

22. Uncross your legs, bring your body forward, and sit over your feet.
23. Inhale. Exhale. With your chest on your thighs the entire time, rise up, straightening your legs as much as your range of motion allows.

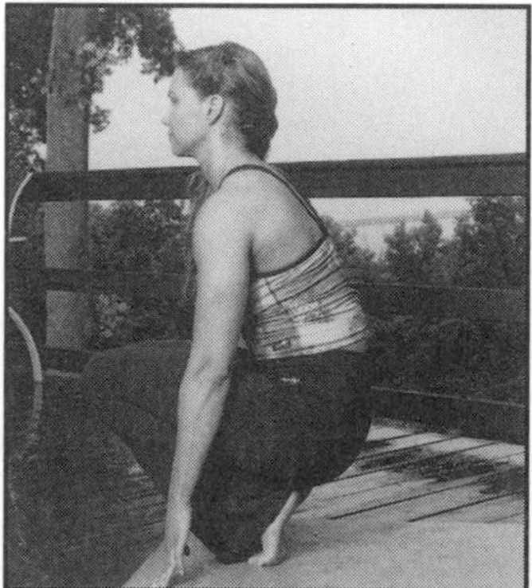

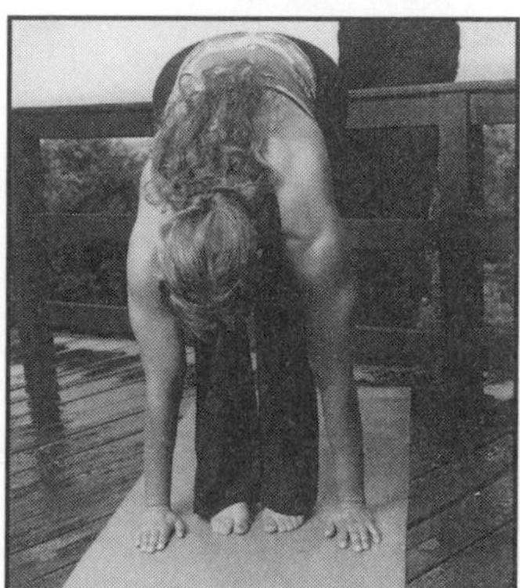

24. Inhale. Exhale and raise your upper body, reaching forward, upward, and then back. Hold for five breaths.
25. Exhale and reach up. Join your hands together and lower them in front to chest level; hold in a prayer pose. Close your eyes and take five deep breaths. Now open your eyes to release the darkness and embrace the light.

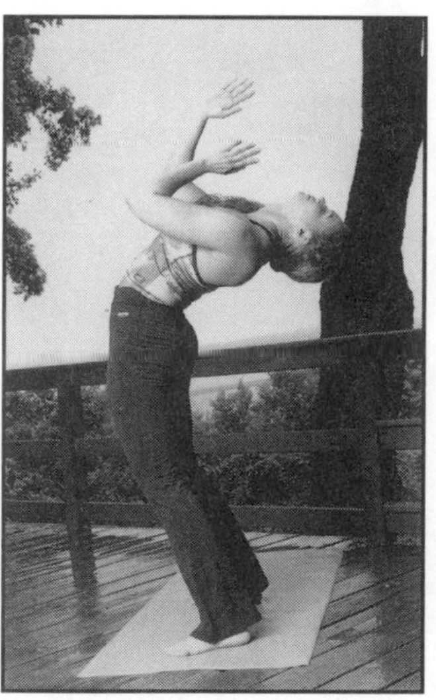

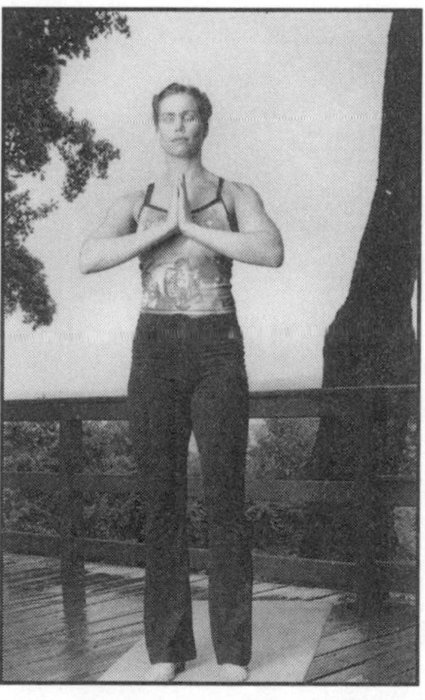

In addition to making you feel great, yoga will also give you the benefits of strength, flexibility, and cardio training. Practicing yoga two to three times a week in addition to your other training will maximize your results and go a long way to increasing your peace of mind.

The Least You Need to Know

- When you practice yoga, you strive to achieve balance between the mind, body, and spirit.
- Learning to use full breaths will automatically increase your energy level.
- When it comes to strength training, flexibility training, and cardio training, yoga does it all.
- A morning yoga practice will energize your day, and an evening practice will release the stress from your day.

Chapter 13

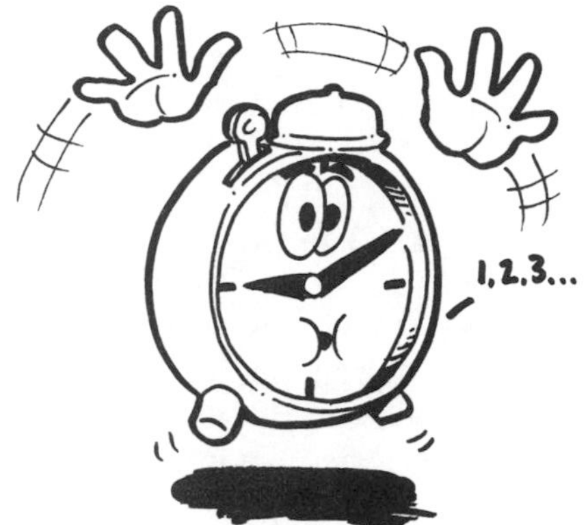

Ten-Minute Ticket to Tone

In This Chapter

- Time-saver tips for faster results
- Quick toning lower-body routine
- Quick toning upper-body routine
- Quick and easy ab routine

The following routines are short, sweet, and serious. The Ticket to Tone Routines can be done alone or together any time for a quick hard-body pump (like before you hit the beach). Adding them to your regular training sessions will raise the intensity and bring new sizzle to your workouts.

My goal was to create nonstop high-rep mini workouts utilizing multiangular movements that can also be combined to create the ultimate 30-minute cutting and shaping workout. Doing a light version of the same muscle group routine later in the day after an intense early training session helps to eliminate next-day soreness.

Just add a warm-up and cool-down, and you have a power-packed mini workout that'll pump your muscles, knock out body fat, and energize your mind and body in as little as 10 minutes.

Time-Saver Form

The three things to always remember when doing these or any other exercise routines are these:

- Form
- Intensity
- Resistance

Always maintain perfect form throughout the exercises. This will give you the maximum results in minimal time and will help prevent injuries. The second key is intensity. You will not benefit from the exercises, even if your form is perfect, if you're not working hard enough. You should be struggling for the last few reps. Several ways to increase the intensity are by slowing the tempo, contracting the muscles at the top of the movement, and increasing the resistance. The only time you increase the resistance level is when you need to increase the intensity. Never sacrifice form simply to lift more weight.

Triple-Crown Leg Routine

I've combined three of my trademark moves—the step-up lunge, the elevated side squat, and the around the world—to form my Triple-Crown Leg Routine. You can do one set to give your legs a quick pump, or experience the full effect with three supercharged sets. All you'll need is a step with risers and hand weights. Raising the elevation of the step will raise the intensity. Start by doing the entire routine with three-pound weights. Increase to a five-pound weight for the second and third sets. For a real challenge, use a 5-pound weight for the first two exercises, and increase to 8 to 10 pounds for the last exercise.

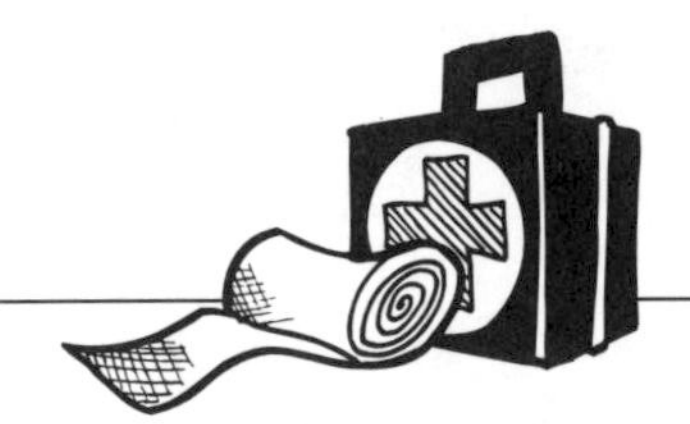

Safety Scoop

Landing softly on your feet when using a step will minimize knee stress.

Find your level in the following table to determine the amount of sets and reps you need to do. Increase to the next level only if your current level is no longer a challenge and you can maintain perfect form at the higher level.

Level	Reps	Sets
Beginner	10	2
Intermediate	15	3
Advanced	20	3

Step-Up Lunge

1. Start by standing behind a step, with your arms by your sides, holding weights if you want.
2. Place your left foot on the step, and lift your right knee as if climbing stairs. (Hint: Lift the knee high for better glute work.)

3. Lower down and lunge back. Curl your left arm when the right knee goes up, and curl your right arm when the right leg lunges back. Repeat for desired reps.
4. Switch sides, and repeat for desired reps. Go directly to the elevated side squat.

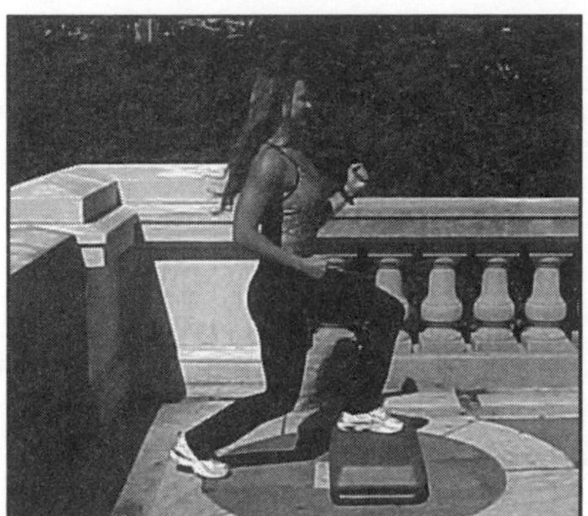
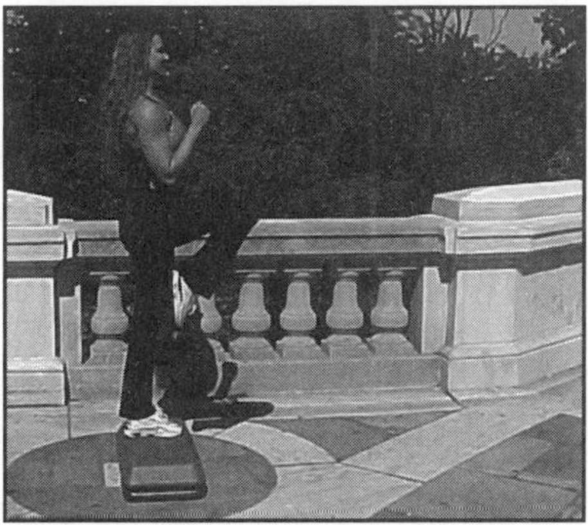

Elevated Side Squat

1. Go to the left side of the step. Start with your left foot on the step and your arms by your sides. Bend at the hips, and squat back until you feel a stretch in your quadriceps.
2 Then shift your weight to your left leg, and rise up on the step while elevating your right leg; arms are out and up to the side. You should be standing with your back straight and your shoulders back.
3. Lower slowly to the starting squat position. Repeat for desired reps. Switch sides and repeat for desired reps. Go directly to the around the world exercise.

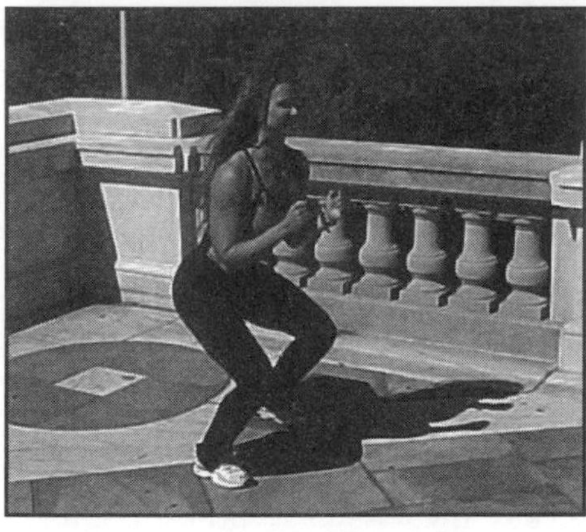
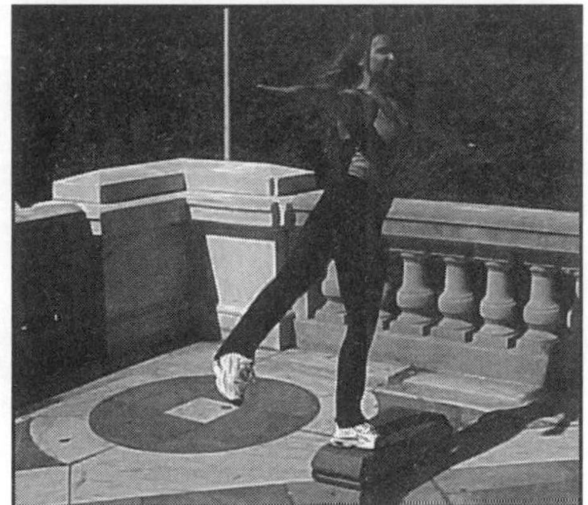

Around the World

1. Start with your left foot on the step and your knee bent so that your knee is directly over your foot and your thigh is parallel to the floor.
2. Now extend your right leg as far back as possible. Your weight should be evenly distributed between the heel of the front foot and ball of the rear. Your upper body should be square over your hips, with a straight back, shoulders back, and arms by your sides, holding weights. (Hint: For higher intensity and maximum results, keep your left knee bent and your thigh parallel to the floor throughout the reps.)
3. Lower and rise on your rear leg for desired reps.
4. Keeping your left foot on the step, turn your body a quarter turn to the right. Your body should be sideways and parallel to the step.
5. Squat down and back, as if you were trying to sit on a stool that is just out of reach. Curl your arms to your shoulders, and your contract biceps at the top position during the squat. Palms should be facing each other.
6. Rise to the starting position. Repeat for desired reps.
7. With your left foot still on the step, turn your body another quarter turn to the right. You should be facing the back, with your arms by your sides and the step behind you. Keeping your upper body erect with shoulders back and chest forward will help your balance.
8. Bend your rear leg, and go as low as your range of motion allows.

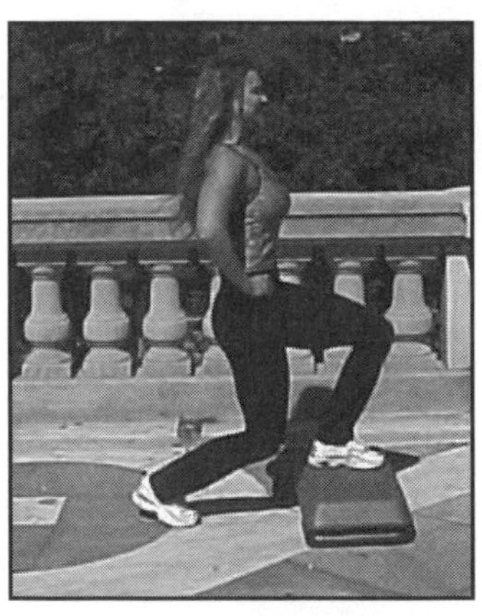

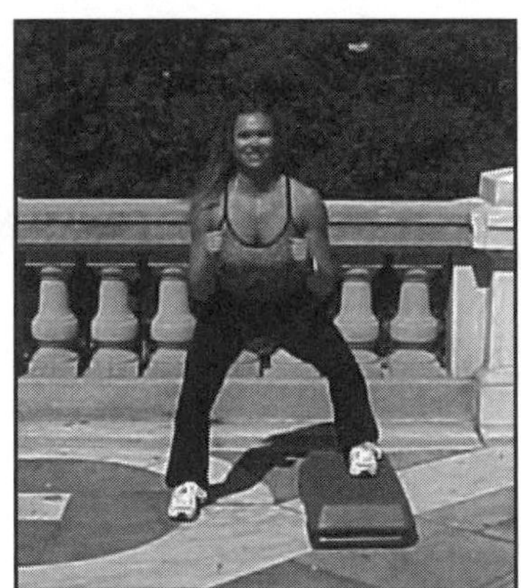

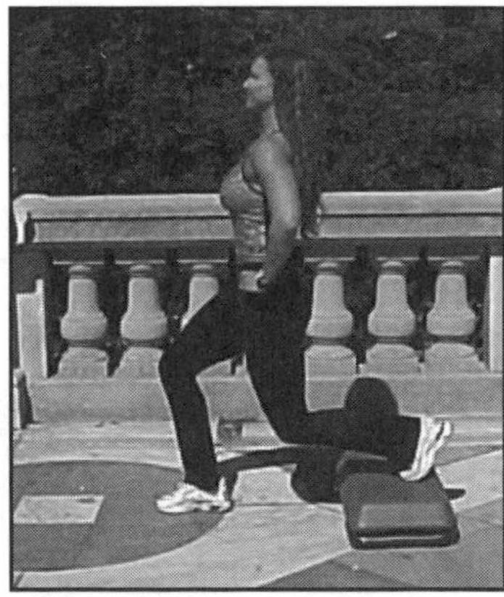

9. Rise to the starting position. Keep your legs bent during entire move. Repeat for desired reps.
10. Now turn your body a quarter turn back to the left, and repeat the squat as in step 4 for desired reps.

11. Finally, turn your body another quarter turn to the left. You should now be facing front again. Repeat the lunge as in step 1 for desired reps.
12. Switch legs and repeat on the other side.

Congratulations! You have just taken your legs around the world and completed my Triple-Crown Leg Routine.

Upper-Body Blast Routine

My Upper-Body Blast Routine utilizes super setting and drop setting techniques so you'll be able to work nonstop and exercise your upper-body muscles in only 10 minutes.

For this routine you'll need a light, a medium, and a heavy set of dumbbells—three pounds, five pounds, and eight pounds—to start. (See the "Dynamite Delt Routine" a little later in this chapter for the vertical raise exercise description and photo. See Chapter 8, "Hard-Body Tower of Power," for all other exercise descriptions and photos.)

Jourdan's Gems

Any time exercise form begins to suffer, it's time to immediately drop to a lighter weight and continue reps at that weight.

Find your level in the following table to know how many sets and reps you need to do. Then do the following exercises in order from start to finish without a rest in between.

- Bent-over row super set—heavy weight
- Forward/reverse flyes—medium or light weight
- Delt press super set—medium to heavy weight
- Lateral raise—medium weight
- Vertical raise—light weight
- Forward curls—medium to heavy weight
- Side curls—medium to heavy weight
- Jcurls—light to medium weight
- Overhead press—medium weight
- Kickback variation—medium or light weight

Level	Reps	Sets
Beginner	10	2
Intermediate	15	3
Advanced	20	3

Dynamite Delt Routine

Whether in a swimsuit or a sweater, you can always spot a great set of shoulders. I'm talking curvaceous and cut. My Dynamite Delt Routine hits the anterior and medial delts from various angles. Working the shoulders from these angles creates a defined and streamlined look. Check the following table to see how many reps and sets you should be doing of the exercises that follow.

Level	Reps	Sets
Beginner	10	2
Intermediate	15	3
Advanced	20	3

1. To do a lateral raise, start with your back straight, your shoulders back, your chest forward, and your arms in front, holding dumbbells.
2. Raise the dumbbells to shoulder height, and tip downward at the top position.
3. Lower slowly and repeat for desired reps. Go to the vertical raise.

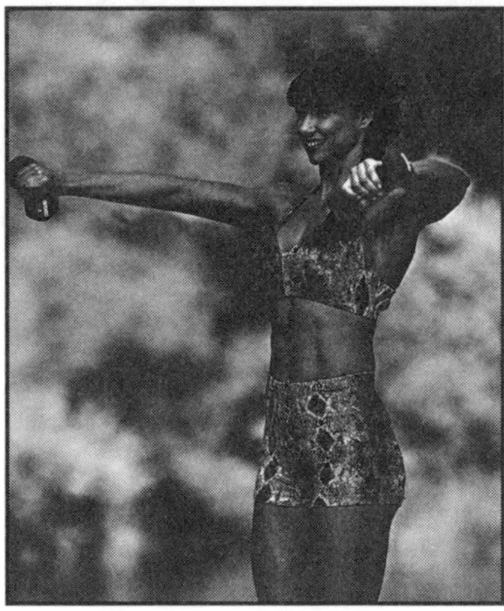

1. To do a vertical raise, straighten your arms, and turn the dumbbells to a neutral position.
2. Raise dumbbells 30° inward to face height.
3. Lower and repeat for desired reps. Go to triangle raise.

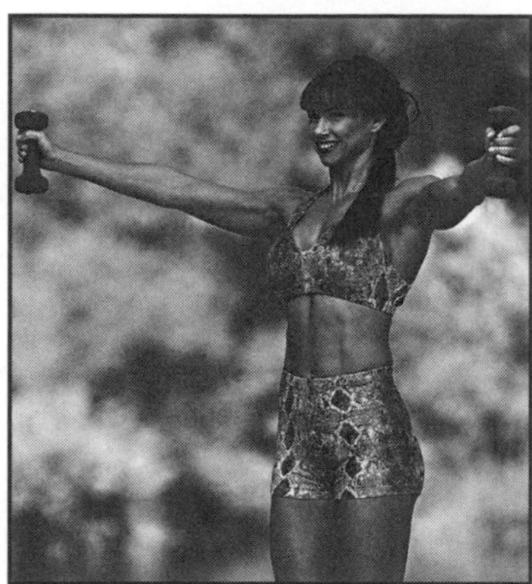

1. To do a triangle raise, keep your arms straight, and raise the dumbbells forward and upward.
2. Turn the dumbbells inward at the top position.
3. Lower and repeat for desired reps.

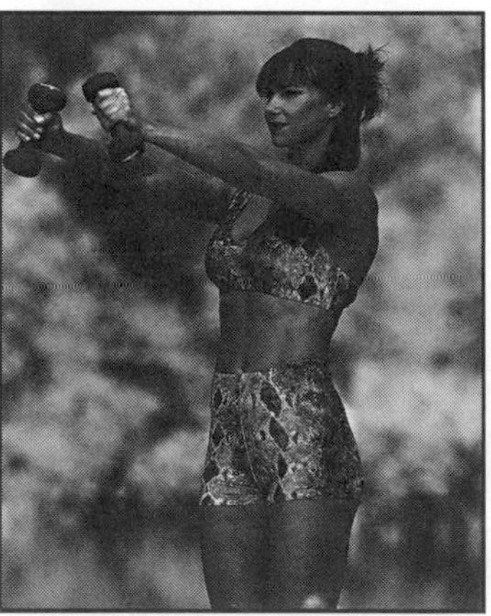

Six-Minute Six-Pack Routine

This whole routine weighs in at a hefty six minutes in length. (There goes the "I don't have time" excuse!) Find your level in the following table to see how many reps you will be doing.

Level	Reps	Hold Count
Beginner	10	10 seconds
Intermediate	15	15 seconds
Advanced	20	20 seconds

1. **Upper ab curl** Lie flat, with your knees bent and your toes raised. (Press the weight into your heels as you curl forward.)
2. Place your hands on either side of your head, with your fingertips touching. Exhale and lift your shoulders off the floor by curling your abs forward.
3. Squeeze the abs for one second, and then lower to the starting position.
4. Repeat for desired reps. Go to the combined crunch.

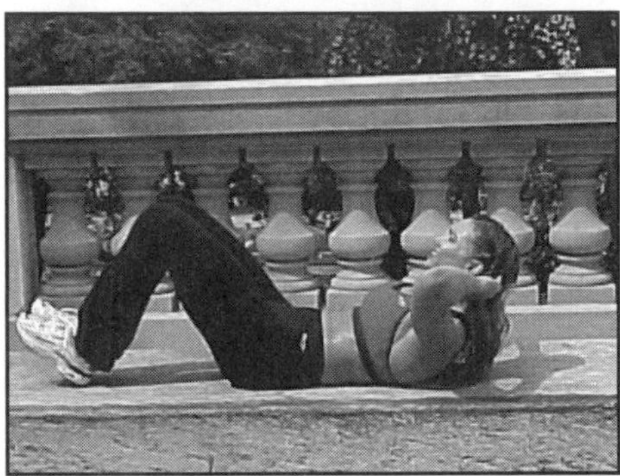

1. **Combined crunch** With your legs up, toes pointed, and fingertips touching your head, exhale and lift both upper and lower abs, squeezing them together in the middle.
2. Hold for one second, and then lower to the starting position.
3. Repeat for desired reps. Go to the knee-up.

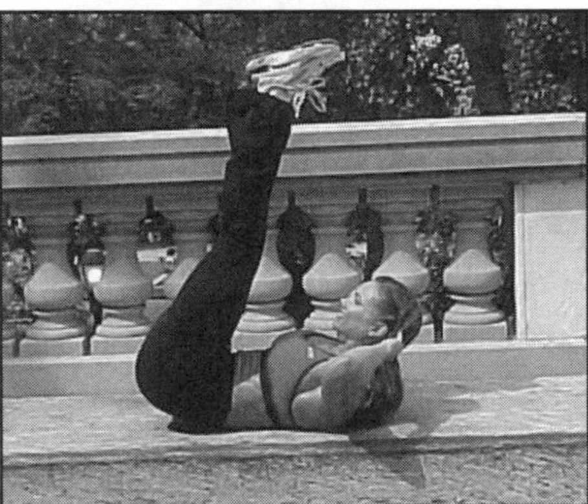

1. **Knee-up** Start by sitting with your hands behind you, with your fingers pointing forward and your elbows flexed.
2. With your legs together, bend your knees and bring them toward your chest.

3. Now extend your legs out at approximately a 45° angle to your upper body.
4. Bring your legs in, and repeat for desired reps. Go to ab balance.

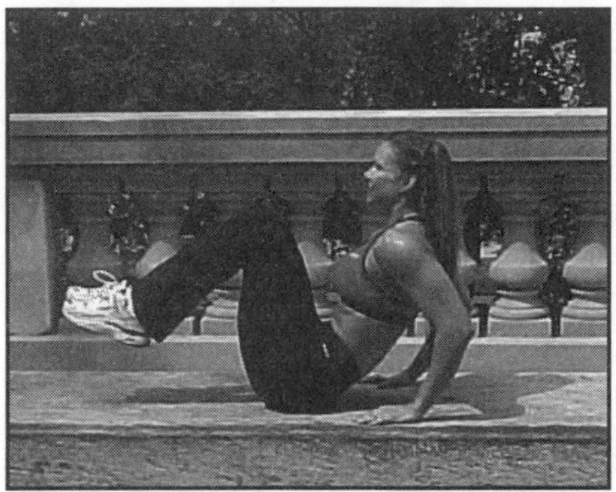

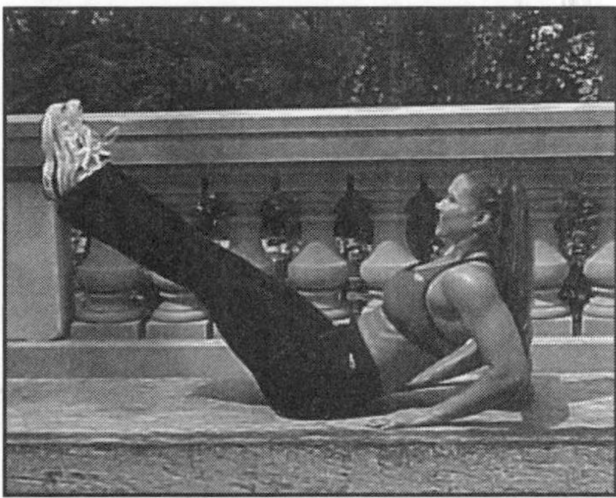

1. **Ab balance** Sit tall, with your legs in and your hands outside your hips.
2. Find a balance point, and then extend both legs forward until they're straight.
3. Raise and extend each arm forward at shoulder height. Hold for desired count, as listed in previous table.

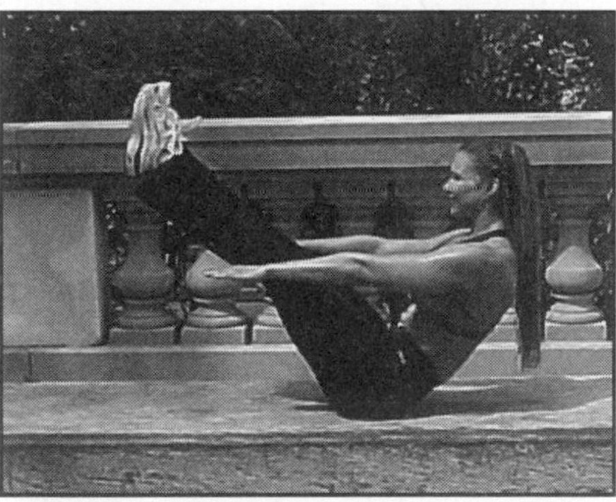

Ten-Minute Travel Routine

Staying swimsuit-lean on vacation is a snap with your gym in a bag and the Ten-Minute Travel Routine. (See Chapter 19, "Home Away from Home," for the complete routine.)

The Least You Need to Know

- Maintaining perfect form, working at maximum intensity, and using enough resistance to challenge your muscles without compromising your form is your ticket to top-level results.
- My Ticket to Tone Routines can help eliminate next-day soreness if done later in the day following an intense workout.
- High-rep nonstop routines that contain multiangular movements make great cutting and sculpting workouts.
- When using a step in your routines, landing softly will minimize knee stress.

Part 3

Body and Soul: Keeping Your Hard Work Hard

The information in this section will maximize your results and give you the knowledge that you need to maintain your hard body at its peak performance level.

Chapter 14, "Fridge Overhaul," shows you how to eat smart instead of dieting. Determining the calories that your body needs to function helps you to calculate the right calories to lose fat, not muscle.

Understanding the risks and taking the necessary steps to avoid them makes your hard-body training safe as well as effective. Chapter 15, "Don't Try This at Home!" shows you how to spot and treat injuries so that you'll know what to do and when.

Learning to relax is just as important as learning to train. Your Hard-Body Hit List is your prescription for pleasure. Turning your home into a minispa so that you can pamper yourself is the goal of my home spa tips.

Staying organized and on top of your hard-body game is easier with the log pages in Chapter 17, "Dear Diary." Cut and copy enough pages to fill your Hard-Body Journal, and you're ready to go.

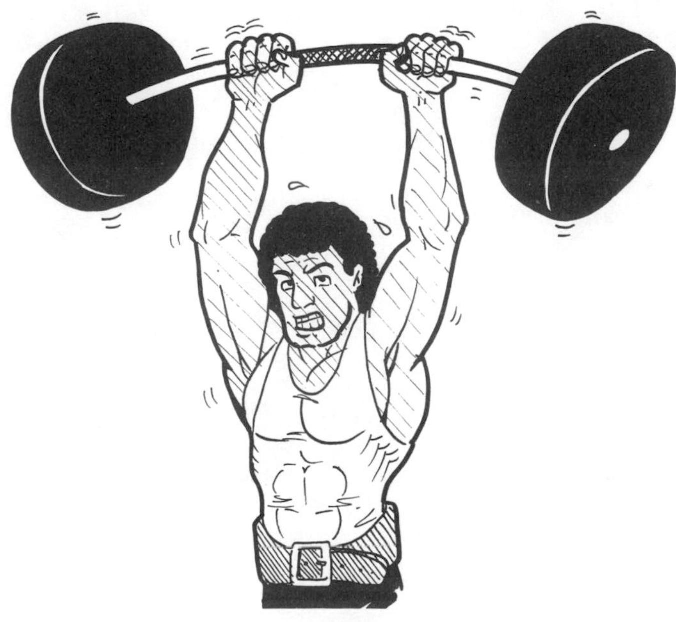

Chapter 14

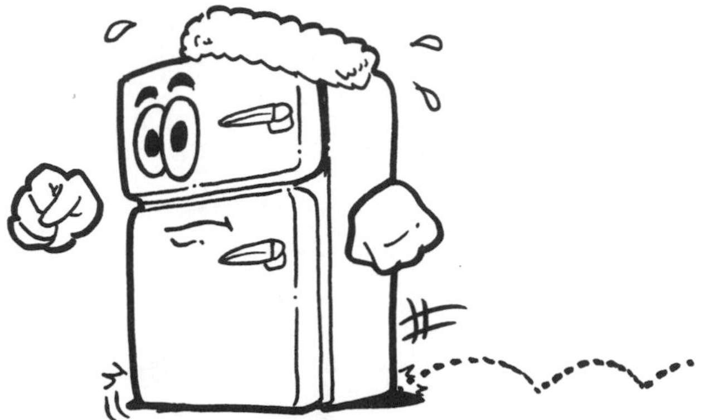

Fridge Overhaul

In This Chapter

- Food full of power rangers
- The not-so-hidden power of protein
- Are carbs the enemy?
- A fat identification program
- Counting calories the BMR way

Eating smart is just as important as training smart. You could have amazing muscles, but no one would know if they were all covered up under a blanket of fat. You could be training like a maniac, but without adequate protein, you couldn't build muscle. You could even be eating and training well, but not drinking enough water will make you retain water and fat.

Treating food like the high-octane fuel that it was designed to be will make you look and feel better then ever before. That's not a bad trade-off for skipping the Twinkies.

Knowing how many calories it takes to maintain your body right now will help you create the right caloric deficit to lose the maximum amount of body fat without losing muscle. You don't have to diet if you simply eat right. The first three letters of the word *diet* spell "die." That should give a clue as to why they don't work.

Hard-Body Power Rangers

Your six hard-body power rangers are found in the food that you eat every day. Together they regulate your growth, supply your energy, and maintain and repair your hard-body's tissue.

The following table lists nutrient names and job descriptions.

Hard-Body Power Rangers

Nutrient	Job Description
Protein	Builds and repairs hard-body tissue Is a major component of enzymes, hormones, and antibodies
Carbohydrates	Are a major hard-body fuel source Provide dietary fiber
Fats	Serve as the main storage form of energy in the body Insulate and protect vital organs Provide fat-soluble vitamins
Vitamins	Help promote and regulate various chemical reactions and bodily processes Help release energy from food
Minerals	Enable enzymes to function Are a component of hormones Are part of bone and nerve impulses
Water	Enables chemical reactions to occur Makes up about 60 percent of your hard body Is essential for life (we can't store or conserve it)

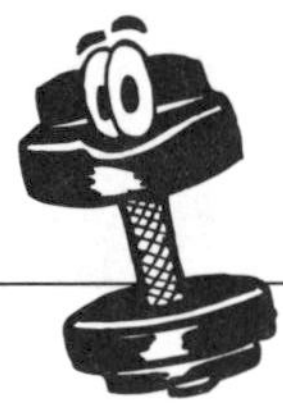

Hard-Body Headliners

Soy protein, which is derived from soybeans, is a complete source of protein, containing all the essential amino acids. The three types of soy include soy protein concentrate, isolated soy protein, and textured soy protein. Isolated soy protein is the best source of protein, containing 92 percent protein.

Power Protein

Protein's main function is to build and repair muscle tissue, ligaments, and tendons. If we don't eat enough protein, we'll start to lose muscle. If we eat too much, the extra will be stored as fat. (Both are good reasons to stay within your protein boundaries.)

The protein that we eat is broken down into amino acids. Proteins from animal sources such as chicken, fish, beef, milk, and eggs have all the essential amino acids and are called complete proteins. Proteins from plant sources are missing one or more amino acids and are called incomplete proteins. They can be made complete proteins by being combined with other foods. Some examples are beans with rice, cereal with milk, peanut butter on bread, and hummus and pita bread.

Choosing low-fat proteins will keep both your calories and your cholesterol level low. Some lean protein options follow:

- Chicken, white meat
- Egg whites, cooked
- Halibut
- Nonfat tofu
- Nonfat, sugar-free yogurt
- Shrimp
- Soybeans
- Tuna
- Turkey, white meat

You should consume about 20 percent of your calories from protein. One gram of protein is equal to 4 calories. So, to find out how many grams of protein you would eat each day, first multiply your daily calories by 20 percent, and then divide that number by 4, as shown:

Total daily calories × .20 = Daily protein calories

Daily protein calories ÷ 4 = Daily grams of protein

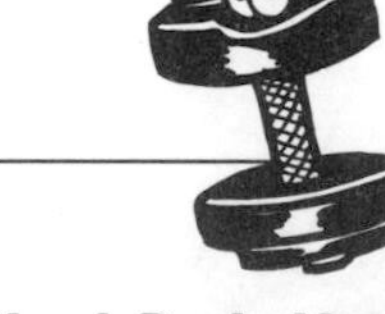

Hard-Body Headliners

The U.S. Department of Agriculture (USDA) says that the average American consumes 20 teaspoons of added sugar each day—that's equivalent to 16 to 20 percent of total calories. That's not hard to believe because many 2-ounce candy bars, 12-ounce sodas, and 1-cup servings of ice cream contain 10 or more teaspoons of added sugar.

The Deal on Dairy

I personally don't eat dairy products and have never felt better. After doing some reading, I found out that we don't have the necessary enzymes (rennin and lactase) to break down and properly digest the casein in milk. The biggest problem with dairy is the formation of mucus. This mucus can zap our energy, attack our immune system, and make weight loss difficult. Cow milk was designed to feed calves (with four stomachs), not us. I'm not telling you that you have to give up dairy, but maybe cut back a little and try some soy-based products as a substitute.

Carbs: Friend or Foe?

A lot of the popular fad diets have turned carbs into enemy number one. Carbohydrates are our energy food. During digestion, the carbs we eat turn into a simple sugar called glucose. Our bodies use this glucose as a fuel source. Any glucose that isn't used right away is stored in our muscles and liver as glycogen.

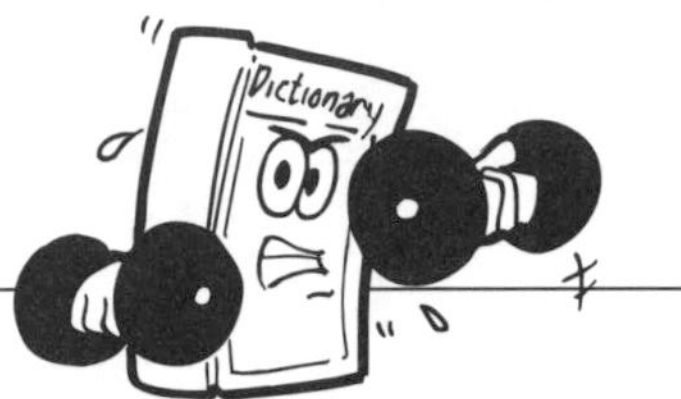

Workout Wisdom

Glucagon is a hormone produced by the pancreas that is responsible for unlocking fat stores. Eating low glycemic foods promotes the production of glucagon by not spiking your insulin levels.

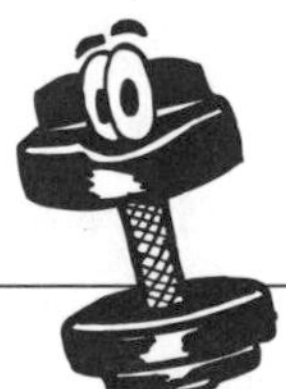

Hard-Body Headliners

The National Research Council recommends eating 20 to 35 grams of fiber a day. Eating more fiber will give you a full feeling sooner so you don't overeat.

There are two types of carbohydrates: simple sugars and complex carbohydrates. Simple sugars are found in fruit, juices, candy, milk, and processed food. Complex carbohydrates are found in whole grains, beans, and vegetables. You should eat more complex carbs than simple sugars because complex carbs have a higher nutrient density (amount of essential nutrients compared to calories).

Simple sugars are easily stored as body fat because of their quick absorption rate. When food is quickly absorbed, your body's insulin level is quickly elevated. You have experienced this if you've ever had a "sugar rush." When your insulin level is high, your body's fat cell enzymes are activated. This means that they go to work moving fat from your blood to your fat storage cells. High insulin levels also stop *glucagon* from coming to the rescue to release your fat prisoners.

Complex carbohydrates take longer to digest, so your energy level is sustained longer and your insulin level remains constant. Complex carbs can be either starchy or fibrous. Starchy carbs include corn, potatoes, rice, and bran. Fibrous carbs include spinach, tomatoes, carrots, and cauliflower.

Fibrous carbs are lower in calories, so you can eat more of them. Complex carbs also provide you with dietary fiber. Eating more fiber will move food through your system quicker so that less can be stored as fat. Fiber leaves you feeling full, so you don't overeat, and it also lowers insulin levels. The following table lists some good sources of dietary fiber.

Hard-Body Fiber Sources

Food	Serving Size	Fiber (grams)
Garbanzo beans	$^{1}/_{2}$ cup	5.0
Corn	$^{1}/_{2}$ cup	4.7
Peas	1 cup	3.2

Food	Serving Size	Fiber (grams)
Brown rice	1 cup	1.6
Edamame	$^{2}/_{3}$ cup	5.0
Lentils	1 cup	2.4
Green apple	1 medium	1.8

Carbohydrates should make up about 60 percent of your calories. Like proteins, a carbohydrate gram is equal to 4 calories. To find your daily gram requirement, multiply your total calories by 60 percent, and then divide that number by 4.

Just Juice It

Going through the produce section these days makes me feel like a kid in a virtual juice candy store. I'm checking out all kinds of "veggies" that I never thought I'd eat, thinking, "I could juice that." Vegetable juicing is one of my all-time best discoveries. Since I started juicing, I have more energy, look younger, and have better skin and hair. Just think about it: Juicing allows you to drink massive amounts of raw, nutrient-dense veggies with all their enzymes intact. No digestion is required, so you get an instant energy boost. Here are some of my favorite juice combos:

- Carrot, apple, ginger (great without ginger, also)
- Jicama, pear, apple
- Carrot, spinach, kale, green bell pepper, ginger
- Apple, $^{1}/_{4}$ lemon with skin, crushed ice (tastes like lemonade)

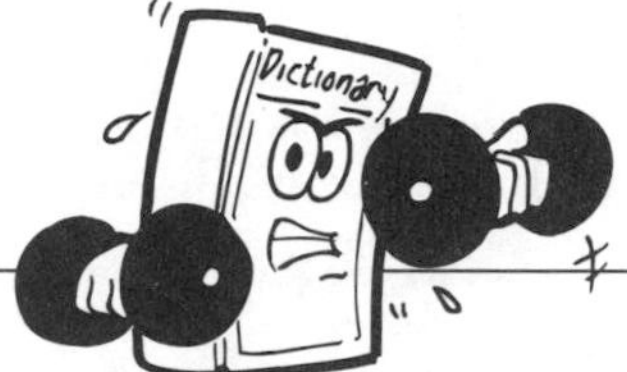

Workout Wisdom

Edamame are soybeans still in the pod. You just boil, drain, and then pop the beans out of the pods for an excellent high-protein snack that has a nutty taste. Edamame can be found in most health food stores.

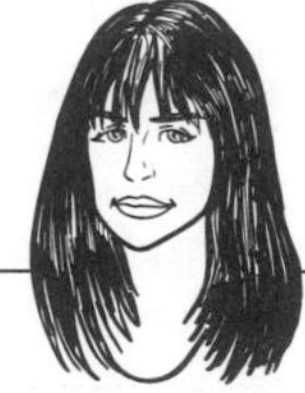

Jourdan's Gems

For amazing energy, have three to four vegetable juices a day. Drink before a meal so that you won't overeat.

Fat: The Good, the Bad, and the Ugly

Fats perform important functions in our bodies, as shown in the following table. Fats can come from both plant and animal sources. But all fats are not created equal, and some are even downright ugly. The following list gives you the lowdown on the good, the bad, and the ugly:

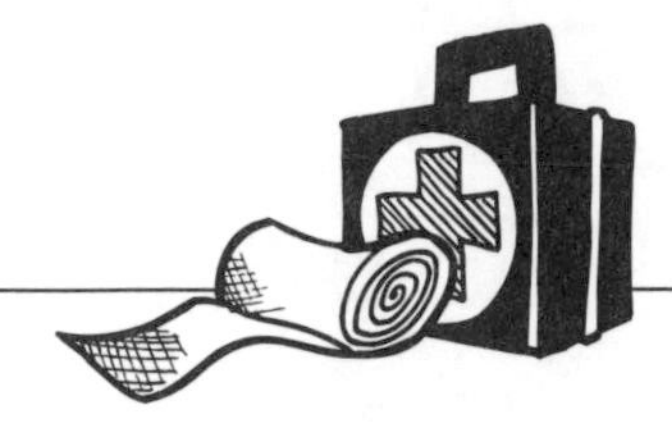

Safety Scoop

Completely eliminating fats from your diet can lead to dry, flaky skin and stiff, painful joints. These symptoms may indicate that your heart, brain, liver, and internal organs are EFA (Essential Fatty Acids) deficient. Good EFA sources include flaxseed oil, linseed oil, and evening primrose oil.

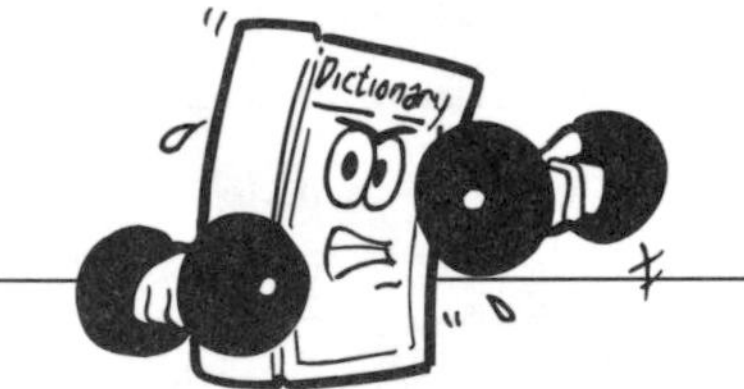

Workout Wisdom

Electrolytes are the minerals sodium, potassium, and chlorine, which are present in the body as electrically charged particles.

- **Polyunsaturated: Omega-3** Found in fish such as salmon and tuna, as well as canola and walnut oil and flaxseed. Enhances the immune system. Also found in dark green, leafy veggies and legumes. Reduces risk of heart disease in animal studies. *Use more.*
- **Polyunsaturated: Omega-6** Found in vegetable oils. Used in salad dressings, mayonnaise, and other processed foods. Increases cholesterol level. Animal studies show cancer risk. *Use less.*
- **Monounsaturated** Found in olive oil, canola oil, nuts, and avocados. Lowers risk of heart disease and cancer, particularly breast cancer. Use olive and canola oils as cooking oil. Consume nuts and avocados in the right calorie amounts.
- **Saturated** Found in fatty meats, high-fat dairy, and poultry. Increases cholesterol levels and risk of heart disease. *Cut way back.*
- **Trans** Found in stick margarine, shortenings, cookies, crackers, commercially fried foods, and anything containing hydrogenated or partially hydrogenated vegetable oil. Increases heart disease risk and breast cancer risk, and enlarges fat cells. *Minimize or avoid.*

Fat should make up about 20 percent of your calories. Fats have a higher caloric value then proteins and carbs. Each gram of fat is equal to 9 calories. To find your daily gram requirement, multiply your total calories by 20 percent, and then divide that number by 9.

Vitamins and Minerals

Vitamins help in the growth of body tissues and are essential for the release of energy. There are two types of vitamins: fat-soluble and water-soluble. Fat-soluble vitamins can be stored in the body, and water-soluble ones cannot.

Minerals are important for bone formation, metabolism, and energy production. *Electrolytes* are responsible for maintaining fluid balance in the body. Sodium, calcium, and chloride are found outside the cell. Potassium, magnesium, and phosphorus are found inside.

Vitamins and Their Functions

Vitamin	Function	Sources	Daily Adult Requirement[a] Men	Women
Thiamin (B_1)	Functions as part of a coenzyme to aid utilization of energy	Whole grains, nuts, lean pork	1.5 mg[b]	1.1 mg
Riboflavin (B_2)	Involved in energy metabolism as part of a coenzyme	Milk, yogurt, cheese	1.7 mg	1.3 mg
Niacin	Facilitates energy production in cells	Lean meat, fish, poultry, grains	19.0 mg	15.0 mg
Vitamin B_6	Absorbs and metabolizes protein; aids in red blood cell formation	Lean meat, vegetables, whole grains	2.0 mg	1.6 mg
Pantothenic acid	Aids in metabolism of carbohydrate, fat, and protein	Whole-grain cereals and breads, dark green vegetables	4–7 mg	4–7 mg
Folic acid	Functions as coenzyme in synthesis of nucleic acids and protein	Green vegetables, beans, whole-wheat products	200 μg	180 μg
Vitamin B_{12}	Involved in synthesis of nucleic acids and red blood cell formation	Only animal foods, not plant foods	2 μg	2 μg
Biotin	Coenzyme in synthesis of fatty acids and glycogen formation	Egg yolk, dark green vegetables	30–100 μg	
C	Aids in intracellular maintenance of bones, capillaries, and teeth	Citrus fruits, green peppers, tomatoes	60 mg	
A	Functions in visual processes; helps with formation and maintenance of skin and mucous membranes	Carrots, sweet potatoes margarine, butter, liver	1000 μg	800 μg[c]
D	Aids in growth and formation of bones and teeth; promotes calcium absorption	Eggs, tuna, liver, milk	5 μg	5 μg
E	Protects polyunsaturated fats; prevents cell membrane damage	Vegetable oils, whole-grain cereals and bread, leafy green vegetables	10 mg	8 mg

continues

Vitamins and Their Functions (continued)

Daily Adult Requirement[a]

Vitamin	Function	Sources	Men	Women
K	Important in blood clotting	Leafy green vegetables, peas, potatoes	80 µg 65 µg	

Notes: [a]*Values are for adults 25 to 50 years of age. The requirements vary for children and pregnant or lactating women.*
[b]*mg = milligram, µg = microgram, IU = international unit.*
[c]*µg vitamin A requirements are expressed in microgram of Retinol equivalents.*

Source: Reprinted, by permission, from E. Howley & B. Franks, Health Fitness Instructor's Handbook, 3rd ed. *(Champaign, IL, Human Kinetics, 1997), 154.*

Minerals and Their Functions

Daily Adult Requirement[a]

Vitamin	Function	Sources	Men	Women
Major Minerals				
Calcium	Bones, teeth, blood clotting, nerve and muscle function	Milk, sardines, dark green vegetables, nuts	800 mg[b]	800 mg
Chloride	Nerve and muscle function, water balance (with sodium)	Table salt	750 mg	750mg[c]
Magnesium	Bone growth; nerve, muscle, and enzyme function	Nuts, seafood, whole grains, leafy green vegetables	350 mg	250 mg
Phosphorus	Bone, teeth, energy transfer	Meats, poultry, seafood, eggs, milk, beans	800 mg	800 mg
Potassium	Nerve and muscle function	Fresh vegetables, bananas, citrus fruits, milk, meats, fish	2000 mg	2000 mg[c]

Vitamin	Function	Sources	Men	Women
Major Minerals				
Sodium	Nerve and muscle function, water balance	Table salt	500 mg	500 mg[c]
Trace Minerals				
Chromium	Glucose metabolism	Meats, liver whole grains, dried beans	.05–.2 mg	.05–.2 mg
Copper	Enzyme function, energy production	Meats, seafood, nuts, grains	1.5–3 mg	1.5–5 mg
Fluoride	Bone and teeth growth	Drinking water, fish, milk	1.5–4 mg	
Iodine	Thyroid hormone formation	Iodized salt, seafood	150 µg	150 µg
Iron	O_2 transport in red blood cells; enzyme function	Red meat, liver, eggs, beans, leafy vegetables, shellfish	10 mg	15 mg
Manganese	Enzyme function	Whole grains, nuts, fruits, vegetables	2.5–5 mg	2.5–5 mg
Molybdenum	Energy metabolism in cells	Whole grains, organ meats, peas, beans	.075–.25 mg	.075–.25 mg
Selenium	Works with vitamin E	Meat, fish, whole grains, eggs	70 µg	55 µg
Zinc	Part of enzymes, growth	Meat, shellfish, yeast, whole grains	15 mg	12 mg

Notes: [a]*Values are for adults 25 to 50 years of age. The requirements vary for children and pregnant or lactating women.*
[b]*mg = milligram, µg = microgram.*
[c]*Minimum requirements for healthy people.*

Source: Reprinted, by permission, from E. Howley & B. Franks, Health Fitness Instructor's Handbook, 3rd ed. *(Champaign, IL, Human Kinetics, 1997), 155.*

Hard-Body Hydrator

If you want to lose more weight, drink more water. Odds are, you don't get nearly enough water every day. You should be drinking at least 8 ounces of water a minimum of eight times a day. If you exercise, drink coffee and alcohol, or take medication, you need even more.

If you want to make sure that you're drinking enough water during your training session, I suggest carrying a medium-size water bottle with you—plan to refill it at least once. You should also carry water with you throughout the day. Sipping water during the day will keep you full so that you eat less and help your liver convert fat into energy.

Not drinking enough water makes you retain water and fat. Muscle cramping can also result from dehydration. Being thirsty or fatigued are signs that you're already dehydrated.

Secrets to Superior Digestion

It doesn't matter how good the food you eat is if your body can't *digest* and assimilate it—you might as well be starving yourself.

The digestive enzymes that are present in raw food are destroyed at temperatures of 118 degrees or above, so most of the food we eat cannot be properly digested. Our sources of backup enzymes aren't enough by themselves to enable us to digest all the cooked food we take in. Signs that our food is not being thoroughly digested include bloating, burping, constipation, flatulence, and feeling tired after a meal.

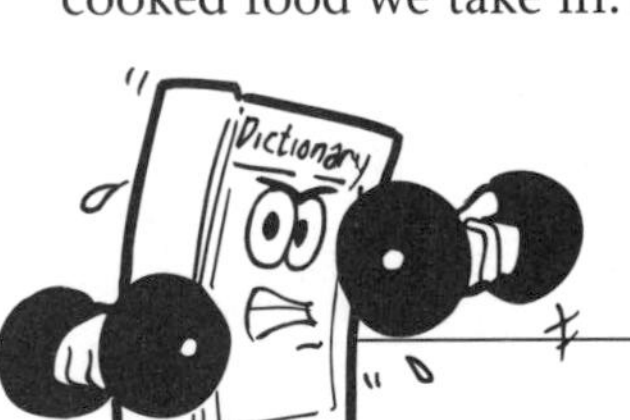

Workout Wisdom

Digestion, which is largely done by enzymes, is the process of breaking down food so it can be absorbed into the bloodstream. Factors such as cooked and processed food, stress, and toxins can interfere with the digestion process.

Taking an antacid will only further disrupt the digestive process. Supplementing is the only way to make sure you have enough enzymes on hand to handle your digestion demands.

With all the products on the market, picking the most effective product can be confusing. You want to make sure the product you choose contains protease to break protein down to amino acids, amylase to break carbohydrates down to disaccharides, lactase and invertase to break disaccharides down to simple sugars, and cellulase to help the body digest fiber.

The only product I've found so far that has all these things and really works for me is manufactured by Optimal Health Systems. I use their "Fitness in a Box" supplement kit, which also comes with a multivitamin antioxidant, fat metabolizer, a protein powder with the right ratio of protein to carbs to fat, and a supplement to increase oxygen at the cellular level. You can check it out at www.optimalhealthsystems.com

Hard-Body Calorie Count

To lose a pound of fat a week, you have to create a deficit of 3,500 calories between diet and exercise. At 500 calories a day, you would have to eat 250 fewer calories and exercise to burn off the other 250 calories. To lose 2 pounds a week, this would be increased to 500 calories each from food and exercise. Any more than this isn't a good idea because you would start to lose some of that valuable hard-body muscle that you worked so hard to build. Losing muscle would also mean that your metabolism would slow down, and I know you don't want that.

If you're trying to lose weight, you should consume between 10 and 15 times your body weight in calories per day. A more accurate way would be to first determine your basal metabolic rate (BMR). Your BMR is the amount of calories that it takes for your body to function. Following are the steps to find your daily calorie requirements, using my numbers as an example:

1. First divide your weight by 2.2 to get your weight in kilograms:

   145 ÷ 2.2 = 66 kilograms

2. Multiply that number by your appropriate BMR factor (men = 1, women = .9):

   66 × .9 = 59.4

3. Multiply that number by 24 (for the hours in a day) to get your BMR:

   59.4 × 24 = 1,425 calories (BMR)

4. To find your activity level energy requirements, multiply your BMR by the appropriate percentage:

   - 40–50 percent of your BMR: sedentary home body (armchair athlete)
   - 55–65 percent of your BMR: lightly active home body (trains up to 1.5 hours week)
   - 65–75 percent of your BMR: moderately active hard-body (trains 1.5–3 hours week)
   - 75–100 percent of your BMR: very active hard-body (trains more than three hours a week)

   1,425 × .75 = 1,068 calories (lower-limit activity level)

   1,425 × 1 = 1,425 calories (upper-limit activity level)

5. Add your BMR and activity level requirements to get your daily calorie requirement:

   1,425 + 1,068 = 2,493 calories

   1,425 + 1,425 = 2,850 calories

So, to maintain my hard-body as is at my current exercise level, I can eat between 2,493 to 2,850 calories a day, depending on my activity level. Cutting my calories too low would slow my metabolism down so that my body would not be able to function at the reduced calorie amount. Knowing this, I can reduce my calories enough to lose weight safely without starving myself. Your body doesn't discriminate between calories from food or exercise, so as long as the week's total adds up to the right number, you can train harder one day and eat less another.

Find your BMR and maintenance calories, and keep these numbers handy in your Home Hard-Body Journal. (See Chapter 17, "Dear Diary," for sample hard-body log pages.)

The Least You Need to Know

- Eating too little protein can lead to muscle loss. Eating too much protein can lead to fat gain.
- Many 2-ounce candy bars, 12-ounce sodas, and 1-cup servings of ice cream contain 10 or more teaspoons of added sugar.
- Not drinking enough water can cause muscle cramping, water retention, and fat retention.
- Losing more than two pounds a week can lead to a loss of lean muscle mass.

Chapter 15

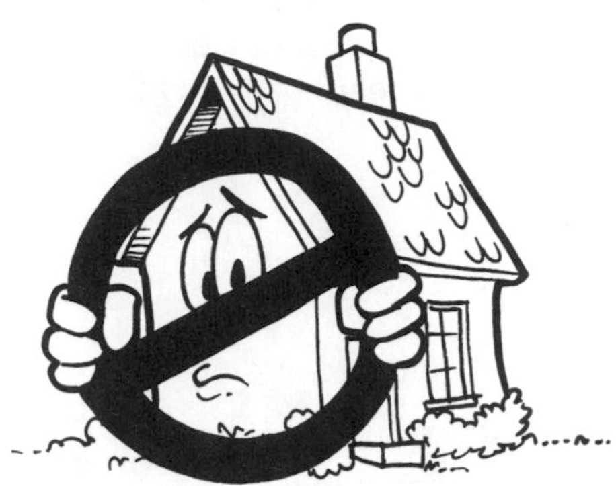

Don't Try This at Home!

In This Chapter

- ➤ Injury risk prevention
- ➤ Spot the signs
- ➤ PRICE to the rescue
- ➤ Injury treatment

The first step to training smart is to understand the risks involved and then to actually take the steps to avoid them. Spotting a pothole in the road doesn't do you any good if you still drive over it. I don't know how many times I have seen someone doing an exercise and thought, "Now there's an accident waiting to happen." Usually it's someone who thinks he or she knows it all (such as those huge guys who bench a thousand pounds and look like muscle in a bowl), or someone who has no clue and is too afraid to ask for help.

After doing a survey to find out some of the most commonly confused exercise safety issues, I put together a simple-to-understand hard-body safety guide that should answer your questions and keep you injury free.

Injury Risk Prevention

Risks can be involved with physical activity. The frequency of injuries can increase when the frequency and intensity of the exercise increases. Being aware of the risks and taking the necessary steps to avoid them will make your hard-body training safe as well as effective.

Factors that can increase the chance of injury include these:

- Exercise intensity maintained at the high end of the target heart rate (THR) too long
- Too little recovery time for your muscles
- Lack of muscle strength
- Imbalance of muscle strength
- Lack of flexibility
- Poor cardio fitness
- Obesity
- Conditions such as asthma or diabetes

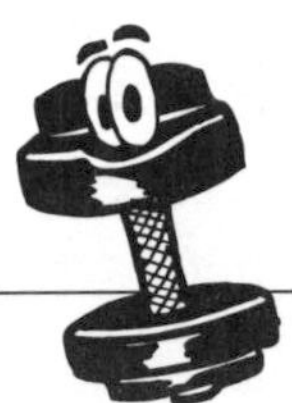

Hard-Body Headliners

Failure to replace worn athletic shoes is a major contributor to leg and lower-back problems.

The following steps will help you avoid possible injury:

- At all times, use correct exercise form.
- Begin each workout with a warm-up and finish each workout with a cool-down.
- Allow muscles enough recovery time between training sessions.
- Work within your fitness level.
- Lower the weight used as soon as exercise form suffers.
- Use proper exercise equipment and maintain it in good condition.
- Follow the directions and safety precautions that come with your equipment.
- Use proper training clothing and footwear.
- Replace footwear when worn.

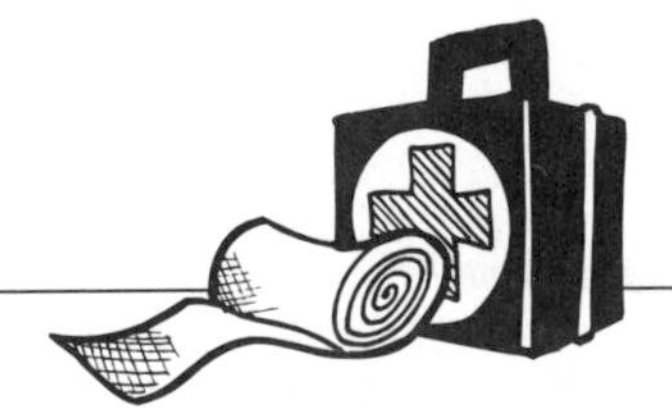

Safety Scoop

It's important to know the difference between muscle soreness and muscle injury. Muscle soreness peaks 24 to 48 hours after the training session and dissipates with use and time.

Tissue Types

Four tissues are involved in musculoskeletal injuries:

- **Muscle.** The shock absorbers for the body. Because of their elasticity, they can handle a great deal of stress. To prevent injury, they need to be strong and flexible.

  A muscle injury can be mild, moderate, or severe. A severe strain would be a rupture or complete tear. As the muscle heals, it forms scar tissue called collagen. This tissue isn't elastic. The unorganized manner in which it's laid out leaves the muscle weak. To organize the collagen and strengthen the muscle, it needs to be stretched and trained with a gradual increase of weight.

- **Tendon.** Connects muscle to bone. Tendons are supplied with less blood, so they heal slower.
- **Ligament.** The nonelastic tissue that connects bone to bone. When stretched out, ligaments allow the joint to move around too much. Strengthening the surrounding muscle tissue prevents this.
- **Bone.** The only tissue that can heal itself with the same type of tissue. Stress fractures (cracks) can occur from abnormal stress. Breaks are known as fractures.

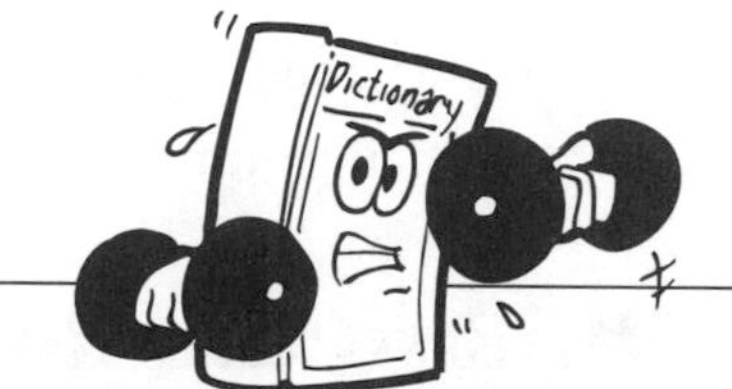

Workout Wisdom

A **strain** is the result of overstretching or tearing a muscle or a tendon.

A **sprain** is the result of overstretching or tearing ligament tissue.

Spot the Signs

When a tissue gets injured, the body immediately sends in the repair crew. This crew, known as the white blood cells, rides the circulatory subway to the inflammation construction site to begin the repair work. The repair site can be recognized by swelling, a black-and-blue mark, pain, and decreased range of motion.

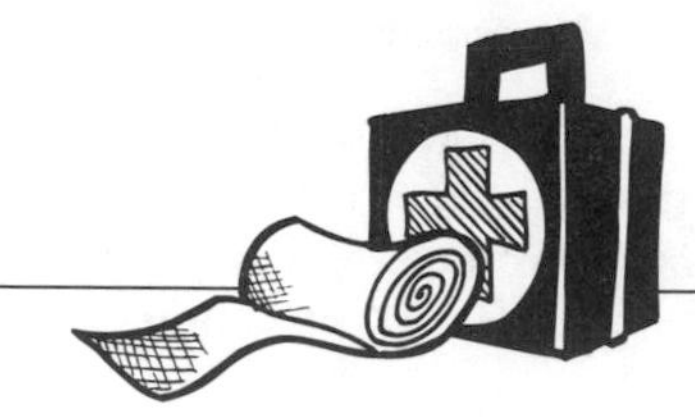

Safety Scoop

Elevate an injured part above the heart to minimize the effect of gravity and reduce bleeding.

Signs and symptoms of tissue injury include these:

- Elevated temperature
- Redness
- Swelling
- Pain that persists when that body part is at rest
- Pain that doesn't go away after warming up
- Increased pain in weight-bearing activities or with movement
- Change in normal bodily functions

PRICE to the Rescue

The American Council of Sports Medicine advocates the *PRICE* method for the treatment of *strains* and *sprains*. The next table outlines soft tissue injuries and their treatment. The second table outlines fractures and their treatment.

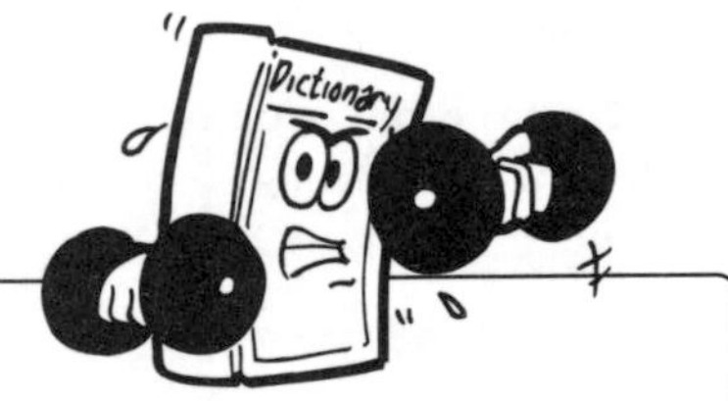

Workout Wisdom

The **PRICE** method is the suggested treatment for strains and sprains: **p**rotection, **r**est, **i**ce, **c**ompression, and **e**levation.

Wounds and skin irritations are other injuries that can be caused by physical activities. The major concern with a wound is to control the bleeding. When that is done, further care steps can be taken. The next table outlines the treatment for wounds. The subsequent table outlines various types of skin irritations and their treatment.

Many common orthopedic problems result from overuse or irritation of a musculoskeletal problem. In the early stages, injury doesn't prevent normal function. If left untreated, this could turn into a severe injury. The next table outlines some common orthopedic problems and their treatment. The subsequent table outlines shin splints and their treatment.

Soft-Tissue Injuries and Their Treatment

Injury	Signs and Symptoms	Immediate Care
Sprain—stretching or tearing of ligamentous tissue **Strain**—overstretching or tearing of a muscle or tendon **Contusion**—impact force that results in bleeding into the underlying tissues; a bruise	1st degree—mild injury resulting in overstretching or minor tearing of tissue. Range of motion is limited. Point tenderness is minimal. No swelling. 2nd degree—moderate injury resulting in partial tearing of tissue. Function is limited. Point tenderness and probable muscle spasm. Range of motion is painful. Swelling and/or discoloration is probable if immediate first-aid care is not given. 3rd degree—severe tearing or rupture of tissue. Exquisite point tenderness. Immediate loss of function. Swelling and muscle spasm likely to be present with discoloration appearing later. Possible palpable deformity.	Protection, rest, ice, compression, and elevation (PRICE) Usual treatment time: 15–20 min. ice bag 5–7 min. ice cup or ice slush How often: Moderate and severe—every hour, or when pain is experienced. Less severe—as symptoms necessitate. Continue with ice treatments at least 24–72 hrs, depending on the severity of the injury. Refer to a physician if function is impaired. Mild to moderate strains—gradual stretching to the point of discomfort is recommended.
Heel bruise (stone bruise)—sudden abnormal force to heel area that results in trauma to underlying tissues		PRICE Pad for comfort when weight bearing is resumed.

Source: Reprinted, by permission, from E. Howley & B. Franks, Health Fitness Instructor's Handbook, 3rd ed. *(Champaign, IL, Human Kinetics, 1997), 410.*

Fractures and Their Treatment

Injury	Signs and Symptoms	Immediate Care
Fracture—disruption of bone with or without loss of continuity or external exposure, ranging from	Acute: Direct trauma to bone resulting in disruption of continuity and immediate disability.	Acute: Control bleeding—elevation, pressure points, direct pressure.

continues

Fractures and Their Treatment (continued)

Injury	Signs and Symptoms	Immediate Care
periosteal irritation to complete separation of bony parts Simple fracture—bone fracture without external exposure	Deformity or bony deviation. Swelling. Pain. Palpable tenderness. Referred pain or indirect point tenderness. Crepitus. False joint. Discoloration—usually becoming apparent later.	Treat for shock. If an open fracture, control bleeding and apply a sterile dressing, prevent further infection; do not move bones back into place. Control swelling with pressure and ice, if wound is closed. Splint above and below the joint and apply traction if necessary. Protect body part from further injury. Refer to physician.
	Chronic: Low-grade inflammatory process causing proliferation of fibroblasts and generalized connective-tissue scarring. Pain progressively worsens until present all the time. Direct point tenderness.	Chronic: Rest. Heat. Refer to physician.

Source: Reprinted, by permission, from E. Howley & B. Franks, Health Fitness Instructor's Handbook, 3rd ed. *(Champaign, IL, Human Kinetics, 1997), 411.*

Treatment of Wounds

Injury	Signs and Symptoms	Immediate Care
Incision—cutting of skin resulting in an open wound with cleanly cut edges; an exposure of underlying tissues.	Smooth edges may bleed freely. Signs of infection (see laceration).	Clean wound with soap and water, moving away from injury site. Minor cuts can be closed with a butterfly bandage or a steri-strip. Apply a sterile dressing.

Injury	Signs and Symptoms	Immediate Care
		Refer to a physician if wound needs suturing (e.g., facial cuts and large or deep wounds) or signs of infection are present.
Laceration—tearing of skin resulting in an open wound with jagged edges and exposure of underlying tissues	Jagged edges may bleed freely. Signs of infection: redness; redness; swelling; increase in skin temperature; tender, swollen, and painful lymph glands; mild ever; and headache.	Soak in antiseptic solution such as hydrogen peroxide to loosen foreign material. Clean with antiseptic soap and water using sterile technique and moving away from the injury site. Apply a sterile dressing. Instruct to seek medical attention if signs of infection are recognized. Usually refer to a physician; a tetanus shot or sutures may be needed. If injury is extensive, control bleeding, cover with thick sterile bandages, and treat for shock. Refer to a physician.
Puncture—direct penetration of tissues by a pointed object	Small opening; may bleed freely Signs of infection (see laceration)	If object is embedded deeply: Protect body part and refer to a physician for removal and care. Treat for shock. Clean around wound,moving away from injury site. Allow wound to bleed freely to minimize risk of infection. Apply a sterile dressing. Puncture wounds are usually referred to a physician. A tetanus shot may be needed. Instruct individual to seek medical attention if signs of infection are present.

continues

Treatment of Wounds (continued)

Injury	Signs and Symptoms	Immediate Care
Abrasion—scraping of tissues resulting in removal of the outer most layers of skin and underlying capillaries	Superficial, reddish, irregular surface Oozing or weeping from the exposure of numerous May contain dirt, debris, or bacteria embedded in tissue	Debride and flush with antiseptic solution such as hydrogen peroxide. Follow with soap-and-water cleansing underlying capillaries Apply a petroleum-based antiseptic agent to keep wound moist. This allows healing to take place from the deeper layers. Cover with nonadherent gauze. Instruct to seek medical help if signs of infection are recognized.
Excessive bleeding—internal or external bleeding that results in massive loss of circulating blood volumes; often results in shock and can lead to death	External hemorrhage **1.** Arterial Color: bright red Flow: spurts, bleeding usually profuse **2.** Venous Color: dark red Flow: steady **3.** Flow: oozing	Elevate affected part above heart. Put direct pressure over the wound, using a sterile compress if possible. Apply a pressure dressing. Use pressure points. Treat for shock. Refer to a physician.
Internal bleeding—bleeding within the deep structures of the body (chest, abdominal, or pelvic cavity) and bleeding of any of the organs contained within these cavities.	Internal hemorrhage—bleeding into chest, abdominal, or pelvic cavity and bleeding of any of the organs contained within these cavities. Generally, there are no external signs. However, any time an individual coughs up blood or finds blood in the urine or feces, internal hemorrhage must be suspected. The signs are also indicative of internal bleeding: Restlessness Thirst Faintness	Treat for shock. Refer to hospital immediately. Don't give water or food.

continues

Injury	Signs and Symptoms	Immediate Care
	Anxiety Cold, clammy skin Dizziness Pulse—rapid, weak, and irregular Blood pressure—significant fall	
Shock caused by bleeding	Restlessness Anxiety Pulse—weak, rapid Skin temperature—cold, clammy, profuse sweating Skin color—pale, later cyanotic Respiration—shallow, labored Eyes—dull Pupils—dilated Thirsty Nausea and possible vomiting Blood pressure—marked fall	Maintain an open airway. Control bleeding. Elevate lower extremities approximately 12 in. (exceptions: heart problems, head injury, or breathing difficulty—place in comfortable position, usually semi-reclining, unless spinal injury suspected, in which case do not move) Splint any fractures. Maintain normal body temperature. Avoid further trauma. Monitor vital signs and record at regular intervals—every 5 min. or so. Do no feed or give any liquids.

Source: Reprinted, by permission, from E. Howley & B. Franks, Health Fitness Instructor's Handbook, 3rd ed. *(Champaign, IL, Human Kinetics, 1997), 412–414.*

Common Orthopedic Problems and Their Treatment

Injury	Common Causes	Signs and Symptoms	Treatment
Inflammatory reactions: **Bursitis**—inflammation of bursa (sac between) a muscle and bone that is filled with fluid, facilitates motion, pads and helps to prevent abnormal function)	Overuse Improper joint mechanics Improper technique Pathology Trauma Infection	Redness Swelling Pain Increased skin temperature over the area of inflammation Tenderness	Ice and rest in the acute stages. If chronic, heat is generally used before exercise or activity, followed by ice after activity.

continues

Common Orthopedic Problems and Their Treatment (continued)

Injury	Common Causes	Signs and Symptoms	Treatment
		Involuntary muscle guarding	Massage Perform muscle strengthening and stretching exercises. Correct the cause of the problem If correction of the cause and symptomatic treatment do not relieve symptoms, referral to a physician is recommended; antiinflammatory medication is usually prescribed.
Capsulitis—inflammation of the joint capsule. **Epicondylitis**—inflammation of muscles or tendons attached to the epicondyles of the humerus **Myositis**—inflammation of voluntary muscle **Plantar fascitis**—inflammation of connective tissue that spans the bottom of the foot			
Tendonitis—inflammation of a tendon (a band of tough, inelastic, fibrous tissue that connects muscle to bone) **Tenosynovitis**—inflammation of a tendonous sheath **Synovitis**—inflammation of the synovial membrane (a highly vascularized tissue that lines articular surfaces)			If disease process or infection is suspected, refer to a physician immediately.
Tennis elbow—inflammation of the musculo-tendonous unit of the elbow extensors where they attach on the outer aspect of the elbow (lateral epicondylitis)	Faulty backhand mechanics—faults may include leading with the elbow, using an improper grip, dropping the racket head, or	Pain directly over the outer aspect of the elbow in region of the common extensor origin Swelling Increased skin temperature-over the area of inflammation	Ice and rest in the acute stages. If chronic, heat is generally used before exercise or activity, followed by ice after activity

continues

Injury	Common Causes	Signs and Symptoms	Treatment
	using a top-spin backhand with a whipping motion.	Pain on extension of the middle finger against resistance with the elbow extended.	Apply deep friction massage at the elbow. Perform strengthening and stretching exercises for the wrist extensors.
	Improper grip size—usually too small Improper hitting—hitting off center, particularly if using wet, heavy balls Overuse of forearm supinators, wrist extensors, and finger extensors	Pain on racket gripping and extension of the of the wrist	Correct the cause of the problem: **1.** Use proper techniques. **2.** Use proper grip size (when racket is gripped, there should be room for one finger to fit in the gap between the thumb and fingers. **3.** Racket should be strung at the proper tension (usually between 50 and 55 lb). **4.** Avoid stiff rackets that vibrate easily. Keep elbow warm, particularly in cold weather. Use a counterforce brace, a circular band that is placed just below the elbow (serves to reduce the stress at the origin of the extensors). If correction of cause and symptomatic treatment do not relieve symptoms, referral to a physician is recommended; anti-inflammatory medication is usually prescribed.
Stress fracture—a bone defect that occurs because of overstress to weight-bearing bones which causes an accelerated rate of remodeling. Inability of the bone to meet the demands of the stress results in a loss of continuity in the bone and periosteal irritation.	Overuse or abrupt change in training program Change in running surface Change in running gait	Referred pain to the fracture site when a percussion test is used (e.g., hitting the heel may cause pain at the site of a tibial stress fracture) Pain usually localized in one spot that is exquisitely tender	Refer to physician; x-ray films should be obtained. Usually no crack is detected in the bone. A cloudy area becomes visible when the callus begins to form. Often this does not show up until 2–6 weeks after the onset of pain. Early detection can usually be made through a bone scan or thermogram.

continues

Common Orthopedic Problems and Their Treatment (continued)

Injury	Common Causes	Signs and Symptoms	Treatment
Tibial stress fractures—more common in individualswith high-arched feet		Pain generally present all the time but increases with weight-bearing activity; no lessening of pain after after warm-up	If a stress fracture is suspected but not diagnosed treat as a stress fracture.
Fibula stress fractures—more common in pronators			Running and other high-stress, weight-bearing activities should not be allowed until the fracture has healed and the bone is no longer tender to palpation. Tibial stress fractures usually take 8–10 weeks to heal; fibula stress fractures take approximately 6 weeks. When acute symptoms have subsided, bicycling and swimming activities can usually be initiated to maintain cardiovascular levels. This should be cleared with the supervising physician. If a specific cause is attributed to the development of a stress fracture, steps should be taken to correct the cause.

Source: Reprinted, by permission, from E. Howley & B. Franks, Health Fitness Instructor's Handbook, 3rd ed. *(Champaign, IL, Human Kinetics, 1997), 424–426.*

Shin-Splint Syndrome

Injury	Common Causes	Signs and Symptoms	Treatment
Shin splints—inflammatory reaction of the musculotendonous unit, caused by over-exertion of muscles during weight-bearing activity. The following conditions must be ruled out: stress fracture, metabolic or vascular disorder compartment syndrome, and muscular strain.	Prominent callus in metatarsal region		Keep callus filed down.
	Fallen metatarsal arch		Wear a metatarsal arch pad.
	Weak longitudinal arch	Lower longitudinal arch on one side in comparison to the opposite side	Conduct strengthening exercises for tow flexors. Wear longitudinal arch tape for support. Wear arch supports.
		Tenderness in arch area	Conduct strengthening exercises for the dorsi-flexors and inverters. Exercise to increase range of motion.
	Poor leg, ankle, and foot flexibility	Muscular imbalance	Avoid hard surfaces.
	Improper running surface		Avoid changing from one surface to another.
	Improper running shoes		Select a shoe with good shock-absorbency qualities; be sure that the shoe is properly fitted.
	Overuse		Be flexible about changing the training program if there are signs that a great deal of physical stress is occurring. Encourage year-round conditioning. Always warm up properly.
	Biomechanical problems or structural abnormalities	Abnormal wear pattern of shoes	Refer to podiatrist or other profes-sional specializing in foot-care; orthotics may not be medicated. Design a special training program to allow for individual differences (e.g., increase intensity of work outs, reduce duration).

continues

Shin-Splint Syndrome (continued)

Injury	Common Causes	Signs and Symptoms	Treatment
	Improper running or skills technique		Correct technique. Perform specific stretching or strengthening exercises as well as technique work.
	Training in poor weather		Use common sense when training Dress properly to maintain warmth. Warm up and cool down properly.

Source: Reprinted, by permission, from E. Howley & B. Franks, Health Fitness Instructor's Handbook, 3rd ed. *(Champaign, IL, Human Kinetics, 1997), 428.*

The Least You Need to Know

- Be aware of injury risks, and take the necessary steps to avoid them.
- Failure to replace worn shoes is a major contributor to leg and lower-back problems.
- Common orthopedic problems can turn serious if left untreated in the early stages.
- Protection, rest, ice, compression, and elevation (PRICE) is the suggested treatment for strains and sprains.

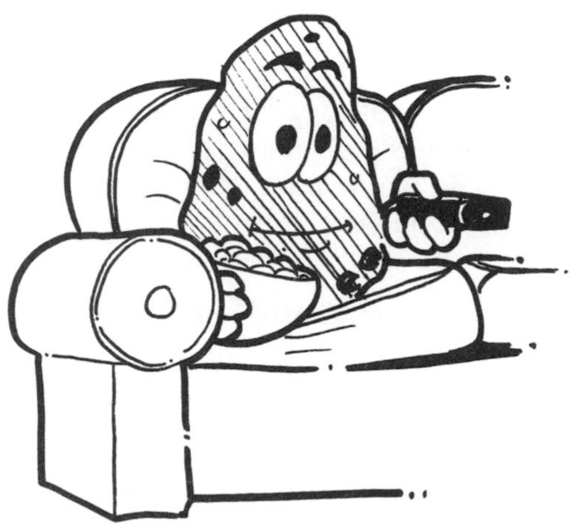

Chapter 16

Return of the Couch Potato

In This Chapter

- Taking a hard-body holiday
- Massaging away your cares
- Visiting the spa in your home

If you can't remember the last time you did something special for yourself, then you need a hard-body holiday. This time is special, so it deserves to be your holiday. Set aside the same time each week so that your holiday can become a weekly self-care celebration.

You can do anything you want with your time (even if it's nothing at all), as long as it makes you feel good about yourself. You are your most prized possession, so it's time you treated yourself that way. My hard-body holiday hit list should give you some R&R ideas to get you started.

Besides feeling good, getting a regular rubdown is good for you and your hard-body results. Getting a massage after a workout can eliminate soreness and speed up the recovery process. If getting pampered in your PJs has your name all over it, then my spa tips will show you how to get the cushy treatment from the comfort of your own home.

Hard-Body Holiday Hit List

Your hard-body holiday can be a couple of hours or a whole day each week that's dedicated to you. This is a mandatory part of your training program, so you should put as much effort into pampering your hard body as you do training it. Your hard-body holiday menu includes one cheat meal of whatever your heart desires in the appropriate portion size.

I've started you off with a few of my favorite R&R activities. Create your own hard-body holiday hit list, and keep it handy. Make it a goal to do everything on your list (at least twice):

- Wear your most comfortable PJs all day.
- Burn your favorite scented candles and/or incense while you listen to your most relaxing CDs. (Nag Champa incense and John Serrie's *Spirit Keepers* are an amazing combination.)
- Turn off the phone, and curl up in your most comfortable chair with that book you've been meaning to read and your favorite herbal tea.
- Go shopping by yourself or with a friend.
- Take a walk in the park, and leave your cell phone at home.
- Play your favorite CD loud, and dance.
- Have brunch with your best friend.
- Get a massage, manicure, pedicure, or facial, or splurge for a day of beauty.
- Watch your favorite old movie.
- Take a bike ride.
- Take a relaxing bath with your favorite bath oils and lighted candles.
- Buy fresh flowers and create arrangements to brighten your rooms.
- Send your mom flowers (just because she'd love it—try iflowers.com for virtual bouquets).
- Meditate.
- Do nothing at all, and love it.
- Stay in bed all day.
- Give that special person a full-body massage with your favorite oils. (Odds are good that he or she will reciprocate.)
- Have breakfast in bed.

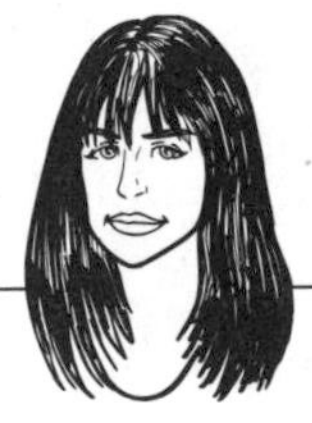

Jourdan's Gems

Whenever you have a great day, write down the activities you did. These will make great additions to your hard-body holiday hit list. Planning your weekly holiday with fun activities will give you something to look forward to and make it easier to do all your weekly workouts.

- Cruise the neighborhood flea markets to find unexpected treasures.
- Do something nice for someone without that person knowing it.
- Bake something.

Massage Magic

Getting a massage is one of my favorite ways to reward myself for all my hard-body training. I make getting a massage a weekly hard-body holiday ritual. It not only makes you feel great (which is reason enough to get one), but it's also good for you (which now makes it a no-brainer). Some of the major benefits include these:

- **Reduced stress.** A massage releases tight muscles and natural *endorphins*. This results in decreased pain, a decreased heart rate, and a sense of calm.
- **Mental sharpness.** The relieved muscle tension allows your blood to flow freely to supply your body with nutrients and oxygen. Your whole system runs more efficiently, and you feel energized.
- **Increased cardio efficiency.** Oxygenated and nutrient-rich blood are circulated more efficiently.
- **Boost for the immune system.** Releasing tight respiratory muscles facilitates more movement throughout the chest cavity and increases lymph flow to aid in killing foreign substances and toxins.
- **Prevention of muscle strain injuries.** Massage increases your flexibility and suppleness.
- **Increased muscle development.** Massage speeds up your post-exercise recovery time so that you can train more often.

When you make an appointment, you need to know the different types of massages that are offered so that you'll be sure to get exactly the type

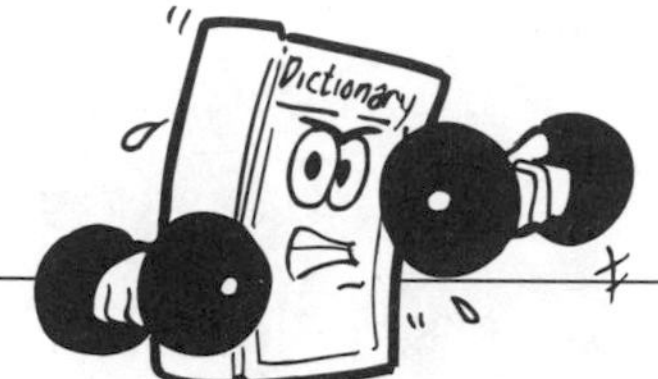

Workout Wisdom

Endorphins are hormones that are found in the brain that reduce the sensation of pain and affect emotions.

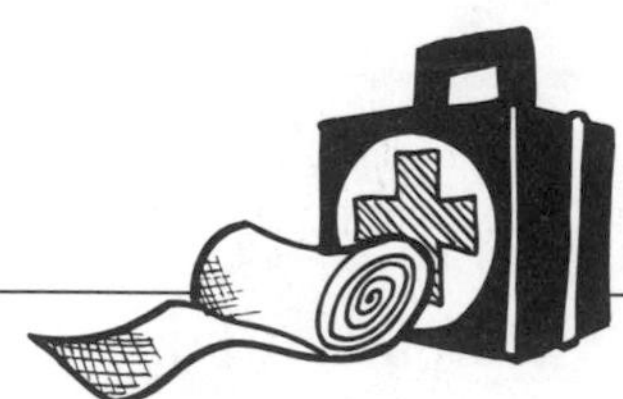

Safety Scoop

To avoid upsetting your stomach because of the kneading and pressure applied to your back, it's best not eat 45 minutes to 1 hour before your massage. It's actually great to exercise before you get your massage in order to remove toxins, eliminate muscle soreness, and speed up recovery time.

of rubdown you want. I say this because a friend once treated me to a massage, and, instead of getting the usual strong hands working out the knots in my back, I got some woman stepping all over my back, legs, and head. (The bar attached to the ceiling over the table should have been my first clue.)

The massage menu options should include the following:

- **Swedish massage** The most popular and well-known type of massage. This technique uses gliding, kneading, and compressing strokes to improve circulation. Deeper strokes can be requested to work out *knots* in your muscles.
- **Shiatsu** Balances the body's life force to keep your systems in balance. Pressure of varying degrees is applied along points throughout the body to encourage balance and energy flow.
- **Reiki** Involves a person called "the healer," who becomes a channeler of universal energy. Deep relaxation and healing are brought about through a traditional pattern of hand positions on the body without pressure.
- **Reflexology** Involves steady pressure applied to specific points on the foot that correspond to different body parts and organs. Freeing blockages in the nervous system stimulates the body's natural healing process.

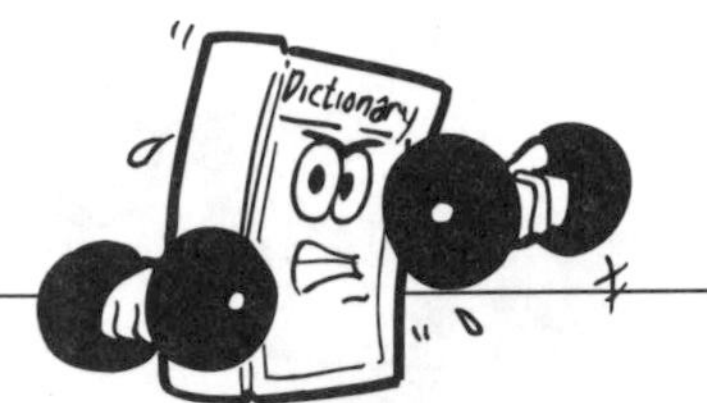

Workout Wisdom

Knots, also known as adhesions, are abnormal joinings of tissues around a site of inflammation. They don't always cause problems, but they can limit flexibility and range of motion.

Home Spa Tips

The following tips and products will give you that spa feeling from the comfort of your own home at a fraction of the price:

- For puffy eyes, place cool cucumber slices over your eyes for 10 minutes or more. Applying heavy oils around the eye area before going to bed can cause eyes to be puffy in the morning.
- Add a few drops of lavender to 4 ounces of distilled water. Use this as an herbal spray for your face throughout the day to replenish lost moisture.
- To add color to your skin, mash a half-cup of strawberries in a blender, and then apply to the face. Leave this on for 10 minutes, and rinse with warm water.
- For the softest skin imaginable, you need to try Body Butter (nut-flavored) from The Body Shop. Use this after you shower, in place of a massage oil, or anytime you want silky, soft skin.

- For a massage oil that smells as good as it feels, try Nature's Massage Oil (Juniper Breeze) from Bath & Body Works.
- I've tried many of the expensive masks, but none have tightened my pores and left my skin as soft as Aztec Secret Indian Healing Clay. You can get a 1-pound jar at the Vitamin Shoppe for about $8.

Home Spa Facial

Getting a facial no longer has to be a luxury for spa goers. Your home spa facial will give your skin the silky feel of a spa facial from the comfort of your own home and at a fraction of the price.

1. Set the mood with scents and sounds. (It's a perfect time for Nag Champa incense and John Serrie's *Spirit Keepers*.)
2. Clean your face first.
3. Steam your face for about 10 minutes to open pores. Simmer two to four tablespoons of dried or fresh peppermint, chamomile, and lavender herbs in two quarts of water. Remove this concoction from heat, and hold your head over it under a towel. Put the herbal water in the refrigerator to cool.
4. Mix Indian Healing Clay with apple cider vinegar, and apply this to your face. Relax for 10 to 15 minutes, or until the mask hardens.
5. Rinse your face with warm water.
6. Rub ice over your face to tighten pores.
7. Use the cooled herbal water as an astringent.
8. Use a moisturizer. (If I plan to be outside, I use a sunblock that's specifically for the face, such as Sea & Ski Faces, with 50 SPF, to protect my skin. I still get color with the 50, so I can't imagine going out without it.)

Having a weekly hard-body holiday will go a long way in helping you maintain balance in your life, and it will give you fun things to look forward to.

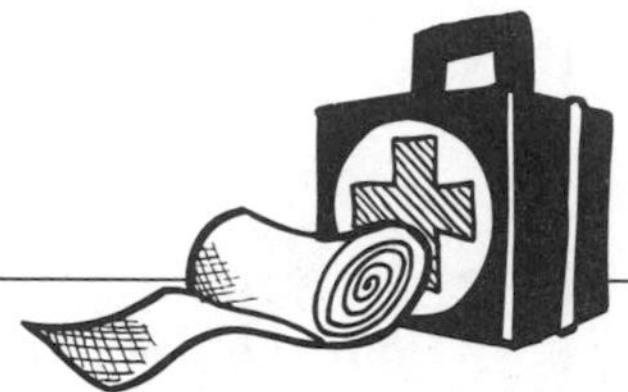

Safety Scoop

If your skin is chapped, take in more water and essential fatty acids. A good source is flaxseed oil capsules or liquid, or Ultimate Oil from Nature's Secret. Avoid saturated and animal fats.

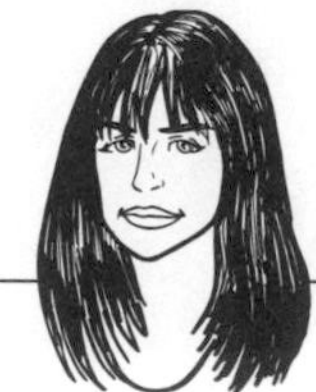

Jourdan's Gems

To soften and nourish your skin, apply a mashed avocado all over your face. Leave it on until it dries, and then rinse your face with warm water. The essential fatty acids and other nutrients help prevent premature wrinkling.

Not only is getting a massage a great way to spend your hard-body holiday, it also removes toxins, helps eliminate muscle soreness, and speeds up recovery time. Finally, the home spa tips are designed to give you that pampered feeling anytime you want or need it. It's a great feeling, so I suggest doing it often.

The Least You Need to Know

- ➤ Take a hard-body holiday every week to recharge your batteries.
- ➤ A massage gives you quicker hard-body results by speeding up post-exercise recovery time so that you can train more often.
- ➤ Spray an herbal mist of lavender oil and distilled water on your face throughout the day to replenish lost moisture.

Chapter 17

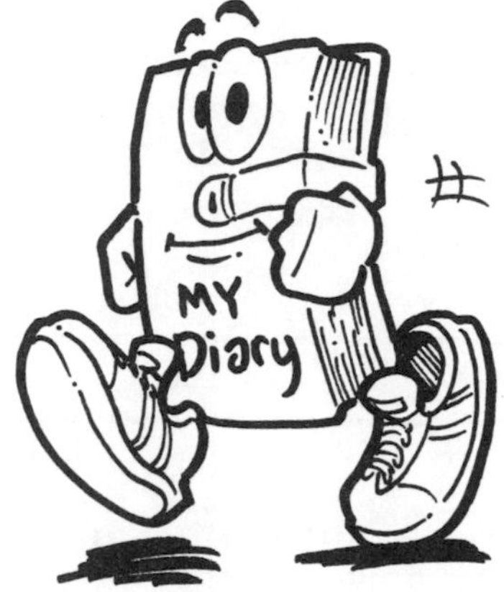

Dear Diary

In This Chapter

- Daily event planner
- Weekly training schedule
- Weight training/cardio log
- Daily food log
- Weekly menu planner

The only way to stay on top of your hard-body game is to be well organized. Your Home Hard-Body Journal will be the guide for your fitness journey. Maximizing your results will be easy because you'll be able to actually see what works and what doesn't.

I've given you some sample log pages to get you started. Simply copy and enlarge the log pages to fit $8^1/_2 \times 11$-inch paper, and then make enough copies (on three-hole paper because punching holes can be a nightmare) to fill your Home Hard-Body Journal.

Daily Planning

Writing down your daily events helps to organize your day and to ensure that you don't miss something important, such as that evening cardio session. I've put together a Hard-Body Daily Planner that you can use in addition to your regular planner. This planner has a place for your business and personal goals. Try to do at least one thing to achieve these goals every day.

Today's Hard-Body Events

Day: **Date:**

Time	Event	Notes and Comments	Time	Event	Notes and Comments
Early morning	______	______	1:00	______	______
7:00	______	______	1:30	______	______
7:30	______	______	2:00	______	______
8:00	______	______	2:30	______	______
8:30	______	______	3:00	______	______
9:00	______	______	3:30	______	______
9:30	______	______	4:00	______	______
10:00	______	______	4:30	______	______
10:30	______	______	5:00	______	______
11:00	______	______	5:30	______	______
11:30	______	______	6:00	______	______
12:00	______	______	6:30	______	______
12:30	______	______	Evening	______	______

Today's Priorities	Business Goals	Personal Goals
____________	____________	____________
____________	____________	____________
____________	____________	____________
____________	____________	____________
____________	____________	____________

Hard-Body Training

Your training schedule and log pages are the meat and potatoes of your Home Hard-Body Journal. Keep your training schedule in the front of your journal. I've combined your strength training and cardio into one two-week log page to make it easier to use. Use one log page for each muscle group trained.

Hard-Body Weekly Training Schedule

Time	Mon.	Tues.	Wed.	Thurs.	Fri.	Sat.	Sun.
6:00 A.M.	____	____	____	____	____	____	____
6:30	____	____	____	____	____	____	____
7:00	____	____	____	____	____	____	____
7:30	____	____	____	____	____	____	____
8:00	____	____	____	____	____	____	____
8:30	____	____	____	____	____	____	____
9:00	____	____	____	____	____	____	____
9:30	____	____	____	____	____	____	____
10:00	____	____	____	____	____	____	____
10:30	____	____	____	____	____	____	____
11:00	____	____	____	____	____	____	____
11:30	____	____	____	____	____	____	____
12:00 P.M.	____	____	____	____	____	____	____
12:30	____	____	____	____	____	____	____
1:00	____	____	____	____	____	____	____
1:30	____	____	____	____	____	____	____
2:00	____	____	____	____	____	____	____
2:30	____	____	____	____	____	____	____
3:00	____	____	____	____	____	____	____
3:30	____	____	____	____	____	____	____
4:00	____	____	____	____	____	____	____
4:30	____	____	____	____	____	____	____
5:00	____	____	____	____	____	____	____
5:30	____	____	____	____	____	____	____
6:00	____	____	____	____	____	____	____
6:30	____	____	____	____	____	____	____
7:00	____	____	____	____	____	____	____
7:30	____	____	____	____	____	____	____
8:00	____	____	____	____	____	____	____

Hard-Body Strength and Cardio Training Log

Muscle Group

Exercise	Date
Pounds	____
Reps	____

continues

Hard-Body Strength and Cardio Training Log (continued)

Muscle Group	
Exercise	**Date**
Pounds	_____
Reps	_____
Pounds	_____
Reps	_____

Target Heart Rate Range

	Beats per Minute	Beats per Six Seconds
55% of your max heart rate	_____	_____
70% of your max heart rate	_____	_____
85% of your max heart rate	_____	_____
	Activity	**Date**
Minutes	_____	_____
Average heart rate	_____	_____
Minutes	_____	_____
Average heart rate	_____	_____
Minutes	_____	_____
Average heart rate	_____	_____
Minutes	_____	_____
Average heart rate	_____	_____

Hard-Body Nutrition

Keeping track of your food intake is the only way that you can be sure you're on the right track. I've divided your daily food log so that you can keep track of your protein, carbs, fats, and water intake. Write down how you felt after a certain meal in the comments section at the bottom of your log page. This way you'll know what meal combinations were hard-body winners.

Your menu planner will save you time by letting you plan your hard-body meals ahead of time. I've also given you a hard-body grocery list to get your "eating smart" shopping started.

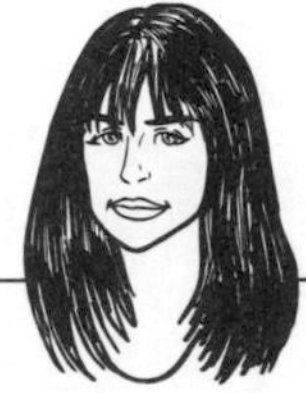

Jourdan's Gems

A meal that leaves you feeling light and energized is a hard-body winner.

Hard-Body Daily Food Log

Protein and carbs = 4 calories per gram

Fat = 9 calories per gram

Alcohol = 7 calories per gram

Date:

Food Eaten	Amount	Protein (g)	Carbs (g)	Fat (g)	Calories
Breakfast	______	______	______	______	______
Time:	______	______	______	______	______
Snack	______	______	______	______	______
Time:	______	______	______	______	______
Lunch	______	______	______	______	______
Time:	______	______	______	______	______
Snack	______	______	______	______	______
Time:	______	______	______	______	______
Dinner	______	______	______	______	______
Time:	______	______	______	______	______
Snack	______	______	______	______	______
Time:	______	______	______	______	______
Water	______	______	______	______	______
Total	______	______	______	______	______

Of the calories consumed, how much was protein? ____________

Of the calories consumed, how much was carbs? ____________

Of the calories consumed, how much was fat? ____________

Comments: ____

Hard-Body Weekly Menu Planner

Mon.	Tues.	Wed.	Thurs.	Fri.	Sat.	Sun.
Breakfast	**Breakfast**	**Breakfast**	**Breakfast**	**Breakfast**	**Breakfast**	**Breakfast**
Calories: ____	Calories: ____	Calories: ____	Calories: ____	Calories: ____	Calories: ____	Calories: ____
Fat grams: ____	Fat grams: ____	Fat grams: ____	Fat grams: ____	Fat grams: ____	Fat grams: ____	Fat grams: ____
Lunch	**Lunch**	**Lunch**	**Lunch**	**Lunch**	**Lunch**	**Lunch**
Calories: ____	Calories: ____	Calories: ____	Calories: ____	Calories: ____	Calories: ____	Calories: ____
Fat grams: ____	Fat grams: ____	Fat grams: ____	Fat grams: ____	Fat grams: ____	Fat grams: ____	Fat grams: ____
Dinner	**Dinner**	**Dinner**	**Dinner**	**Dinner**	**Dinner**	**Dinner**
Calories: ____	Calories: ____	Calories: ____	Calories: ____	Calories: ____	Calories: ____	Calories: ____
Fat grams: ____	Fat grams: ____	Fat grams: ____	Fat grams: ____	Fat grams: ____	Fat grams: ____	Fat grams: ____
AM Snack	**AM Snack**	**AM Snack**	**AM Snack**	**AM Snack**	**AM Snack**	**AM Snack**
Calories: ____	Calories: ____	Calories: ____	Calories: ____	Calories: ____	Calories: ____	Calories: ____
Fat grams: ____	Fat grams: ____	Fat grams: ____	Fat grams: ____	Fat grams: ____	Fat grams: ____	Fat grams: ____
PM Snack	**PM Snack**	**PM Snack**	**PM Snack**	**PM Snack**	**PM Snack**	**PM Snack**
Calories: ____	Calories: ____	Calories: ____	Calories: ____	Calories: ____	Calories: ____	Calories: ____
Fat grams: ____	Fat grams: ____	Fat grams: ____	Fat grams: ____	Fat grams: ____	Fat grams: ____	Fat grams: ____
% calories from fat: ____	% calories from fat: ____	% calories from fat: ____	% calories from fat: ____	% calories from fat: ____	% calories from fat: ____	% calories from fat: ____
Weekly Total	Calories: ____	Fat grams: ____	% calories from fat: ____			

Hard-Body Grocery List

Dairy and Substitutes

- ❑ Eggs
- ❑ Low-fat milk
- ❑ Low-fat yogurt
- ❑ Low-fat cottage cheese
- ❑ Soy milk
- ❑ Soy cheese
- ❑ ___________
- ❑ ___________

Protein

- ❑ Chicken
- ❑ Turkey
- ❑ Beef
- ❑ Fish
- ❑ Tofu
- ❑ Soy protein powder
- ❑ Veggie burgers
- ❑ Textured soy protein
- ❑ Soybeans
- ❑ ___________
- ❑ ___________

Fruit

- ❑ Apples
- ❑ Bananas
- ❑ Berries
- ❑ Grapefruit
- ❑ Grapes
- ❑ Lemons
- ❑ Limes
- ❑ Melon
- ❑ Oranges
- ❑ Pears
- ❑ ___________
- ❑ ___________

Vegetables

- ❑ Broccoli
- ❑ Cabbage
- ❑ Carrots
- ❑ Cauliflower
- ❑ Celery
- ❑ Cucumbers
- ❑ Garlic
- ❑ Lettuce
- ❑ Mushrooms
- ❑ Onions
- ❑ Peppers
- ❑ Potatoes
- ❑ Radishes
- ❑ Spinach
- ❑ Tomatoes
- ❑ Yams
- ❑ ___________
- ❑ ___________

Breads

- ❏ Stone-ground bread
- ❏ Whole-wheat pita
- ❏ ___________
- ❏ ___________

Dry Goods

- ❏ Oatmeal
- ❏ Beans/lentils/peas
- ❏ Brown rice
- ❏ Gelatin
- ❏ ___________
- ❏ ___________

Canned Goods

- ❏ Applesauce
- ❏ Fruit
- ❏ Mushrooms
- ❏ Stewed tomatoes
- ❏ Tomato paste
- ❏ Tomato sauce
- ❏ Low-sodium tuna
- ❏ Vegetables
- ❏ ___________

Frozen Foods

- ❏ Vegetables
- ❏ Frozen dinners

Baking Goods

- ❏ Baking soda
- ❏ Baking powder
- ❏ Salt
- ❏ Peppers
- ❏ Nuts
- ❏ Raisins
- ❏ Vanilla
- ❏ Dried herbs
- ❏ Spices
- ❏ ___________
- ❏ ___________

Condiments

- ❏ Oil
- ❏ Vinegar
- ❏ Low-sugar ketchup
- ❏ Mustard
- ❏ Olives
- ❏ Pickles
- ❏ Salsa
- ❏ Salad dressing
- ❏ Low-sodium soy sauce
- ❏ Honey
- ❏ Sugar-free jam
- ❏ Peanut butter
- ❏ Sugar-free syrup
- ❏ ___________

Beverages

- ❑ Coffee
- ❑ Tea
- ❑ Fruit juice
- ❑ Mineral water
- ❑ ___________
- ❑ ___________
- ❑ ___________

If this seems like too much work, then you can use a journal that's already set up and ready to go on my Web site, www.teamjourdan.com. In addition to enough log pages for 30 days, I've added a motivational thought for each day and calorie charts for hard-body foods, fast foods, and frozen foods.

The Least You Need to Know

- ➤ Planning your daily events keeps you on top of your goals.
- ➤ A training log charts your progress and alerts you when you need to vary your routine.
- ➤ Writing down how you feel after a meal in your daily food log lets you know which meal combinations are hard-body winners.
- ➤ Time-saver tools such as the hard-body weekly meal planner and a grocery list make it easier for you to spend more of your valuable time enjoying your hard-body results.

Part 4

Expanding Your Hard-Body Horizons

This section shows you that your hard-body training doesn't have to stop at your front door. Chapter 18, "Taking It to the Streets," covers hard-body cardio roadwork and includes a complete routine for cross-training in the park.

Taking your hard body on the road for business or pleasure is easy with your travel workout and gear in a bag. My vacation tips will help maximize your hard-body fun in the sun.

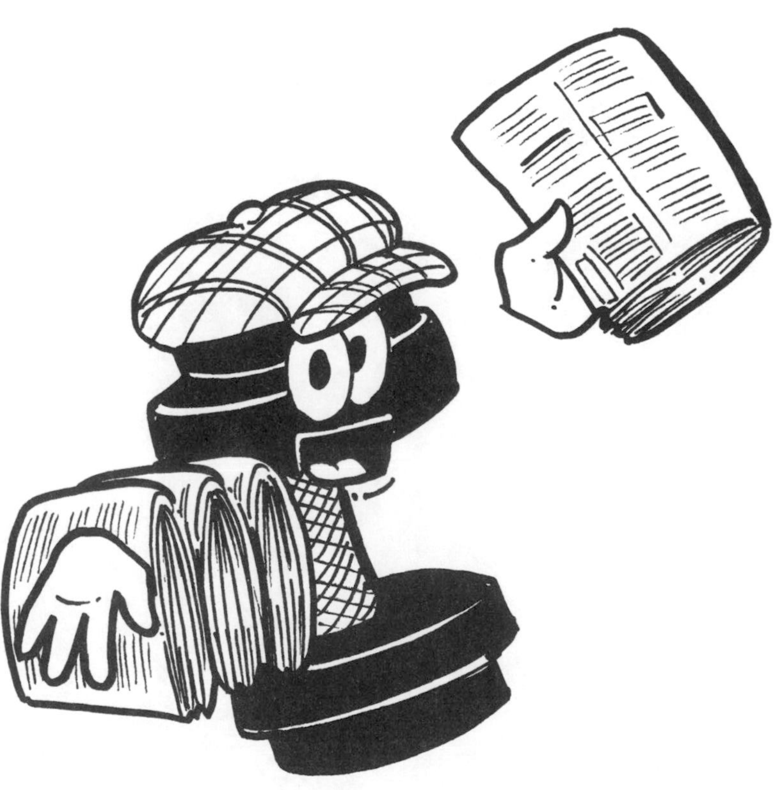

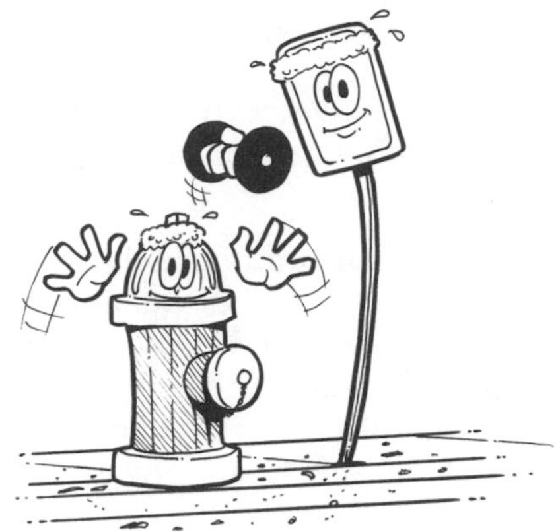

Chapter 18

Taking It to the Streets

In This Chapter

- Hard bodies hit the road
- Six-week hard-body running program
- Cross-training in the park

Your hard-body training gym doesn't have to end at your front door. Extending your training area to include backyards, neighborhood sidewalks, nearby parks, and school playing fields will give you numerous new hard-body workout options.

Lacing up your shoes and hitting the road for sprint work is a great way to keep your legs toned and trim. The six-week hard-body running program will make your transition from walking to running smooth and shin splint-free.

Training in a park is like being in a cross-training candy store. There is a gold mine of training gear around every corner just sitting there waiting for you. With all the conditioning choices, doing the same workout twice is never an option.

Hard Bodies Hit the Road

To give your cardio training more variety, you might want to give your treadmill the day off and take a brisk walk or run through the neighborhood. A nearby park can become a perfect outdoor setting for your hard-body training.

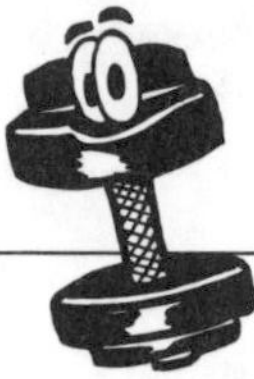

Hard-Body Headliners

Running burns about 100 calorie per mile and 300 calories for an easy 30-minute run.

Running is a great way to tone your leg muscles and burn fat. If you're not a seasoned runner, then you need to gradually incorporate running into your program. Doing too much too soon can easily result in shin splints.

An easy way to increase your running ability is to incorporate running intervals into your walking sessions. Gradually increase the time you spend running and decrease the time you walk until you are able to run continuously for 30 minutes. The following table outlines your six-week hard-body running program.

Hard-Body Running Program

Week	1	2	3	4	5	6
Warm-up						
Walk	10 minutes	10 minutes	8 minutes	5 minutes	5 minutes	5 minutes
Run	1 minutes	2 minutes	3 minutes	4 minutes	5 minutes	6 minutes
Walk	2 minutes	1 minutes	2 minutes	3 minutes	4 minutes	4 minutes
Total intervals	3	3	3	3	2	2
Cool-down walk	10 minutes	10 minutes	8 minutes	5 minutes	5 minutes	5 minutes

Cross-Training in the Park

Some of my favorite cardio sessions have been in the park. By using ordinary objects found in the park and then adding your own unique combination of strengthening exercises, you can turn an ordinary cardio session into an ultimate conditioning workout. Blazing your own cardio trail can make cardio an adventure to look forward to.

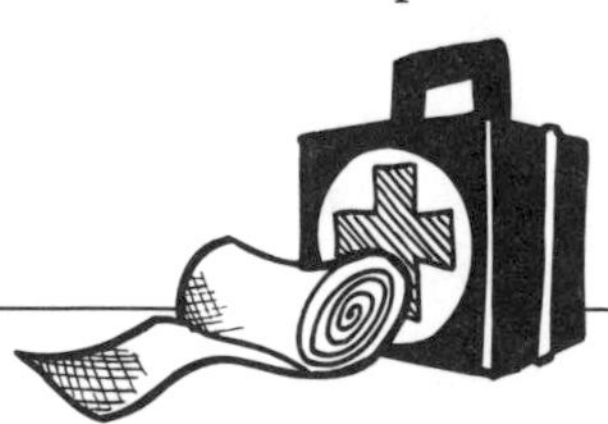

Safety Scoop

Side stitches (cramps) are usually a result of shallow breathing or dehydration. Taking several deep breaths through your nose and exhaling through your mouth can bring quick relief.

Warm Up and Stretch

My warm-up is an easy-paced jog to the park. When I find a scenic and relaxing spot, I stop and stretch.

Quadriceps Stretch

1. Start standing with your back straight. While holding on to a rail, bend your knee, reach back, and grasp your foot behind you.

2. With your knees together, push forward with your hip as you gently pull your foot back. Hold the stretch.
3. Release and repeat on your other side.

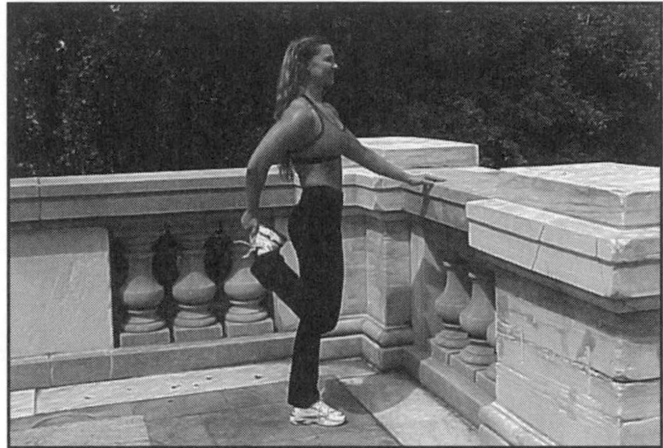

Hamstring Stretch

1. Place your leg on a rail, and turn your body to face your foot.
2. Reach forward, bring your chest as close to your thigh as possible, and hold the stretch.
3. Release and repeat on the other side.

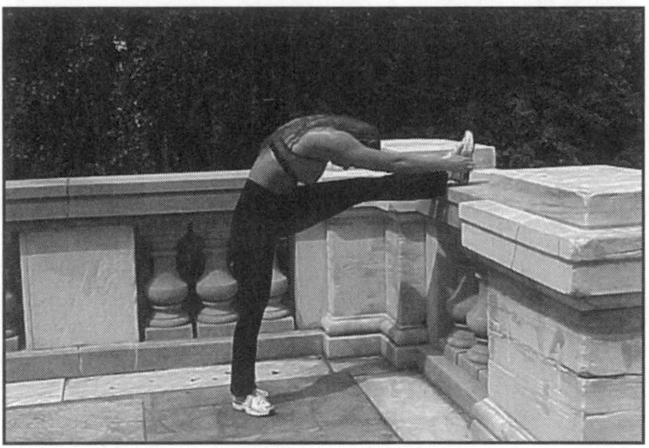

Side Bend

1. With your leg still on the rail, turn your body outward away from your leg.
2. Bend sideways, reaching overhead toward your foot, and hold the stretch.
3. Repeat on the other side.

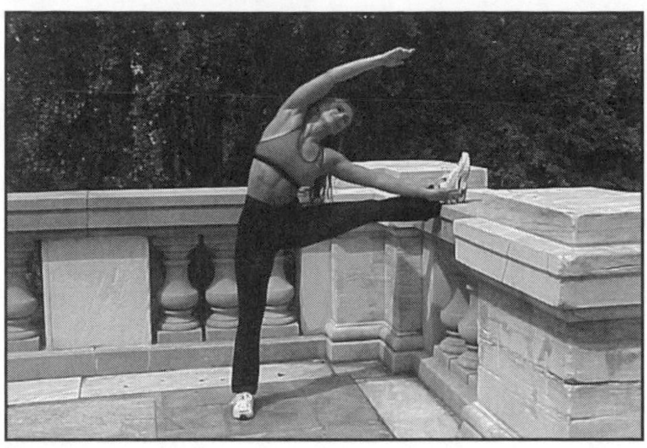

Butterfly Stretch

1. Sit tall, with your back straight and your shoulders back.
2. Grasp your feet in front of you, and pull in as you try to touch your knees to the floor. Hold the stretch.

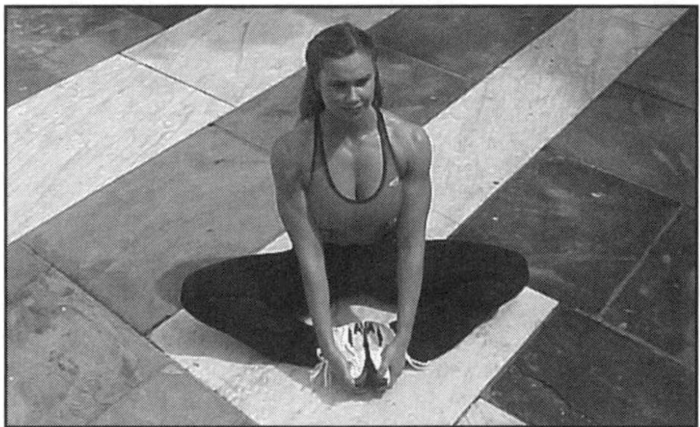

Abdominals

I then continue with a light jog until I find a flat bench wide enough to do my ab training. I like to jog for approximately 10 minutes between my stretch and ab training.

Lower Ab Lift

1. Lie flat on a bench, with your legs straight up and your hands by your sides.
2. Using your ab muscles, lift your lower body a couple of inches off the bench, hold for one second, and lower to the starting point.
3. Repeat for desired reps. Go to the crunch.

Crunch

1. Bring your hands to the sides of your head. Knees should be bent, with toes up.
2. Exhale and lift your shoulders off the bench as you press your weight into your heels. (Doing this will enable you to work the lower abs as well.) Hold for one second and lower to the starting point.
3. Repeat for desired reps. Go to the combined crunch.

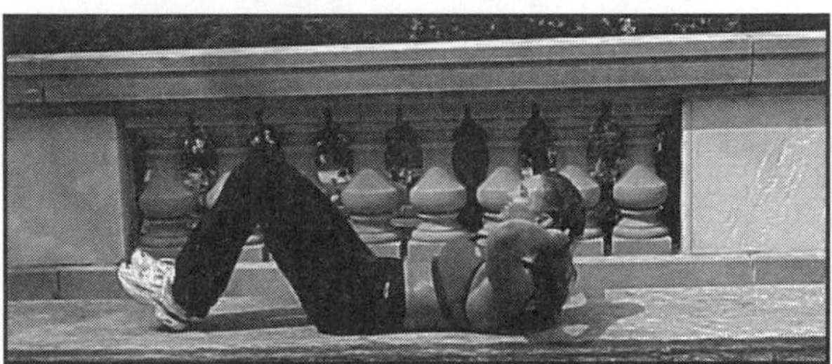

Combined Crunch

1. Bring your legs straight up again. Exhale and lift both your upper and lower body.
2. Contract your abs for one second, and lower to the starting point.
3. Repeat for desired reps.

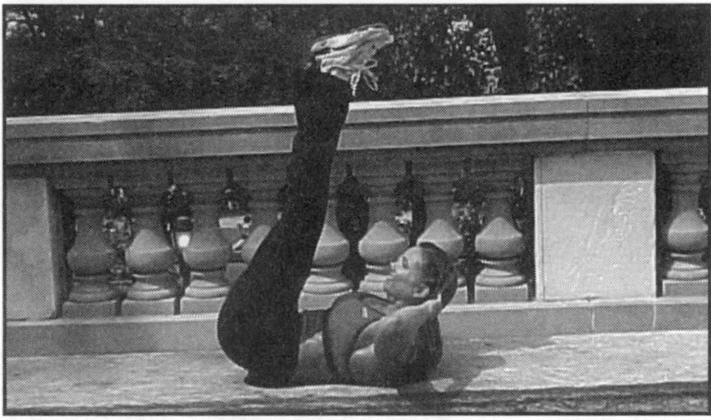

Interval Sprints

I look for a clear path or bridge to do my interval sprint work. I do five intervals, but you can start with three if you're not accustomed to interval training.

1. Sprint across the length of a bridge (I look for a length of approximately 100 yards. Another option would be to use a stop watch or second hand on a regular watch and sprint for 30 seconds.)
2. Jog back at an easy pace.

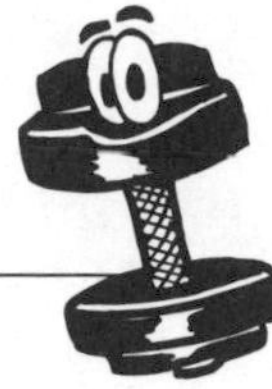

Hard-Body Headliners

Sprinting increases leg development, boosts metabolism, and speeds up fat loss.

Push-Ups

When I finish my intervals, I find a place along the railing and do three sets of push-ups. Do as many reps as possible (AMRAP) until you reach 20.

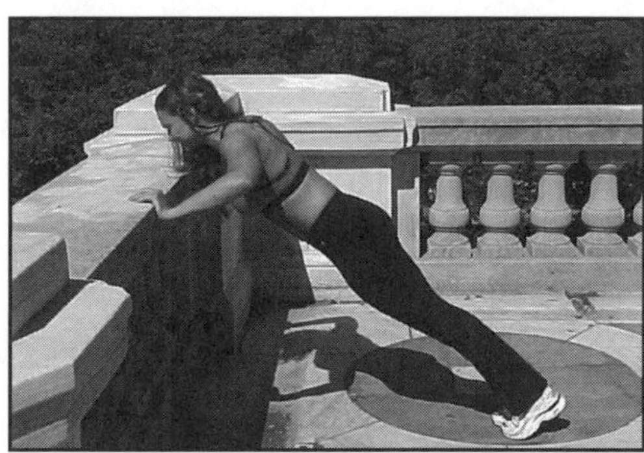

With your hands shoulder-width apart, lower yourself until your chest almost touches the railing, and then press up. Repeat for desired reps.

Elevation Work

I now look for a hill or a tall set of stairs to do my elevation work. Start with two sets and work up to five sets, up and back.

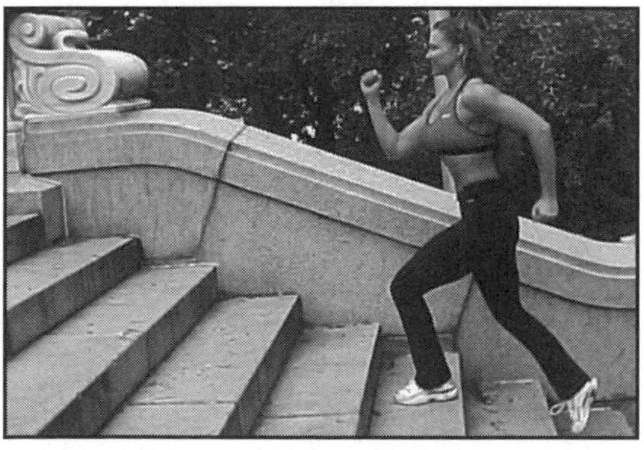

Take the stairs up two at a time for a better butt workout.

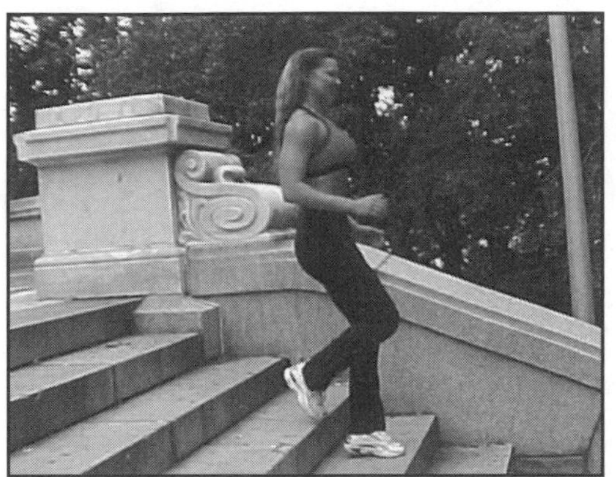

Jog down at an easy pace. Repeat for desired sets.

Triceps Dip

After my hill work, I do more strength training. There are usually plenty of places to do dips. Do AMRAP.

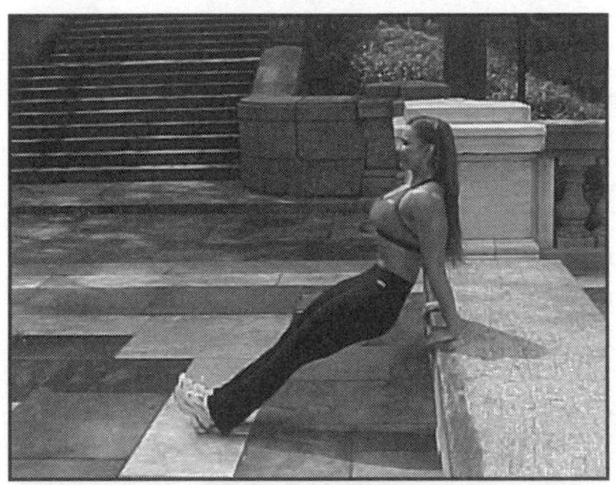

Start with your hands outside your hips, and your fingers forward, grasping the edge of the wall. Legs are extended straight in front of you. (Those with less upper-body strength can bend their knees.)

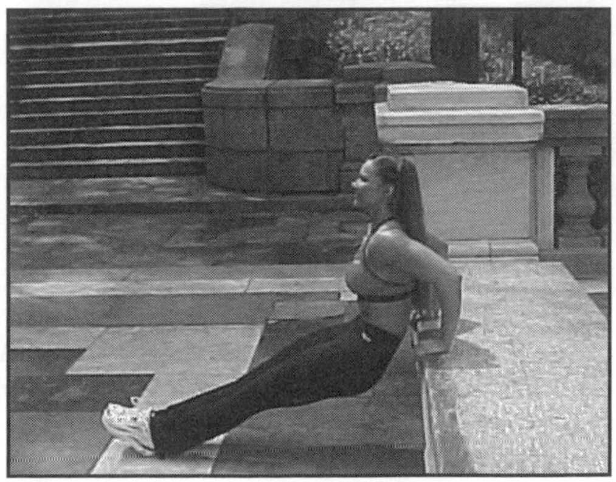

Keeping your butt close to the wall, bend your elbows and lower your body until you feel a stretch, and then press up. Repeat for desired reps.

Elevated Side Squats

I find a bench or a low wall to do my final strength move, elevated side squats. Work up to 20 reps on each side.

1. Start with your right foot on a bench. Bend at your hips, and squat back until you feel a stretch in your quads.
2. Shift your weight to your right foot, and raise yourself up until you're standing straight. Raise your left leg and arms as you rise up.
3. Lower slowly so that you land softly, and then repeat for desired reps.

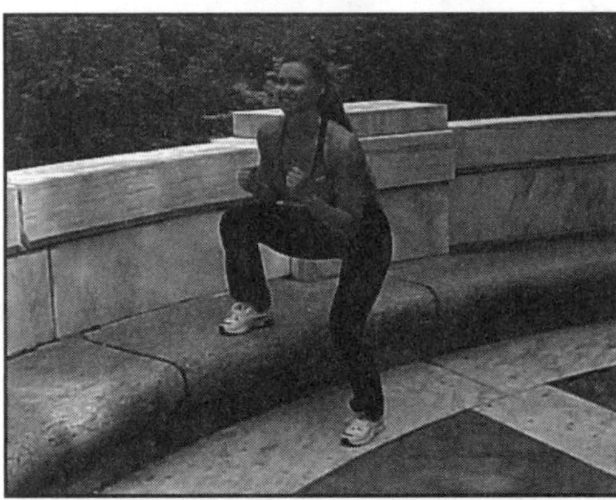

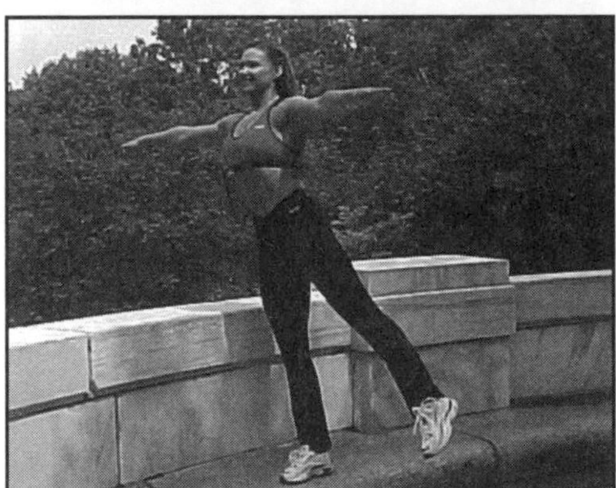

Cool Down and Stretch

I now do a light jog for about five minutes until I find a cool place to do my stretching exercises. Take 5 to 10 minutes and thoroughly stretch the muscles of your body. When you finish stretching, find a comfortable spot and just sit still for a while. Use this time to connect with your spirit.

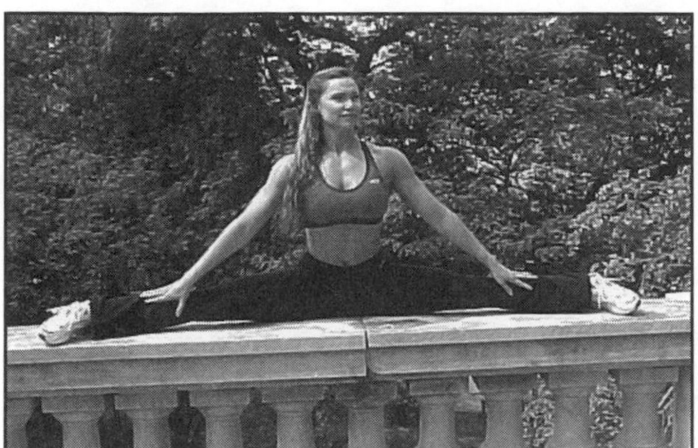

Taking in the park view after my training session. (Don't try this at home.)

The Least You Need to Know

- Side stitches are usually a result of shallow breathing and dehydration. Taking several deep breaths through your nose and exhaling through your mouth can bring quick relief.
- Sprinting increases leg development, boosts metabolism, and speeds up fat loss.
- Running burns around 100 calories per mile.
- You can get a complete conditioning workout by using ordinary objects found in a park.

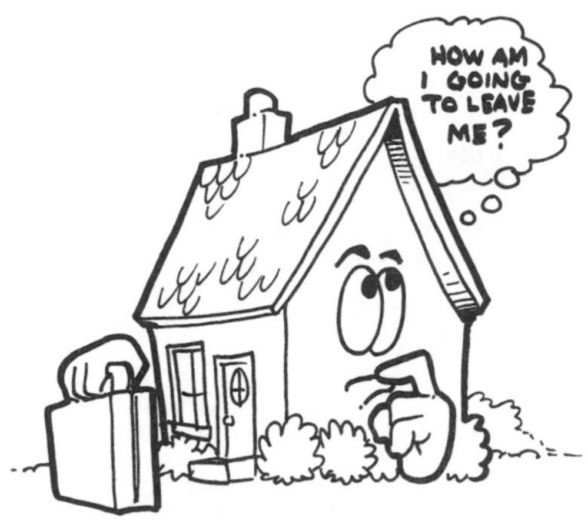

Chapter 19

Home Away from Home

In This Chapter

- Travel cardio options
- Resistance bands that rock
- Hard-body travel workout
- Hard-body vacation tips

Vacations or business trips don't mean that all that hard-body hard work has to go to waste. With a little ingenuity (this chapter has you covered on that one) and your hard-body journal, you'll be well-equipped to handle whatever workout obstacles you might face on the road.

If you think that training on the road means lugging a suitcase full of dumbbells, you'll be jazzed when you see my workout-in-a-bag gear (leave the extra space for cool travel souvenirs). *Quick* and *easy* are the words that describe your hard-body travel workout. (For more quick and easy routines, see Chapter 13, "Ten-Minute Ticket to Tone.")

My vacation tips are designed to keep your hard body looking good, so when you hear someone say, "Did you see that hot body?" smile—they'll be talking about you.

Travel Cardio

Scheduling your cardio work while traveling isn't that tough if you realize that any time you're moving, you have an opportunity to do some cardio. You might have to extend the time and step up the pace a little, but there is no downside to getting to your meeting early, taking a longer walk on the beach, or power shopping. (Turning shopping into an event to burn calories always makes me feel better about the money I spent.) The following are a few suggestions to get you started on burning those calories:

- Sightsee on foot.
- Jog on a beach. (For a real challenge, run on soft sand.)
- Swim laps in a pool before breakfast. (See Chapter 10, "Home Is Where the Heart Gets Fit," for cardio-maximizing tips.)
- Check out the hotel gym for cardio gear.
- Dance until dawn.
- Power shopping (shopping at a brisk pace for a period of time without taking a break to sit).
- Take a walk after dinner.

Resistance Bands Rock

You have to love exercise equipment that can fit in a 6"-by-6" bag. That resistance bands can give you a good workout in a short amount of time is just the cherry on top.

When you're on the road and want to get a good workout, a resistance band rocks for these reasons:

- It's so small that you can fit it in the tiniest of bags, making it ideal for travel.
- You can do a large variety of exercises with it.
- The bands come in different resistance levels, so you can't outgrow them.
- They're inexpensive, so you can spend your valuable cash on important stuff, such as an outfit to show off your new hard body.

Hard-Body Travel Moves

This time-saver routine will give your muscles the perfect pump before you hit the beach, the slopes, the shops, or the boardroom.

Start with a brief warm-up like a brisk walk or light jog for 5–10 minutes. Attaching the bands to the leg cuffs of the "Burke Spencer's Personal Trainer" during the warm-up will increase the intensity and burn more calories. After the warm-up, attach the hand grips to the bands and do the following exercises in the order shown, with no rest in between, for one giant set. This way you'll get your heart going, giving you a cardio boost and a full-body muscle workout in one shot. Work up to 20 reps for each move. Finishing your workout with my yoga cool-down in Chapter 12, "Have Floor, Will Lotus," will get you energized and ready to go.

Squat Press

This exercise works the quads, the hamstrings, the glutes, the lower back, the delts, and the triceps.

1. Start by standing on a resistance band with your feet hip-width apart and your arms by your sides, palms up, holding the ends of the band.
2. With your shoulders back and your chest forward, inhale and squat back, as if sitting in a chair, while curling your arms up to your shoulders.
3. Next, exhale and rise, extending your arms overhead while turning your palms until they face forward.
4. Lower slowly, and repeat for desired reps. Go to the row/x-cross.

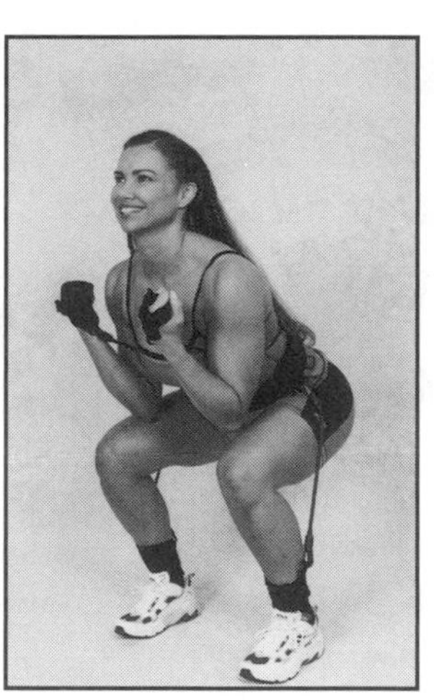

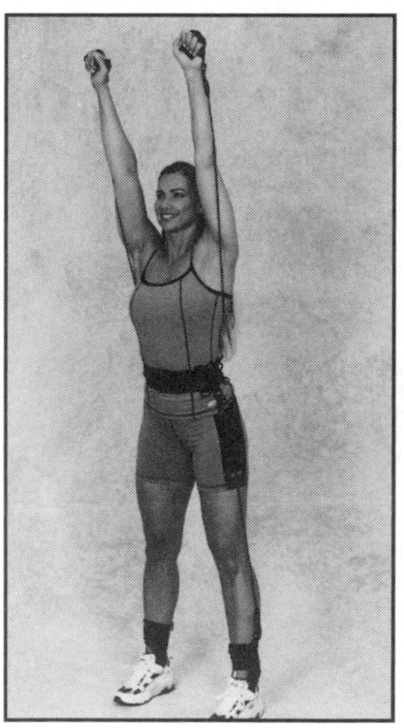

Row/X-Cross

This exercise works the upper back and the rear delts.

1. Start with your feet on a resistance band and your back straight, and bend slightly forward from your waist. Keep your abs tight and your shoulders back.

2. With the band crossed in front, pull up and back, leading with your elbows. Row back as far as you can without moving your shoulders, contract back at top position, and return to start.
3. Next, stand up straight and extend your arms up and out. The band should be in the shape of a giant X.
4. Lower slowly and repeat for desired reps. Go to the one-arm chest lift.

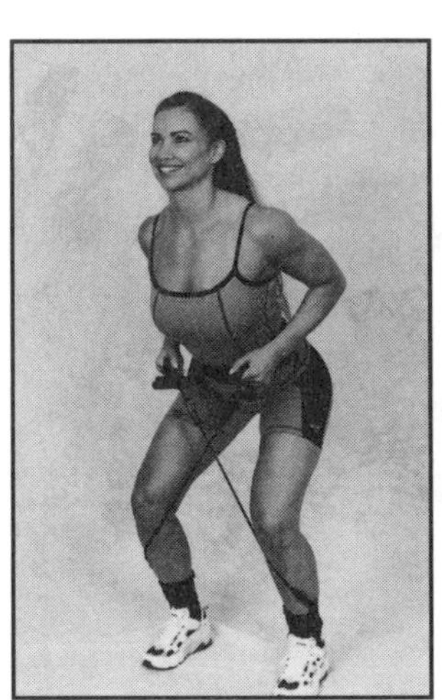

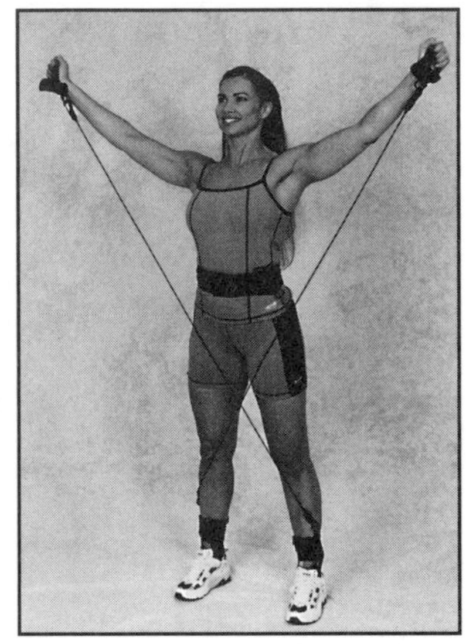

One-Arm Chest Lift

This exercise works the pectorals and the anterior delts.

1. Start by standing with your feet on a resistance band, hip-width apart. With a straight back, abs tight, and shoulders back, place one hand on your hip and one straight by your side, holding the band with your palm up.
2. Exhale, and extend your straight arm up and across your body.
3. Lower slowly, and repeat for desired reps. Switch arms and repeat on your other side. Go to the upright row/lateral raise.

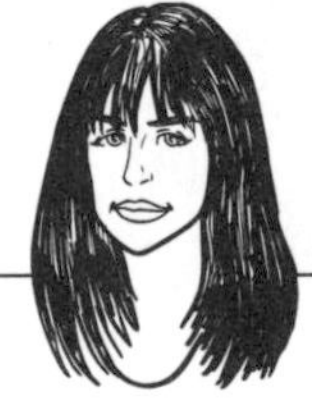

Jourdan's Gems

During the chest lift, be sure that the shoulder of the stationary arm does not go back as you lift the band. For maximum intensity, push your shoulder slightly forward while you lift the band.

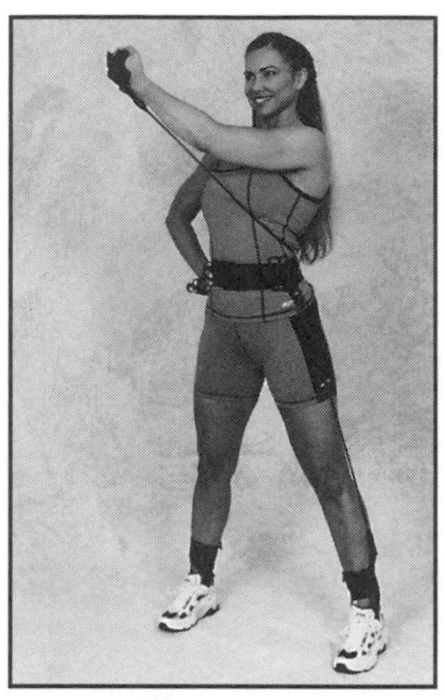

Upright Row/Lateral Raise

This exercise works the anterior and the medial delts.

1. Start by standing with your feet on a resistance band, hip-width apart. With a straight back, abs tight, and shoulders back, raise the band up to your shoulders so that your elbows are out to the side.
2. Lower slowly to the starting position.
3. Raise the band out to the side, with your arms straight but not locked, until you reach shoulder height.
4. Lower slowly to the starting position, and repeat the entire move for desired reps. Go to the overhead press/kick back.

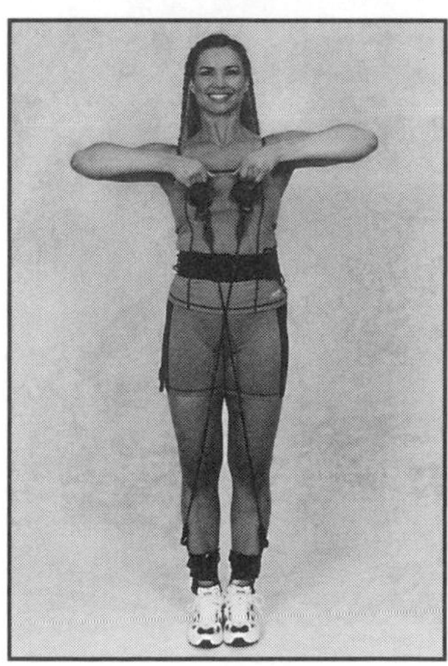

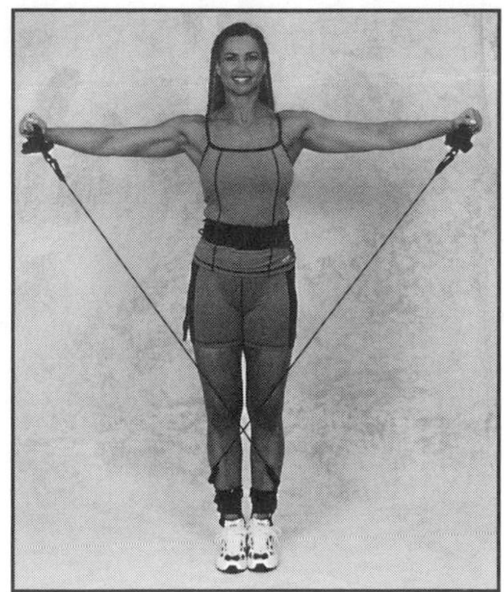

Overhead Press/Kick Back

This exercise works the triceps.

1. Stand with your back straight and one foot behind you on a resistance band. With both hands, raise the band straight up, and then lower it behind your head.
2. Raise the band up so that your arms are straight above your head but not locked. Lower and repeat for desired reps.
3. Then, with a flat back, bend at your waist and bring your arms into your sides, with your elbows back.
4. Straighten your arms behind you while rotating them midlift so that your palms face up at the top position. Contract the triceps and lower slowly to the starting position. Repeat for desired reps. Go to the forward/side curl.

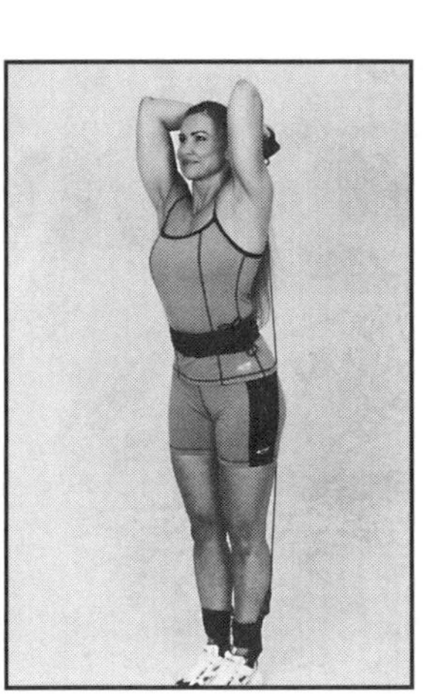

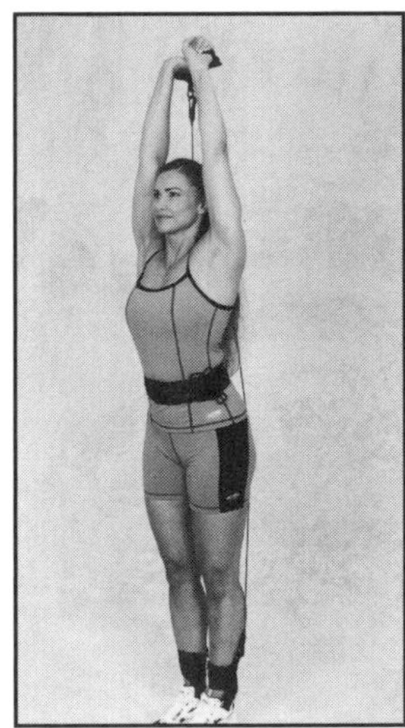

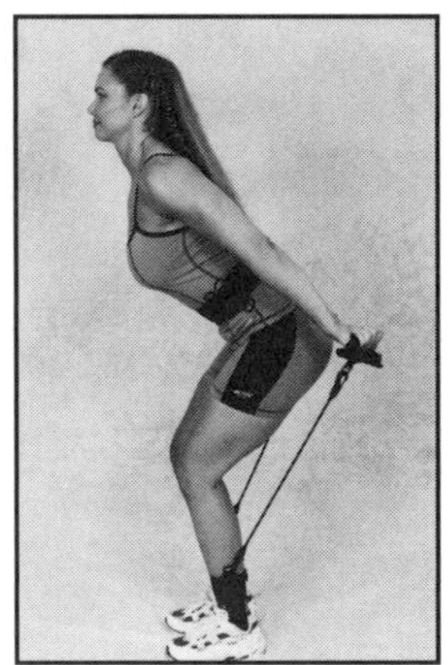

Forward/Side Curl

This exercise works the biceps.

1. Stand with your feet on a resistance band, hip-width apart. With your back straight, shoulders back, arms by your sides, and palms up, curl your arms up to your shoulders.
2. Contract your biceps at the top position. Lower slowly to the starting position. Repeat for desired reps.
3. Then turn your arms out to the sides and curl your arms up to your shoulders. Lower and repeat for desired reps.

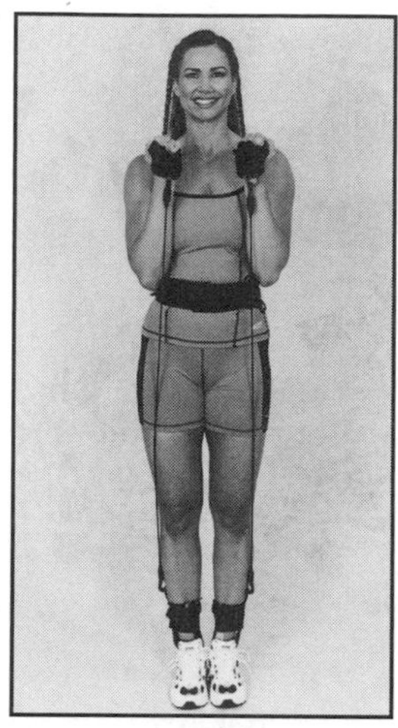

Hard-Body Vacation Survival Tips

After all your hard work, the following tips will maximize your fun in the sun and give you more time to strut your new hard body.

- **Sexy skin.** Add a little almond oil to your suntan lotion. Not only will it leave your skin extra soft, but almond oil has a skin-tightening effect. This will help your skin look extra-toned over your muscles.
- **Beach breakfast tip.** Try watermelon for breakfast. It tastes great and it's refreshing, light, and packed with nutrients. Best of all, watermelon acts as a natural diuretic, so you'll look your leanest when you hit the beach.
- **Protect yourself.** Nothing ages the skin faster than the sun. Try to avoid the rays completely from 11 A.M. to 2 P.M. (I know, it's prime tanning time.) At least put on some lotion with 35 SPF during that time to protect yourself. Trust me, you'll still get tan.
- **Party smart.** Vacation may mean party time galore, but alcohol robs your skin of moisture (unattractive); stresses your heart, liver, and kidneys (unhealthy); slows down your muscle-building progress (so uncool), fills your body with empty calories (unflattering); and loosens up your inhibitions (unwise). So, toss a lime and a stir stick in a club soda (that'll

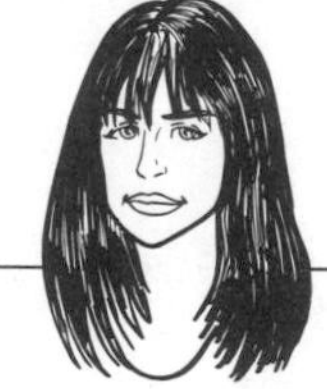

Jourdan's Gems

You can spend less time tanning and use some tan-in-a-bottle instant tanner to get that deep, dark, tropical tan. Doing this will give you more time for fun-in-the-sun activities.

solve the dilemma of what to do with your hands), and try having a spectacular time sober. (Hey, it's one sure way of knowing that the hottie you were talking to last night was really hot.)

The Least You Need to Know

- Travel cardio options include sightseeing on foot, running on the beach, doing laps in the pool, dancing until dawn, and using the cardio gear in the hotel gym.
- Resistance bands can give you a great workout while on vacation, without taking up valuable souvenir space in your luggage.
- Adding almond oil to your suntan lotion will leave your skin extra soft and toned because almond oil has a skin-tightening effect.
- Alcohol can slow your hard-body muscle-building results.

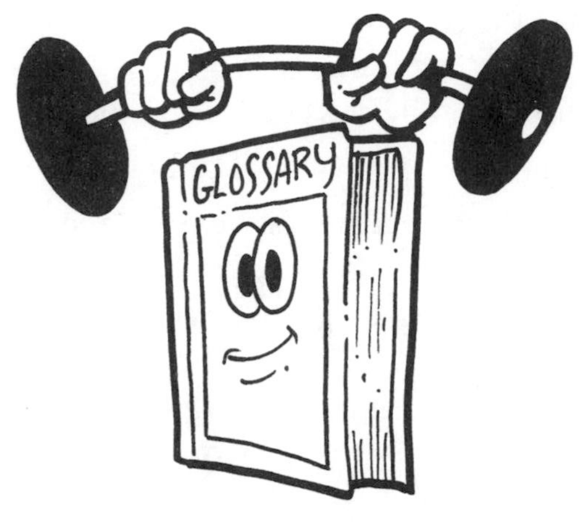

Glossary

abdominals (abs) The four-paired muscles in the front and side wall of your midsection (internal oblique, external oblique, *transverse abdominis,* and *rectus abdominis*).

abduction Movement of a body part away from the middle of the body; opposite of adduction.

adduction Movement of a body part toward the middle of the body; opposite of abduction.

adenosine triphosphate (ATP) A phosphate molecule required to provide energy for your body's functions. ATP is produced aerobically and anaerobically and is stored in the body.

adipose tissue Fatty tissue made up of fat cells.

aerobic With, or in the presence of, oxygen.

aerobic system The metabolic pathway that, in the presence of oxygen, uses glucose for energy production.

amino acids Building blocks of protein.

AMRAP Abbreviation for "as many reps as possible."

anaerobic Without the presence of oxygen; this type of activity doesn't require oxygen.

anaerobic glycolysis The metabolic pathway that uses glucose for energy production without oxygen.

anterior Anatomical term meaning front. Opposite of posterior.

atrophy Decrease in muscle size. Opposite of hypertrophy.

ballistic High-impact, jerking movements.

ballistic stretch A high-force, short-duration stretch using rapid bouncing movements.

basal metabolic rate (BMR) The energy that your body uses at rest to function.

biceps Muscle group in the front part of your upper arm that bends the elbow.

body composition Makeup of body in terms of percentage of fat-free mass and body fat.

body mass index (BMI) A measure of body height and weight to determine level of obesity.

calorie The amount of heat needed to raise the temperature of one kilogram of water 1° Celsius.

carbohydrate Nutrient that provides your body with energy.

chamber In martial arts, the position that your leg goes to before you kick, and the position that your leg goes to after completing the kick before it lands on the ground.

closed-chain exercise (CCE) Exercise in which the postural co-contractors, stabilizers, and neuromuscular system are trained at the same time, and in which the end of the movement chain is fixed against an object such as the floor to support the weight of the body. Examples are squats and lunges.

compound movement Exercise that involves the movement of more then one joint at a time. Examples are squats, lat pull-down, and chest press.

concentric contraction When the muscle shortens because the muscle force is greater then the resistive force. An example is the lifting phase of a curl.

core stabilizer muscles Abdominal and lower-back muscles.

dehydration Having a less then optimal level of body water.

delayed-onset muscle soreness (DOMS) Muscle soreness that happens 24 to 48 hours after an intense exercise session. Thought to be the result of microscopic tears in muscle or connective tissue.

deltoids (delts) Shoulder muscles that are divided into three sections: anterior, medial, and posterior.

drop setting Technique used to raise the intensity of an exercise. You do AMRAP at one weight and then immediately drop down to a lighter weight and do AMRAP at that weight.

eccentric contraction Lengthening of the muscle because muscle force is less than resistive force. An example is the lowering phase of curl.

endocrine system Organs and tissues in the body that release hormones to regulate growth, development, tissue function, and many processes of metabolism.

endorphins Hormones in the brain that reduce the sensation of pain and affect emotions.

fast-twitch fiber Large muscle fiber that is characterized by its fast contraction speed and high anaerobic capacity.

glucagon Hormone produced by the pancreas that is responsible for unlocking fat stores.

glucose A simple sugar that is a vital energy source in the body. It's made from the breakdown of carbohydrates.

***gluteus maximus* (glutes)** Your largest butt muscle (*gluteus medius* and *minimus* are the smaller ones). These muscles are responsible for hip extension.

glycogen The storage form of glucose in the muscles and liver.

hamstrings (hams) Muscles of the back of the upper leg, made up of the *biceps femoris,* the *semitendinosus,* and the *semimembranosus*. These muscles bend the knee and extend the hip.

hypertrophy Increase in muscle size.

incomplete proteins Foods that contain less than the 9 to 10 essential amino acids.

intensity Stress on the body during exercise. This indicates how hard your body should be working.

interval training Short high-intensity exercise periods alternated with periods of rest.

isolation exercise Exercise that uses only one joint and that focuses on one muscle.

isometric contraction A contraction in which a muscle exudes force but does not change in length. An example is pushing against a wall.

lactic acid A waste product of anaerobic energy production that causes muscle fatigue.

***latissimus dorsi* (lats)** The large muscles of the middle and upper back.

ligaments Connective tissue that connects bone to bone.

minerals Organic substances needed in diet in small doses to help regulate bodily functions.

muscle fiber A muscle cell.

obesity Having too much body fat.

open-chain exercise (OCE) Exercise in which a muscle group is isolated to function alone and in which the end of the movement chain is open, or free. An example is leg extension.

opposite muscle groups Front and back muscle arrangement of the trunk and limbs. Examples are the chest and back, biceps and triceps, and quads & hams.

pectorals (pecs) The large muscles of the chest.

posterior Anatomical term meaning back. Opposite of anterior.

PRICE Suggested treatment for strains and sprains: protection, rest, ice, compression, and elevation.

prime-mover muscle The muscle that contracts concentrically to accomplish movement in any given joint.

pronation Position of forearm with palm facing down or back. Opposite of supination.

protein An essential nutrient made up of 22 amino acids that builds and repairs body tissues.

quadriceps (quads) Muscle of the front of the upper thigh: *rectus femoris, vastus lateralis, vastus medialis,* and *vastus intermedius*. These muscles are responsible for extending (straightening) the knee.

range of motion (ROM) The movement from the beginning to the finishing point of an exercise.

repetition (rep) Doing an exercise one time. A group of reps done in a row is called a set.

sedentary Not active; a couch potato.

set A series of reps done in a row.

SITS muscles Four muscles of the rotator cuff: *supraspinatus, infraspinatus, teres minor,* and *subscapularis*.

slow-twitch fiber A muscle fiber characterized by its slow speed of contraction and high aerobic capacity.

sprain Overstretching or tearing of ligament tissue.

split training Training method in which a body is hypothetically divided into different parts, with each part trained on different days.

stabilizer muscles Muscles that stabilize one joint so that a desired movement can be done by another joint.

strain Overstretching or tearing of a muscle or tendon.

super setting Technique used to raise the intensity of an exercise. Two exercises are done back-to-back, with no rest in between.

target heart rate (THR) The number of heartbeats per minute that indicate appropriate exercise intensity levels.

tendon Strong connective tissue that attaches a muscle to a bone.

triceps Muscles of the back of the upper arm that extend (straighten) the elbow.

vitamins Organic compounds that function as body regulators—either water-soluble or fat-soluble.

Appendix B

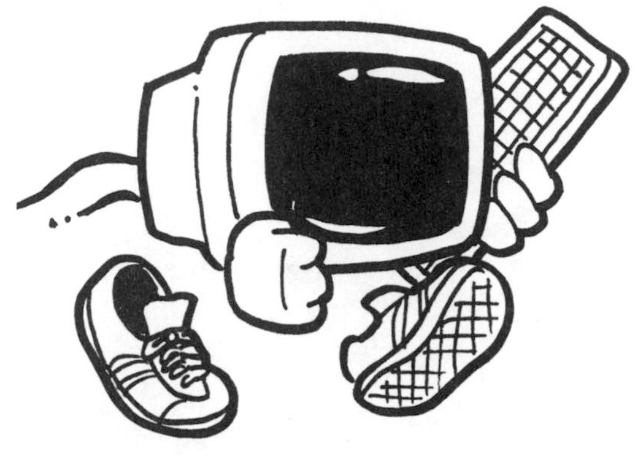

Resources

American College of Sports Medicine (ACSM)
P.O. Box 1440
Indianapolis, IN 46206-1440
317-637-9200
www.acsm.org

American Council on Exercise (ACE)
5820 Oberlin Ave., Suite 102
San Diego, CA 92121-3787
1-800-825-3636
www.acefitness.org

Boxergenics
1-800-848-8244
www.boxergenics.com

Burke Spencer USA, Inc.
1-888-862-8753
www.burkespencer.com

Century Martial Arts Supply
1-800-626-2787
www.centuryma.com

Collage Video
1-800-433-6769

Fitness First
1-800-421-1791
www.fitness1st.com

Fitter International Inc.
1-800-348-8371
www.fitter1.com

Fogdog Sports
1-800-624-2017
www.fogdog.com

Hotskins Bodywear
224 Main St.
Venice, CA 90291
1-800-468-0065
www.hotskins.com

K-Time Productions
www.kicktime.com

Nike
1-800-806-6453
www.nike.com

Ogio Sport
1-800-922-1944
www.ogio.com

Optimal Health Systems
1-800-890-4547

Phyzex Technologies
905-812-4997
www.phyzex.com

Power Blocks
1-800-446-5215
www.powerblock.com

Ringside
877-426-9464
www.ringside.com

Rykä
1-800-848-8698

The Sports Authority
1-888-801-9164
www.sportsauthority.com

SPRI Products
1-800-222-7774
www.spriproducts.com

Team Jourdan Inc.
www.teamjourdan.com

Workout Partners Fitness
www.workoutpartnersfitness.com

Index

A

B

C

D

F

G

M

N–O

S

T

U

V–W

Y–Z

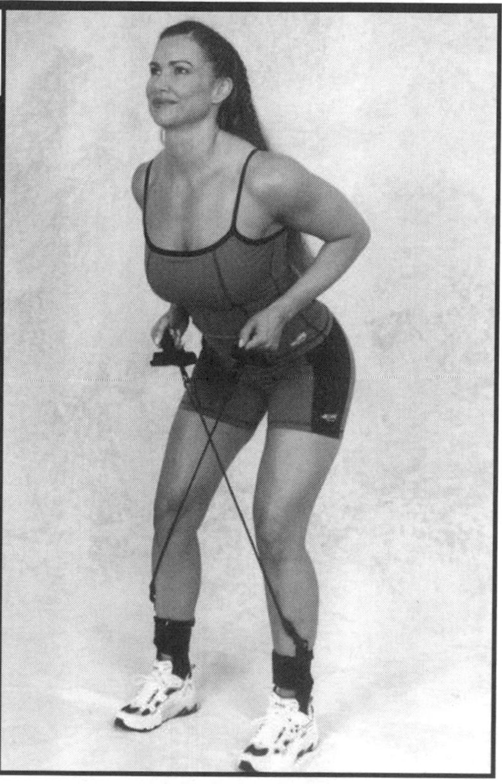